# Recent Advances in
# PAEDIATRIC ANAESTHESIA

# Recent Advances in
# PAEDIATRIC ANAESTHESIA

*Editors*

**Sukhminder Jit Singh Bajwa**
Consultant Anaesthesiologist
Ex-Professor and Head
Bajwa Nursing Home, Patiala
Department of Anaesthesia
Gian Sagar Medical College and Hospital
Patiala, Punjab, India
Honorary Secretary, ISA National

**Madhuri Kurdi**
Professor and Head
Department of Anaesthesia
Karnataka Medical College and
Research Institute
Hubballi, Karnataka, India

**Indu M Sen**
Professor
Department of Anaesthesia
and Intensive Care
Post Graduate Institute of Medical
Education & Research (PGIMER)
Chandigarh, India

**Suvarna Kaniyil**
Professor
Department of Anaesthesiology
Government Medical College
Wayanad, Kerala, India

**Mukesh Kumar Prasad**
Professor and Head
Department of Anaesthesia,
Critical Care and Pain Medicine
Teerthanker Mahaveer Medical College
Moradabad, Uttar Pradesh, India

**Ridhima Sharma**
Associate Professor
Department of
Anaesthesiology and Critical Care
All India Institute of Medical Sciences
Nagpur, Maharashtra, India

*Foreword*

**Dr J Balavenkatasubramanian**

JAYPEE

**JAYPEE BROTHERS MEDICAL PUBLISHERS**
*The Health Sciences Publisher*
**New Delhi | London**

**Jaypee Brothers Medical Publishers (P) Ltd**

**Headquarters**
EMCA House, 23/23-B
Ansari Road, Daryaganj
New Delhi 110 002, India
Landline: +91-11-23272143, +91-11-23272703
+91-11-23282021, +91-11-23245672
e-mail: jaypee@jaypeebrothers.com

**Corporate Office**
4838/24, Ansari Road, Daryaganj
New Delhi 110 002, India
Phone: +91-11-43574357
Fax: +91-11-43574314
e-mail: jaypee@jaypeebrothers.com

**Overseas Office**
JP Medical Ltd
83 Victoria Street, London
SW1H 0HW (UK)
Phone: +44-20 3170 8910
e-mail: info@jpmedpub.com

**EU GPSR** Authorised Representative
Logos Europe, 9 rue Nicolas Poussin
17000, La Rochelle, France
Phone: +33 (0) 6 67 93 73 78
e-mail: contact@logoseurope.eu

Website: www.jaypeebrothers.com
Website: www.jaypeedigital.com



**Inquiries for bulk sales may be solicited at:** jaypee@jaypeebrothers.com

***Recent Advances in Paediatric Anaesthesia***

*First Edition:* **2026**

ISBN: 978-93-7202-153-0

*Printed at: Samrat Offset Pvt. Ltd.*

# Contributors


**Aavula Muralidhar**
Professor and Head
Department of Anaesthesiology
Gandhi Medical College
Hyderabad, Telangana, India

**Aditi Jain**
Assistant Professor
Department of Anaesthesiology
Postgraduate Institute of Medical
Education and Research
Chandigarh, India

**Akshita Singla**
Assistant Professor
Department of Anaesthesiology
Mahatma Gandhi Medical College
Jaipur, Rajasthan, India

**Amrita Rath**
Associate Professor
Department of Anaesthesia
and Critical Care
Banaras Hindu University
Varanasi, Uttar Pradesh, India

**Anil Kumar MR**
Professor
Department of Anaesthesiology
JSS Medical College
Mysore, Karnataka, India

**Anita Malik**
Former Professor and Head
Department of Anaesthesia
and Critical Care
King George Medical University
Lucknow, Uttar Pradesh, India

**Anita Shirley Joselyn**
Professor
Department of Anaesthesia
Christian Medical College, Vellore
Vellore, Tamil Nadu, India

**Anjolie Chhabra**
Professor
Department of Anaesthesia
All India Institute of Medical Sciences
New Delhi, India

**Anju Gupta**
Associate Professor
Department of Anaesthesiology, Pain
Medicine and Perioperative Care
All India Institute of Medical Sciences
New Delhi, India

**Ankit Desai**
Founder Director
Children's Anaesthesia Services
Mumbai, Maharashtra, India

**Anudeep Jafra**
Associate Professor
Department of Anaesthesia and
Intensive Care
PGIMER
Chandigarh, India

**Aruna Parameswari**
Professor and Head
Department of Anaesthesiology and
Pain Medicine
Sri Ramachandra Institute of Higher
Education and Research (SRIHER)
Chennai, Tamil Nadu, India

**Avnish Bharadwaj**
Professor and Head
Department of Anaesthesiology
Mahatma Gandhi Medical College
Jaipur, Rajasthan, India

**B Vishnu Mahesh Babu**
Professor
Department of Anaesthesiology
GSL Medical College
Rajahmundry, Andhra Pradesh, India

**Banashree Mandal**
Professor
Department of Anaesthesia and Intensive Care
Postgraduate Institute of Medical Education and Research
Chandigarh, India

**Bhavna Gupta**
Associate Professor
Department of Anaesthesia
All Institute of Medical Sciences, Rishikesh
Rishikesh, Uttarakhand, India

**Deepshikha R**
Assistant Professor
Sri Ramachandra Institute of Higher Education and Research (SRIHER)
Chennai, Tamil Nadu, India

**Dilip Chavan**
Director
Children's Anaesthesia Services
Mumbai, Maharashtra, India

**Dinesh Gunasekaran**
Senior Consultant
Paediatric Anaesthesia
GKNW Hospital
Coimbatore, Tamil Nadu, India

**Divya Jain**
Professor
Department of Anaesthesia and Intensive care,
Postgraduate Institute of Medical Education and Research
Chandigarh, India

**Ekta Rai**
Senior Professor and Head
Department of Anaesthesiology
Christian Medical College
Vellore, Tamil Nadu, India

**Geeta Kamal**
DMS, Senior Specialist and Head
Department of Paediatric Anaesthesiology
Chacha Nehru Bal Chikitsalaya Super Speciality (Autonomous) Children Hospital
New Delhi, India

**Geeta Singariya**
Senior Professor
Department of Anaesthesiology and Critical Care
Dr SN Medical College
Jodhpur, Rajasthan, India

**Gita Nath**
Senior Consultant Anaesthesiologist and Intensivist
Rainbow Children's Hospital and Birthright
Hyderabad, Telangana, India

**HM Krishna**
Professor and Head
Department of Anaesthesiology
All India Institute of Medical Sciences
Mangalagiri, Andhra Pradesh, India

**Ina Smriti**
Professor
Department of Anaesthesiology
University Malaya
Kuala Lumpur, Malaysia

**Indrani Hemantkumar**
Professor and Head
Department of Anaesthesia
Symbiosis Medical College for Women
Pune, Maharashtra, India

**Indu M Sen**
Professor
Department of Anaesthesia and Intensive Care
Post Graduate Institute of Medical Education & Research (PGIMER)
Chandigarh, India

**Jeetinder Kaur Makkar**
Professor
Department of Anaesthesiology
Postgraduate Institute of Medical Education and Research
Chandigarh, India

**Kajal Jain**
Professor
Department of Anaesthesiology
Postgraduate Institute of Medical Education and Research
Chandigarh, India

**Khushboo Mehta**
Senior Resident
Department of Anaesthesia and Intensive Care
VMMC and Safdarjung Hospital
New Delhi, India

**Madhuri Kurdi**
Professor and Head
Department of Anaesthesia
Karnataka Medical College and Research Institute
Hubballi, Karnataka, India

**Malavika Kulkarni**
Professor and Head
Department of Anaesthesiology
Kasturba Medical College, Manipal Academy of Higher Education
Manipal, Karnataka, India

**Manoj Kumar**
Associate Professor
Anugrah Narayan Magadh Medical College and Hospital
Gaya, Bihar, India

**Mayank Kumar**
Additional Professor
Department of Anaesthesiology,
All India Institute of Medical Sciences
Raipur, Chhattisgarh, India

**Milon V Mitragotri**
Assistant Professor
Department of Anaesthesiology
Karnataka Medical College and Research Institute
Hubballi, Karnataka, India

**Mridul Dhar**
Associate Professor
Department of Anaesthesiology
All India Institute of Medical Sciences
Rishikesh, Uttarakhand, India

**Mridul Dua**
Consultant
Department of Paediatric Anaesthesia and Acute Pain Services
Bai Jerbai Wadia Hospital for Children
Mumbai, Maharashtra, India

**Mukesh Kumar Prasad**
Professor and Head
Department of Anaesthesia,
Critical Care and Pain Medicine
Teerthanker Mahaveer Medical College
Moradabad, Uttar Pradesh, India

**Nandini Dave**
Senior Consultant and Head
Department of Anaesthesia, NH-SRCC Children's Hospital
Mumbai, Maharashtra, India

**Narendra Tajne**
Senior Consultant
Department of Paediatric Anaesthesia
Kanchi Kamakoti CHILDS Trust Hospital
Chennai, Tamil Nadu, India

**Navdeep Sethi**
Director and Head (Anaesthesia)
Yashoda Superspeciality and Cancer Hospital
Ghaziabad, Uttar Pradesh, India

**Neerja Bhardwaj**
Ex-Professor and Head
Department of Anaesthesia and Intensive Care
Postgraduate Institute of Medical Education and Research
Chandigarh, India

**Neeru Sahni**
Additional Professor
Department of Anaesthesia and Intensive Care
PGIMER
Chandigarh, India

**Nidhi Bhatia**
Professor
Department of Anaesthesiology
Postgraduate Institute of Medical Education and Research
Chandigarh, India

**Parul Jindal**
Professor of Anaesthesia
Himalayan Institute of Medical Science
Dehradun, Uttarakhand, India

**Payal Jain**
Professor
Department of Anaesthesia, Critical Care and Pain Medicine
Teerthanker Mahaveer Medical College
Moradabad, Uttar Pradesh, India

**Pooja Bihani**
Associate Professor
Department of Anaesthesiology and Critical Care
All India Institute of Medical Sciences
Bhubaneswar, Odisha, India

**Poonam Motiani**
Professor
Department of Paediatric Anaesthesia
Postgraduate Institute of Child Health
Noida, Uttar Pradesh, India

**Pradnya Sawant**
Head of Department of Paediatric Anaesthesia
Course Director: Fellowship in Paediatric Anaesthesia
Department of Paediatric Anaesthesia and Acute Pain Services
Bai Jerbai Wadia Hospital for Children
Mumbai, Maharashtra, India

**Pratheeba Natarajan**
Professor and Head
Department of Anaesthesia
Indira Gandhi Medical College and Research Institute
Puducherry, India

**Preethy J Mathew**
Professor
Department of Anaesthesia and Intensive Care
PGIMER, Chandigarh
Department of Anaesthesia and Perioperative Care
University of California
San Francisco, USA

**Priya Rudingwa**
Additional Professor
Department of Anaesthesiology and Critical Care
JIPMER
Puducherry, India

**Priyanka Pavithran**
Senior Consultant
Department of Anaesthesiology
Aster MIMS
Calicut, Kerala, India

**R Jayanthi**
Senior Consultant in Paediatric Anaesthesia
Kanchi Kamakoti CHILDS Trust Hospital
Chennai, Tamil Nadu, India

**(Brig) Rahul Yadav**
Director and Commandant
159 General Hospital
Ferozepur, Punjab, India

**Rakhee Goyal**
Director Anaesthesia
Madhukar Rainbow Children's Hospital
New Delhi, India

**Raksha Kundal**
Associate Professor
Department of Anaesthesiology
All India Institute of Medical Sciences
Vijaypur, Jammu, India

**Ranjith Karthekeyan**
Professor and Head
Department of Cardiac Anaesthesia
Sri Ramachandra Medical College and Research Institute
Chennai, Tamil Nadu, India

**Ranju Singh**
Director Professor
Department of Anaesthesiology
Lady Hardinge Medical College
New Delhi, India

**Richa Saroa**
Professor
Department of Anaesthesia and Intensive Care
Government Medical College and Hospital (GMCH)
Chandigarh, India

**Ridhima Sharma**
Associate Professor
Department of Anaesthesiology and Critical Care
All India Institute of Medical Sciences
Nagpur, Maharashtra, India

**Ruchi Gupta**
Professor and Head
Department of Anaesthesia
SGRDIMSR
Amritsar, Punjab, India

**S Ramesh**
Senior Consultant and Head
Paediatric Anaesthesia
Kanchi Kamakoti CHILDS Trust Hospital
Chennai, Tamil Nadu, India

**S Sanjay Prabhu**
Consultant Paediatric Anaesthetist
Department of Paediatric Anaesthesia
Apollo Children's Hospital
Chennai, Tamil Nadu, India

**Sangeeta Khanna**
Senior Director
Department of Anaesthesia
Medanta Institute of Critical Care and Anaesthesiology
Gurugram, Haryana, India

**Sanjeev Palta**
Professor and Head
Department of Anaesthesia and Intensive Care
Government Medical College and Hospital
Chandigarh, India

**Sapna Bathla**
Professor
Department of Anaesthesia and Intensive Care
VMMC and Safdarjung Hospital
New Delhi, India

**Sarvjeet Kaur**
Professor and Head
Department of Anaesthesiology
Guru Gobind Singh Medical College and Hospital
Faridkot, Punjab, India

**Shamshad Beegum TS**
Professor and Head
Department of Anaesthesiology
MES Medical College
Perinthalmanna, Kerala, India

**Shelly Rana**
Professor and Head
Department of Anaesthesia
Dr Rajendra Prasad Govt Medical College
Kangra, Himachal Pradesh, India

**Shikha Gupta**
Professor
Department of Anaesthesiology
Dayanand Medical College
Ludhiana, Punjab, India

**Shikha Sharma**
Professor
Department of Anaesthesia and Critical Care
Acharya Shri Chander College of Medical Sciences
Jammu, India

**Shilpa Goyal**
Professor
Department of Anaesthesiology and Critical Care
All India Institute of Medical Sciences
Jodhpur, Rajasthan, India

**Shilpa Kedarishetty**
Consultant Anaesthesiologist
Rainbow Children's Hospital and Birthright
Hyderabad, Telangana, India

**Shilpa Tiwaskar**
Consultant Anaesthesiologist
Bhaktivedanta Hospital, Mira Road East
Thane, Maharashtra, India

**Shwethashri K**
Associate Professor
Department of Neuroanaesthesia and Neurocritical Care
NIMHANS
Bangalore, Karnataka, India

**Smriti Anand**
Professor
Department of Anaesthesia and Critical Care
Maharishi Markandeshwar Medical College and Hospital
Solan, Himachal Pradesh, India

**Sripriya R**
Additional Professor
Department of Anaesthesia
All Institute of Medical Sciences
Mangalagiri, Andhra Pradesh, India

**Subrahmanyam Maddirala**
Senior Consultant
Anaesthesiologist and Head
Department of Anaesthesiology
Rainbow Children's Hospital and Birthright
Hyderabad, Telangana, India

**Sujata Chaudhary**
Director Professor and Head
Department of Anaesthesiology and Intensive Care
Vardhman Mahavir Medical College and Safdarjung Hospital
New Delhi, India

**Sukhminder Jit Singh Bajwa**
Consultant Anaesthesiologist
Ex-Professor and Head
Bajwa Nursing Home, Patiala
Department of Anaesthesia
Gian Sagar Medical College and Hospital
Patiala, Punjab, India
Honorary Secretary, ISA National

**Sunidhara P Reddy**
Consultant
Anaesthesiologist
Rainbow Children's Hospital and Birthright
Hyderabad, Telangana, India

**Suvarna Kaniyil**
Professor
Department of Anaesthesiology
Government Medical College
Wayanad, Kerala, India

**Swati Daftary**
Chief Anaesthesiologist and Clinical Coordinator
Department of Anaesthesiology and Pain Management
Sir HN Reliance Foundation Hospital and Research Centre
Mumbai, Maharashtra, India

**Swati Jindal**
Associate Professor
Department of Anaesthesia,
Government Medical College and Hospital
Chandigarh, India

**Vanita Ahuja**
Professor
Department of Anaesthesiology and Critical Care
Government Medical College
Chandigarh, India

**Varun Byrappa**
Professor and Head of ICU
Department of Emergency Medicine
Kempegowda Institute of Medical Sciences
Bengaluru, Karnataka, India

**Vibhavari Naik**
Senior Consultant
Department of Oncoanaesthesia, Pain and Palliative Medicine
Basavatarakam Indo-American Cancer Hospital and Research Institute
Hyderabad, Telangana, India

# Foreword by the Chancellor, CISA

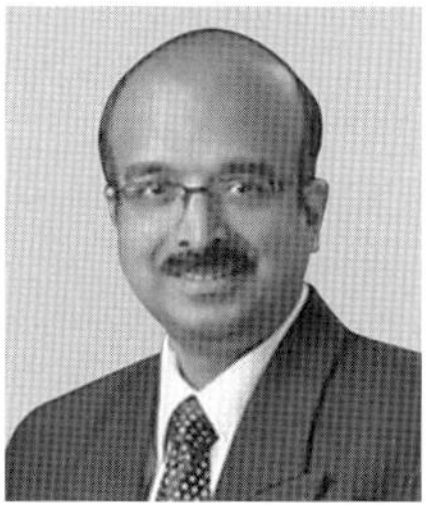

I deem it a great honour to write the Foreword to the book "Recent Advances in Paediatric Anaesthesia." I heartily congratulate all the contributors of this well-curated book for sharing their expertise and experiences. This evidence-based book will add to the global literature and be a treasure house for all those who want to know the intricacies of paediatric anaesthesia.

The contents of the book are very rich, inclusive and holistic. It gives insights into all the facets of paediatric anaesthesia including the management of critically ill in resource-limited settings, crisis management in elective and emergency settings, the possible new curriculum, research and communication skills among others. I am also extremely happy that this is the maiden initiative of the College of Indian Society of Anaesthesiologists to create several updates in several superspecialities of anaesthesia.

I extend my sincere thanks to the Academic Secretary of College of ISA, Dr Sukhminder Jit Singh Bajwa, for spearheading this initiative. This would be an excellent resource to postgraduates in anaesthesia, paediatrics, emergency medicine, and neonatology apart from the several paramedical students, including physician assistants, nurses and anaesthesia and emergency medicine technicians.

Gratitude goes to all those who are responsible for creating this enriching book.

Best regards,

**Dr J Balavenkatasubramanian**
Senior Consultant and Academic Director
Department of Anaesthesia and Perioperative Care
Ganga Medical Centre and Hospitals Pvt Ltd, Coimbatore, Tamil Nadu, India
President, Indian Society of Anaesthesiologists (2024–2025)
Secretary, World Federation of Society of Anaesthesiologists (2024–2026)
Immediate Past President, Asian Oceanic Society of Regional Anaesthesia
Educational Committee Member, World Federation of Society of Anaesthesiologists (2020–2026)
National Chairman, Academy of Regional Anaesthesia of India
Member, ASRAPM Newsletter Committee
Course Director of the following:
Aeasculap Academy Ganga Hospital Regional Anaesthesia Guidance Centre
WFSA-GANGA Hospital Regional Anaesthesia Fellowship
Postdoctoral Fellowship in Nerve Block and Pain Management, Dr MGR Medical University

# Message from the Vice Chancellor, CISA

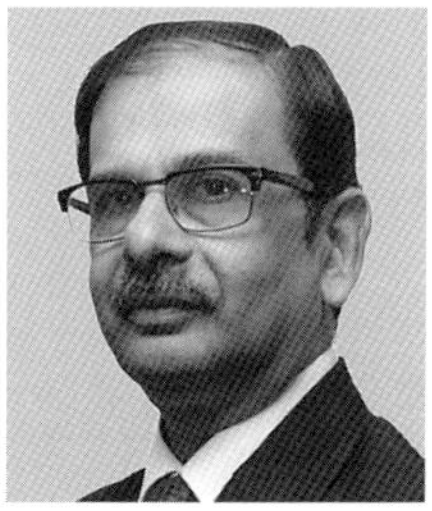

It is indeed my privilege to write this message for "Recent Updates in Paediatric Anaesthesia". It is indeed a special book as it is the first publication to be launched under the aegis of the College of the Indian Society of Anaesthesiologists (CISA) that was formed in November 2023 to co-ordinate the academic activities of the ISA. The editors, Drs Sukhminder Jit Singh Bajwa, Madhuri Kurdi, Indu Sen, Mukesh Prasad, Suvarna Kaniyil and Ridhima Sharma, have done a commendable job in assembling over 23 chapters written by multiple eminent authors. The book covers all major aspects of the principles and practice of paediatric anaesthesia and will be of great interest to postgraduate students and specialists as well the occasional paediatric anaesthesiologist. Apart from the chapters on clinical management, the sections on the role of soft skills and consent in paediatric anaesthesia, communication with children that presents distinct challenges, the rights of children, the ethical conduct of anaesthetic practice and education and research in paediatric anaesthesia are extremely important and relevant in today's times.

"Recent Updates in Paediatric Anaesthesia" has been a labour of love for the subject and for teaching for the editors. I congratulate the editors and authors for this book. It will be a must-read for every postgraduate student as well as practitioner and will find itself on the shelves of every medical library. I extend my best wishes to all the authors, and especially the editors.

**Dr J V Divatia** MD FICCM
Head, Critical Care,
Lilavati Hospital and Research Centre
Mumbai, Maharashtra, India
Immediate Past-President, Indian Society of Anaesthesiologists
Vice-Chancellor, College of the Indian Society of Anaesthesiologists

# Message by the Pro Vice Chancellor, CISA

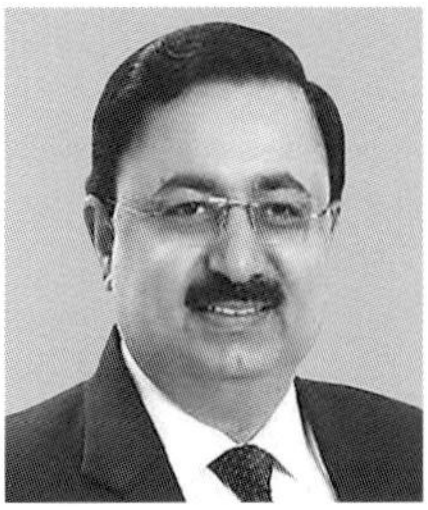

Dear ISAians,

It is a pleasure to pen down this message for the first textbook on "Update in Paediatric Anaesthesia", being published by the College of Indian Society of Anaesthesiologists (CISA). CISA is an academic vision come true. It was born just some time back, and this book is one of the baby academic steps of CISA. It truly reflects the goals and vision of CISA. ISA has always strived to achieve academic excellence and spread the light of knowledge among its members. CISA will be a great help in this endeavour and will carry the torch of knowledge throughout the country and beyond.

The intelligent planning, good foresight, and quality work have culminated in the production of this book. I appreciate the editorial team of this book and all the authors who have contributed to the various chapters through their vast knowledge and skills. I acknowledge their hard work and dedication.

I wish CISA all the very best. Long live CISA! Long live ISA!

**Dr Naveen Malhotra**
President Elect, ISA National Pro Vice Chancellor, CISA

# Message by Dean (Publication of Textbooks, Monographs, etc.), CISA

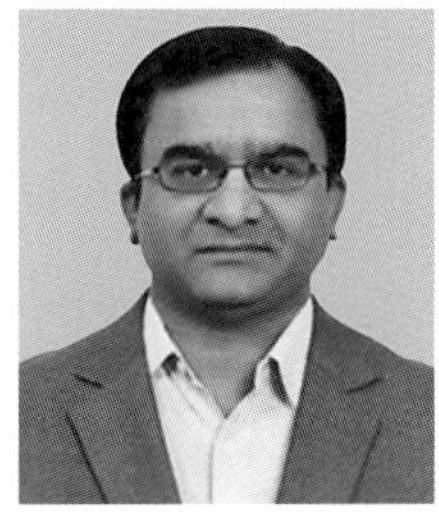

I am pleased to write the foreword to this book. This is the first book under the Deanery of Textbooks and Monogram of the College of Indian Society of Anaesthesiologists (CISA).

This is an excellent book with solid resource for trainees. This book provides a useful refresher of knowledge for experienced clinicians and an excellent starting point for the novice in paediatric anaesthesia.

Each chapter is written by an expert sharing a wealth of practical experience. Every topic is unique, from topics ranging from paediatric airway management to cardiac arrest in paediatrics and NORA in paediatrics, ethics and communication skills.

I appreciate the efforts of all the contributing authors. My sincere thanks go to Chancellor of CISA Dr Bala Venkat Subramaniam Sir, Vice-Chancellor Dr JV Divatia Sir, Pro-Chancellor Dr Naveen Malhotra Sir and Honorary Secretary, ISA National Dr Sukhminder Jit Singh Bajwa Sir, who played an important role in bringing out this book.

**Dr Rama Krishna Reddy Mudiganti**
Dean, College of Indian Society of Anaesthesiologists (T&M Deanery)
Governing Council Member, ISA National
Professor and Medical Superintendent
PMRIMS, Hyderabad

# Message by the Academic Secretary, CISA

ISA Indian Society of Anaesthesiologists

CISA College of Indian Society of Anaesthesiologists

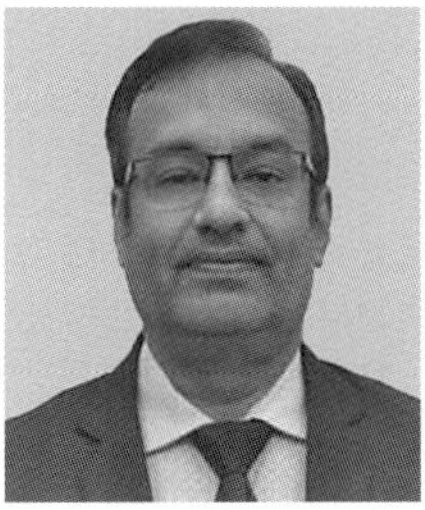

My dear colleagues of the Indian Society of Anaesthesiologists,

Warm greetings from ISA National Headquarters!

The publication of this book by the newly instituted College of Indian Society of Anaesthesiologists (CISA) is a proud and satisfying moment for me. This book is the first of a series of books of the CISA that will cover speciality topics and marks the onset of a new era of meaningful and useful academic publications by the CISA.

Dreams are often pleasant. But they will fade off if not properly captured and nourished to stay as realities or memories. As I have always said, when I took over as Honorary Secretary, ISA National, I had vivid academic dreams and the publication of these books was one of those which probably arose from my passion for scientific writing and publications. One has to be patient and work relentlessly to pursue one's dream and make it a reality. I did just that and was fortunate to have been backed by a similar-minded team of editors, authors and reviewers who have worked hard and meticulously in the making of this scholarly masterpiece. I heartily congratulate each and every one of them.

Paediatric anaesthesia is a speciality that is needed for almost every postgraduate student and anaesthesia practitioner. This book brings to you latest updates on the management of the airway in children, the perils of facing perioperative adverse events, the challenges of massive blood transfusion and enhanced recovery after surgery in children, the tumultuous moments of facing perioperative emergencies and trauma in children, the intricacies of anaesthetising children for airway surgeries and laparoscopic surgeries and the dilemmas of paediatric perioperative fluid management. It provides practical tips for the practitioner administering paediatric anaesthesia in the resource-limited set-ups and also touches upon the finer aspects of training, research and education in paediatric anaesthesia.

The making of this book was possible only because of the support of the Chancellor, Vice Chancellors, the Dean of Textbooks and Monographs section of CISA and the entire Governing Council of ISA. This book is a testament to the unique academic vision of CISA and heralds the onset of an interesting journey of CISA academics filled with neatly organised academic activities of different specialities of our subject including CMEs, conferences, webinars, curriculae, publications and guidelines, all ensembled under one roof. I am sure that this book will be a 'super hit' and spread the rich aroma of paediatric anaesthesia to the postgraduate students, superspeciality students, postgraduate teachers and practitioners of our nation and beyond.

Long Live CISA academics!

Long Live ISA!

**Dr Sukhminder Jit Singh Bajwa**
Honorary Secretary, ISA National

# Preface

We are pleased to present Recent *Paediatric Anaesthesia Update 2024–25*, a comprehensive volume that brings together current perspectives, emerging advancements, and critical discussions in the field of paediatric anaesthesia. This book has been carefully curated to serve as an essential resource for paediatric anaesthesiologists involved in the perioperative care of infants and children.

The field of paediatric anaesthesia continues to evolve rapidly, driven by advancements in technology, refined surgical techniques, and a growing body of clinical research. This edition addresses a wide range of key topics, including updates in airway management, perioperative cardiac arrest, and minimally invasive surgical procedures in paediatric patients.

Recognising the increasing complexity of paediatric care, this volume also covers specialised areas such as ex utero intrapartum treatment (EXIT) procedures, massive transfusion protocols, fluid management strategies, and enhanced recovery after surgery (ERAS) programs. Furthermore, it explores advances in pharmacological therapies, including the safe use of vasopressors, inotropes, and total intravenous anaesthesia, along with the prevention and management of local anaesthetic toxicity.

In addition to clinical topics, the book addresses essential aspects of practice that are often underrepresented in traditional literature. These include the management of emergencies in non-operating room settings, trauma care, and approaches to anaesthesia in resource-constrained environments. Dedicated chapters also focus on soft skills, patient consent, paediatric patient rights, and ethical considerations in both clinical practice and research, reflecting the importance of a holistic, patient-centred approach. The evolving educational landscape of paediatric anaesthesia is also explored, offering insight into curriculum advancements and training methodologies.

This volume is intended to support anaesthesiologists, surgeons, critical care physicians, and all practitioners engaged in paediatric perioperative care. We hope that the content of this book will not only enhance clinical knowledge but also inspire further research, innovation, and excellence in paediatric anaesthesia.

We extend our heartfelt appreciation to all contributing authors and reviewers for their expertise, dedication, and commitment to advancing the field.

**Editorial Team**
*Recent Paediatric Anaesthesia Update 2024–25*

# Contents

# Plate 1

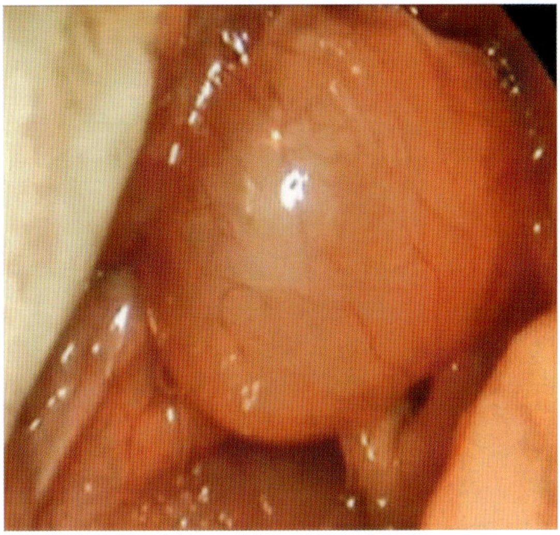

**Fig. 1:** Vallecular cyst ***(Chapter 3)***.

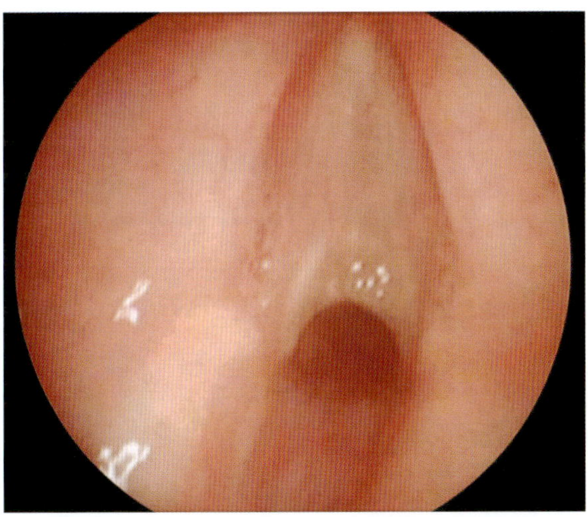

**Fig. 2:** Laryngeal web ***(Chapter 3)***.

## Plate 2

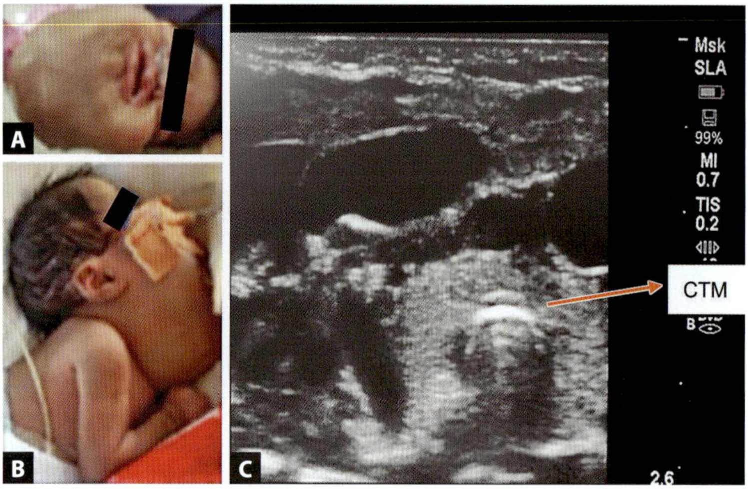


**Figs. 4A to C:** Cystic hygroma *(Chapter 3)*.

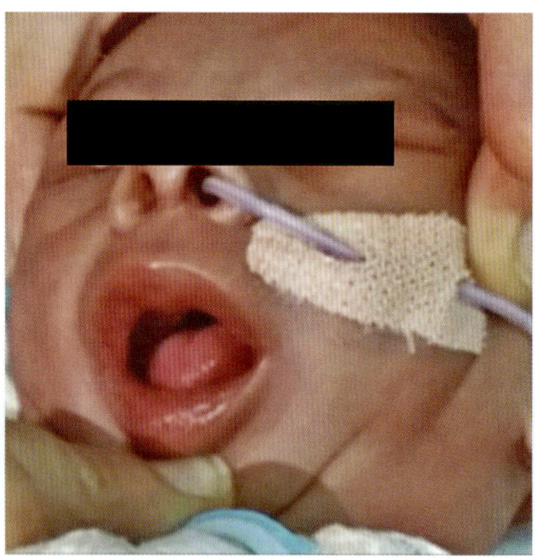

**Fig. 5:** Multiple birth defects *(Chapter 3)*.

## Plate 3

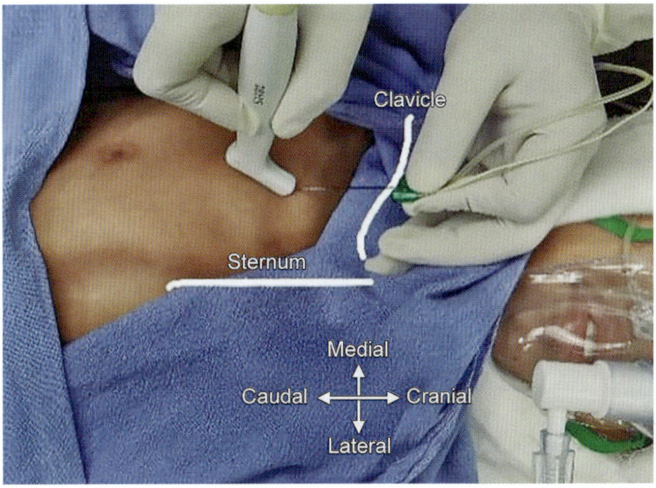


**Fig. 1:** Patient image and needle position for PEC block. (PEC: pectoral nerve) ***(Chapter 8)***.

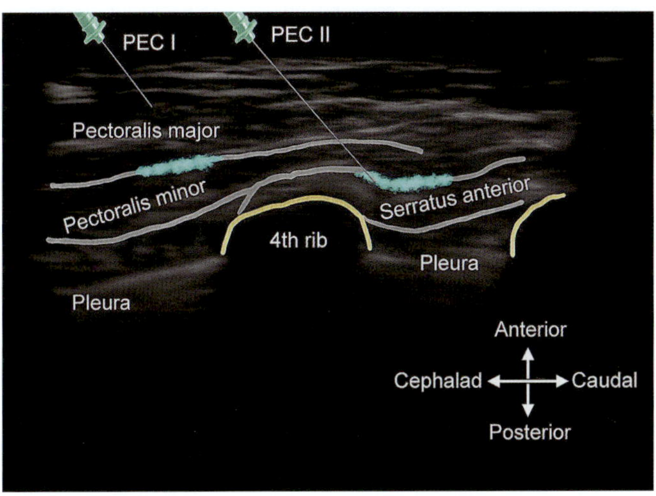


**Fig. 2:** Ultrasound image of PEC block ***(Chapter 8)***.

## Plate 4

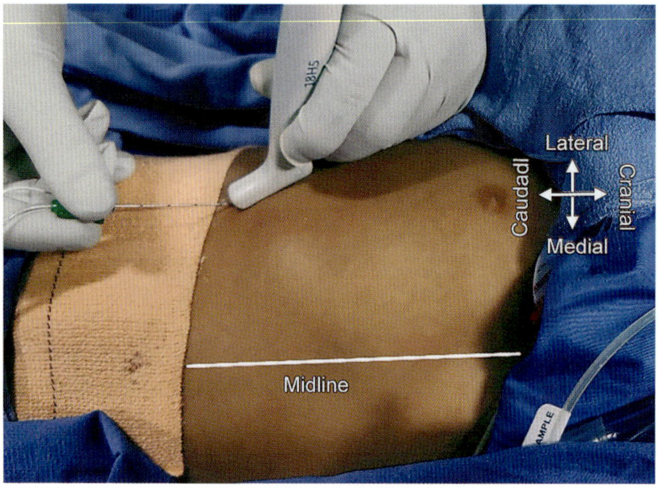


**Fig. 3:** Patient image and needle position for M-TAPA block. (M-TAPA: modified thoracoabdominal paravertebral) ***(Chapter 8)***.

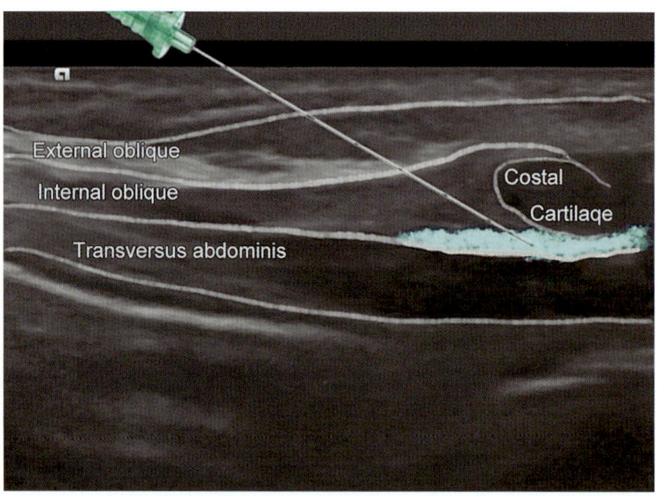


**Fig. 4:** Ultrasound image of M-TAPA block ***(Chapter 8)***.

## Plate 5

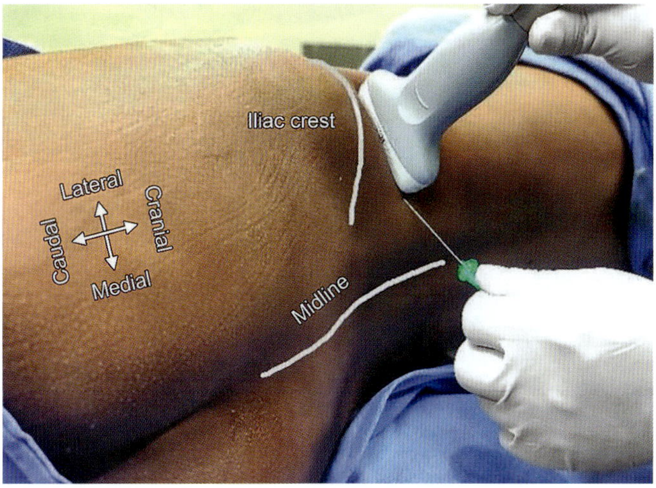


**Fig. 5:** Patient image and needle position for QL block. (QL: quadratus lumborum) ***(Chapter 8)***.

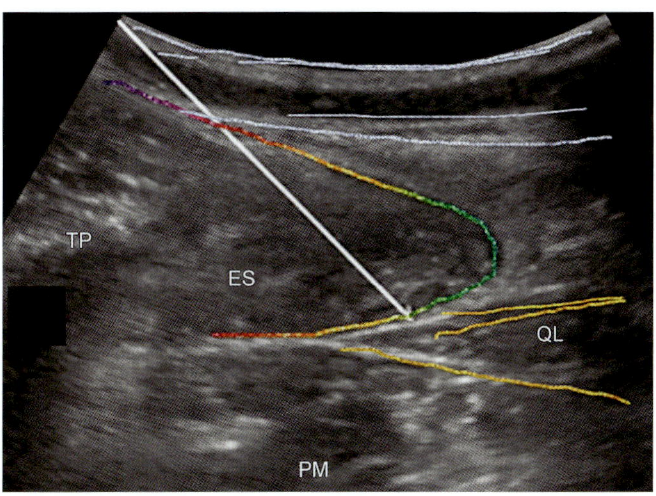


**Fig. 6:** Ultrasound image of QL block. (ES: erector spinae; PM: psoas major; QL: quadratus lumborum; TP: transverse process) ***(Chapter 8)***.

## Plate 6

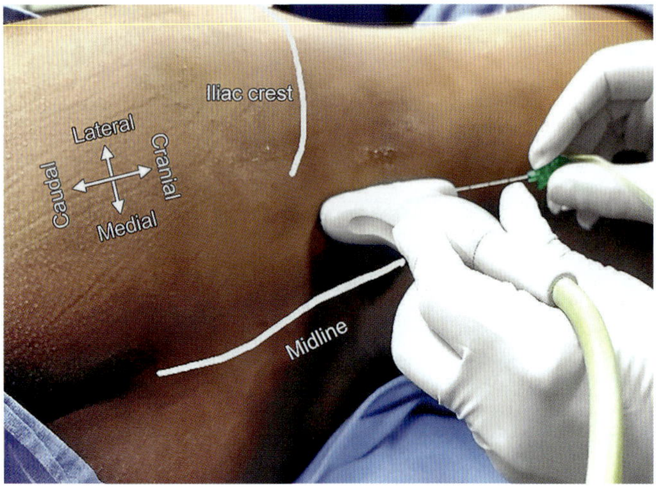


**Fig. 7:** Patient image and needle position for ESP block. (ESP: erector spinae plane) ***(Chapter 8)***.

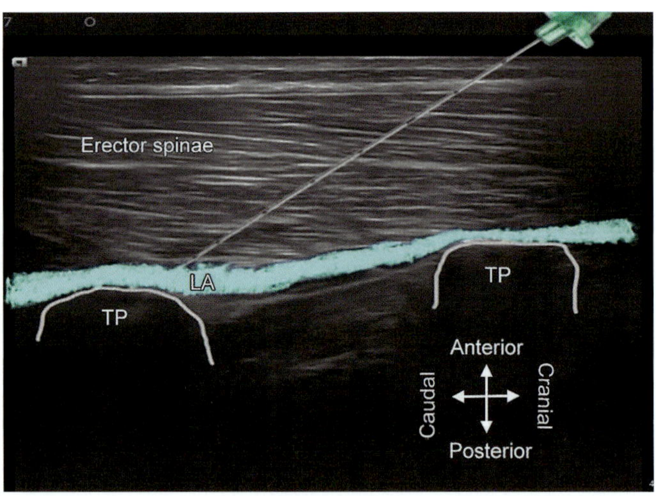


**Fig. 8:** Ultrasound image of ESP block. (ESP: erector spinae plane; LA: local anaesthetic; TP: transverse process) ***(Chapter 8)***.

## Plate 7

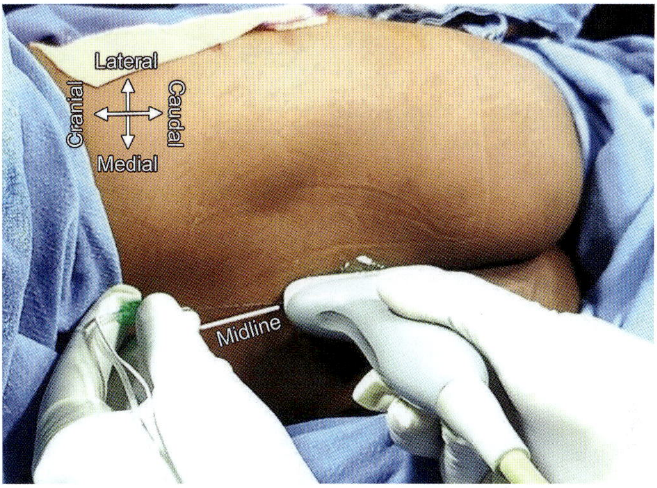


**Fig. 9:** Patient image and needle position for sacral erector spinae plane block ***(Chapter 8)***.

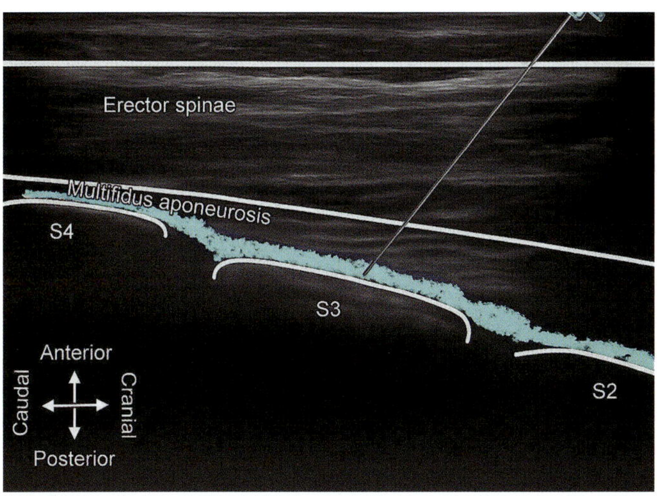


**Fig. 10:** Ultrasound image of sacral erector spinae plane block ***(Chapter 8)***.

## Plate 8

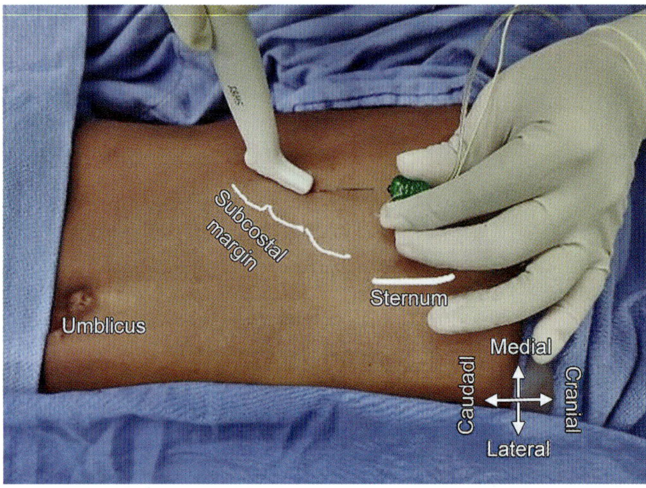


**Fig. 11:** Patient image and needle position for EOIP block. (EOIP: external oblique intercostal plane) ***(Chapter 8)***.

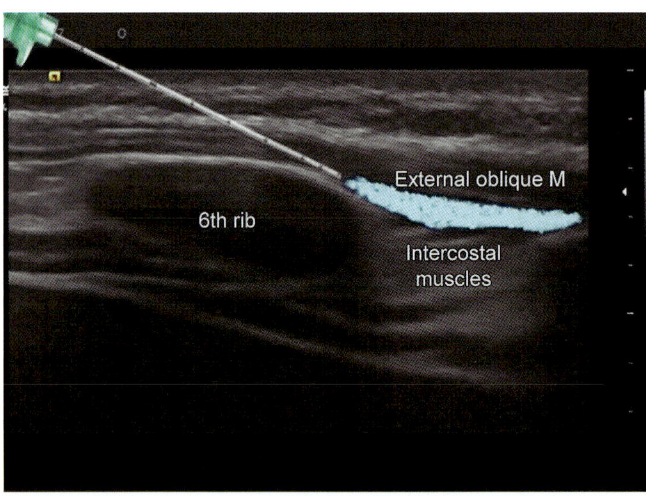


**Fig. 12:** Ultrasound image of EOIP block ***(Chapter 8)***.

## Plate 9

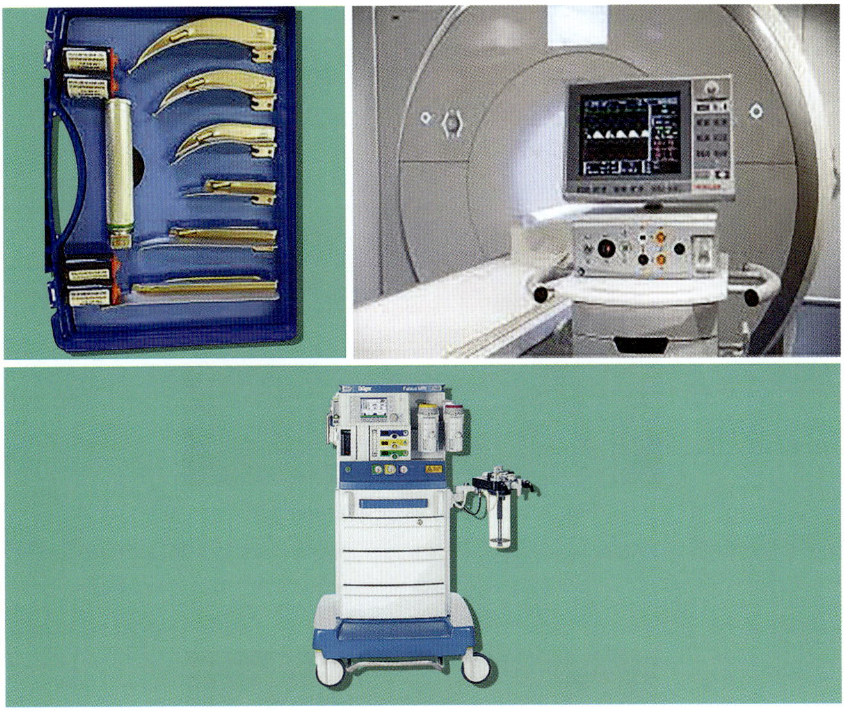

**Fig. 1:** Magnetic resonance imaging (MRI) compatible laryngoscope with blades, MRI compatible pulse oximeter and workstation ***(Chapter 13)***.

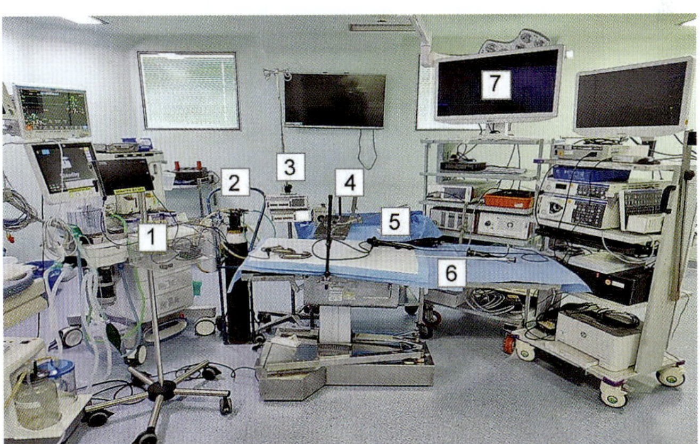


**Fig. 1:** Operation theatre setup for airway procedure. All airway equipment is kept ready in the operating theatre. 1. Videolaryngoscope, 2. Jet ventilation apparatus, 3. Total intravenous anaesthesia, target controlled infusion pumps, 4. Laryngostat, 5. Fibreoptic bronchoscope, 6. Rigid bronchoscope/telescope. 7. Monitors with recording facility. ***(Chapter 17)***.

# Plate 10

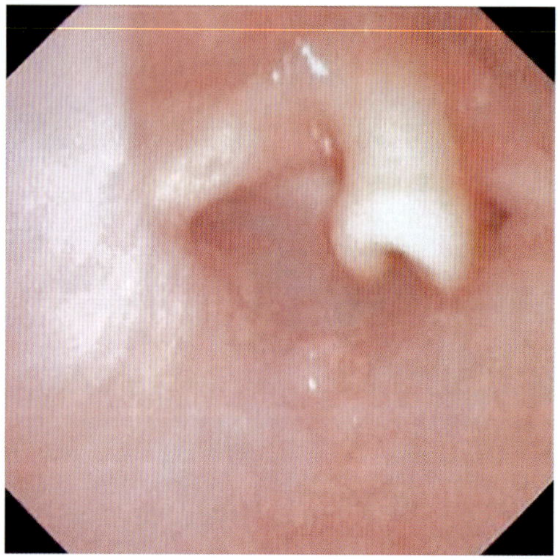

**Fig. 2:** Laryngomalacia *(Chapter 17)*.

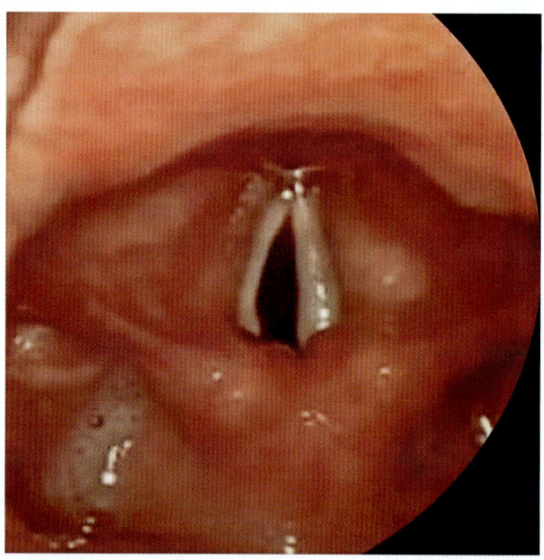

**Fig. 3:** Unilateral (right) vocal cord palsy *(Chapter 17)*.

# Plate 11

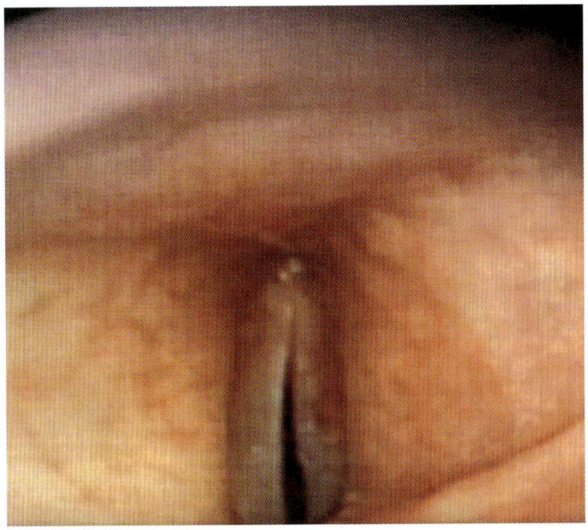

**Fig. 4:** Bilateral vocal cord paralysis ***(Chapter 17)***.

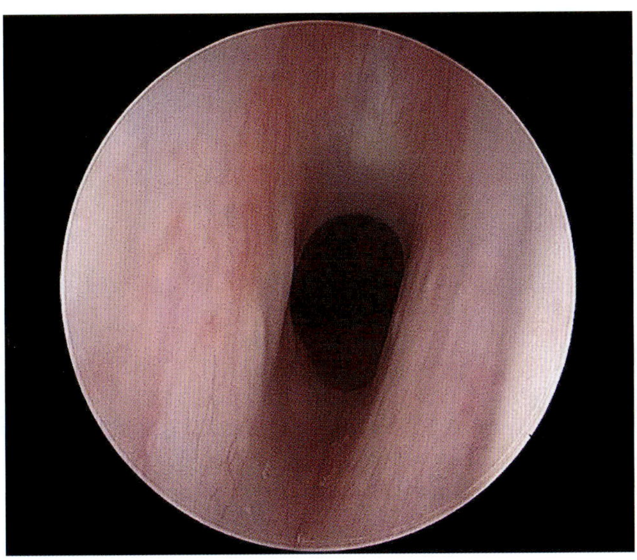

**Fig. 5:** Subglottic stenosis ***(Chapter 17)***.

# Plate 12

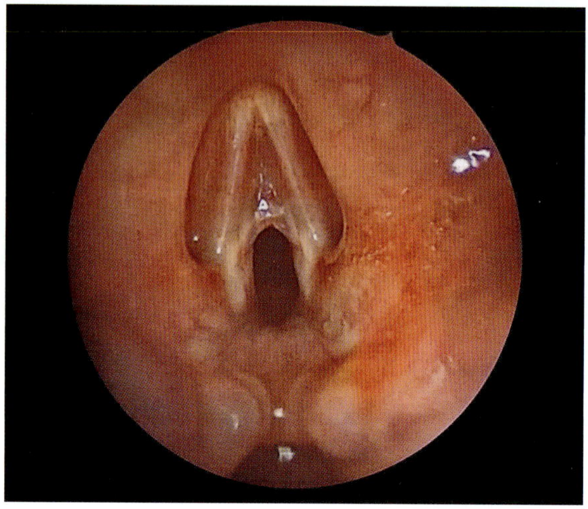

**Fig. 6:** Laryngeal web *(Chapter 17)*.

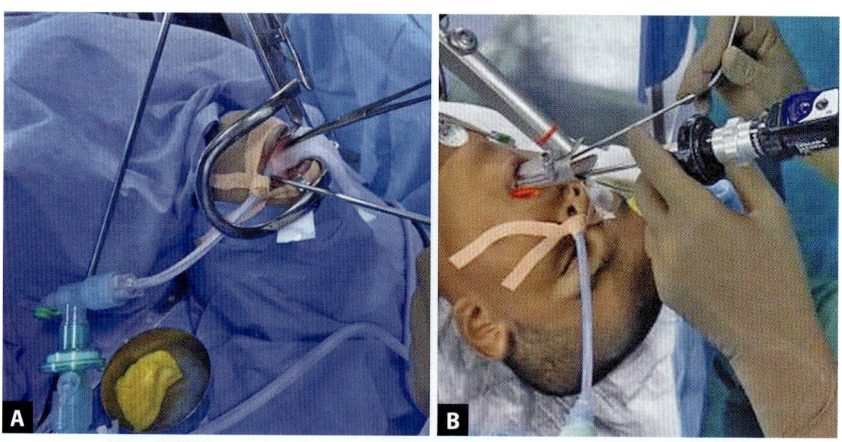


**Figs. 7A and B:** (A) Conventional technique: oral intubation with a small endotracheal tube; and (B) Tubeless technique with nasopharyngeal airway and high-flow oxygen *(Chapter 17)*.

## Plate 13

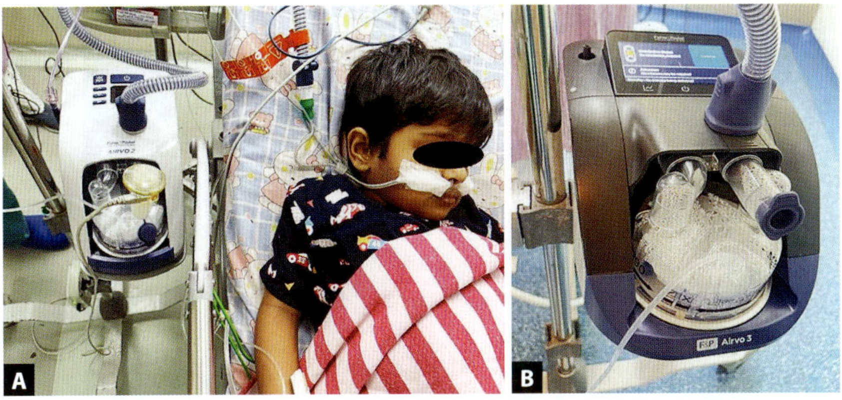


**Figs. 8A and B:** (A) Patient connected to the THRIVE apparatus via nasal cannula and (B) AIRVO 3 (Fisher and Paykel) delivering up to 70 L/min flow with a humidifier (THRIVE device). (THRIVE: transnasal humidified rapid insufflation ventilatory exchange) ***(Chapter 17)***.

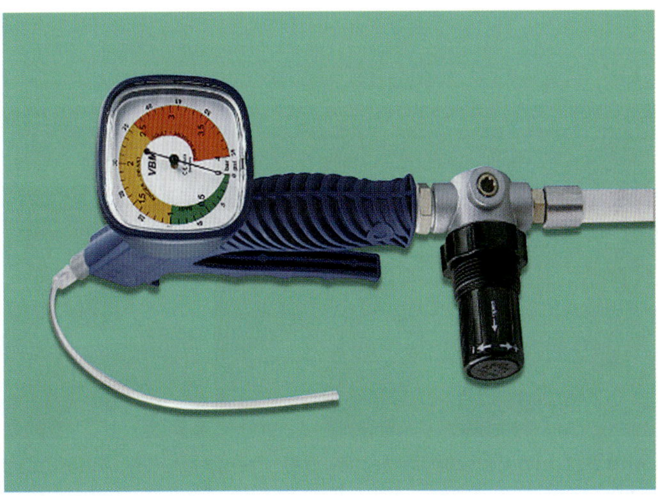


**Fig. 9:** VBM Manujet (VBM Medizintechnik GmbH, Germany). Jet ventilator device showing the pressure gauge, toggle switch and catheter ***(Chapter 17)***.

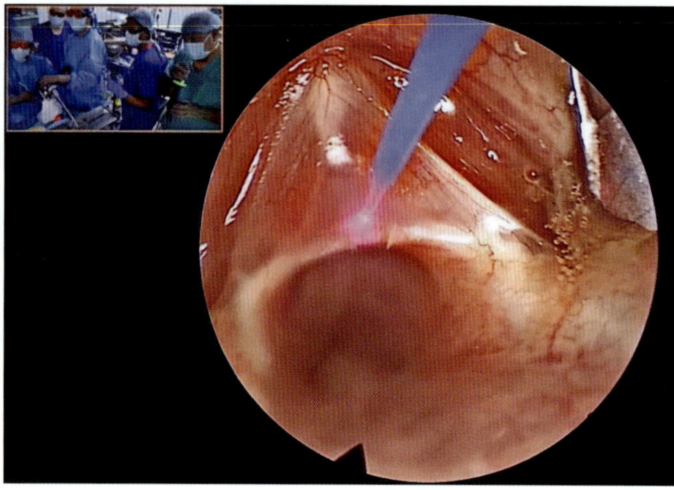

**Fig. 10:** Use of laser for division of laryngeal web ***(Chapter 17)***.

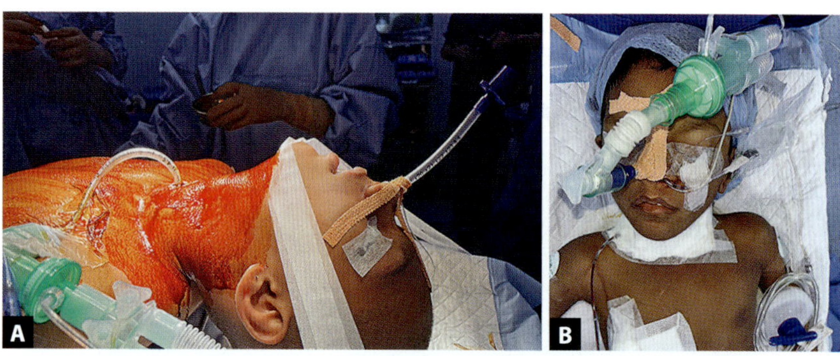

**Figs. 11A and B:** *Laryngotracheal resection:* (A) Preoperatively: A nasotracheal tube is inserted and kept above. Ventilation is maintained via tracheostomy through a flexometallic tube; (B) Postoperatively: Child is ventilated via the nasotracheal tube which also acts as a stent ***(Chapter 17)***.

## Plate 15

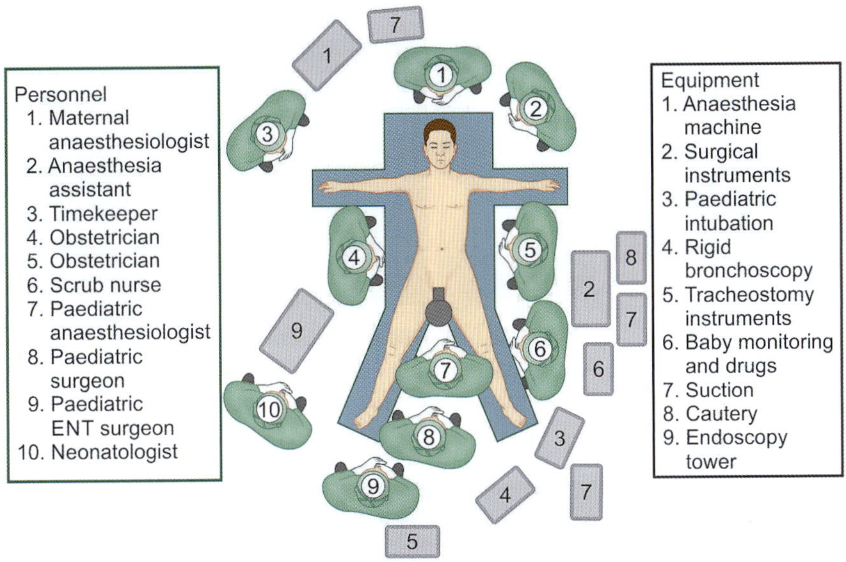


**Fig. 2:** Arrangement of personnel and equipment for EXIT procedure. (ENT: ear, nose and throat; EXIT: ex utero intrapartum treatment) ***(Chapter 18).***

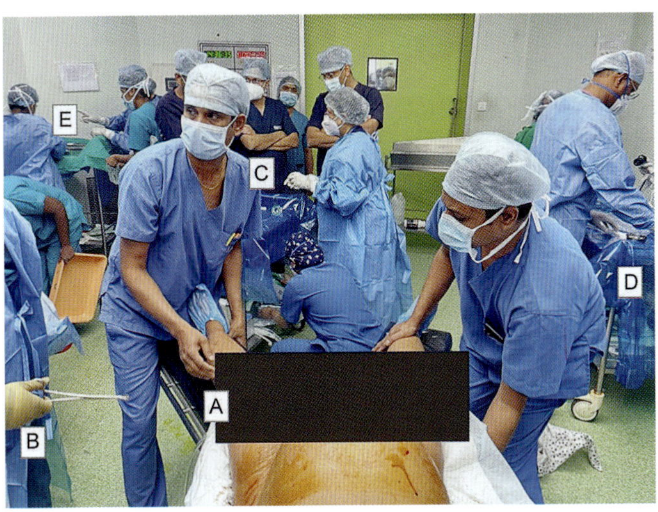


**Fig. 3:** Preparation for EXIT procedure. (A) Patient is positioned in lithotomy; (B) Surgeon is ready to operate; (C) Airway trolley; (D) Bronchoscopy trolley; (E) Tracheostomy trolley. (EXIT: ex utero intrapartum treatment) ***(Chapter 18).***

# Plate 16

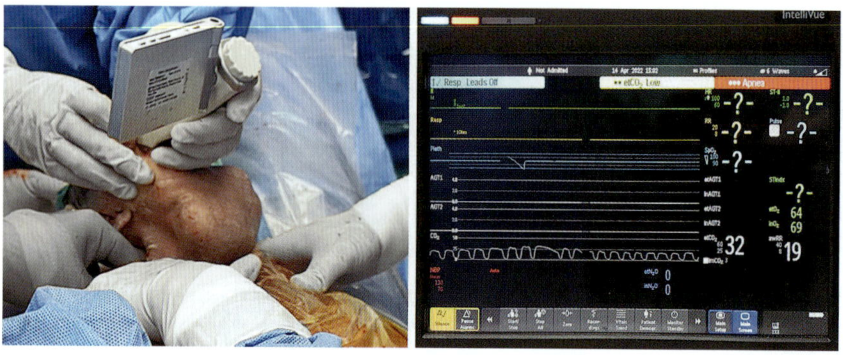


**Fig. 4:** Securing airway during EXIT.
(EXIT: ex utero intrapartum treatment) ***(Chapter 18)***.

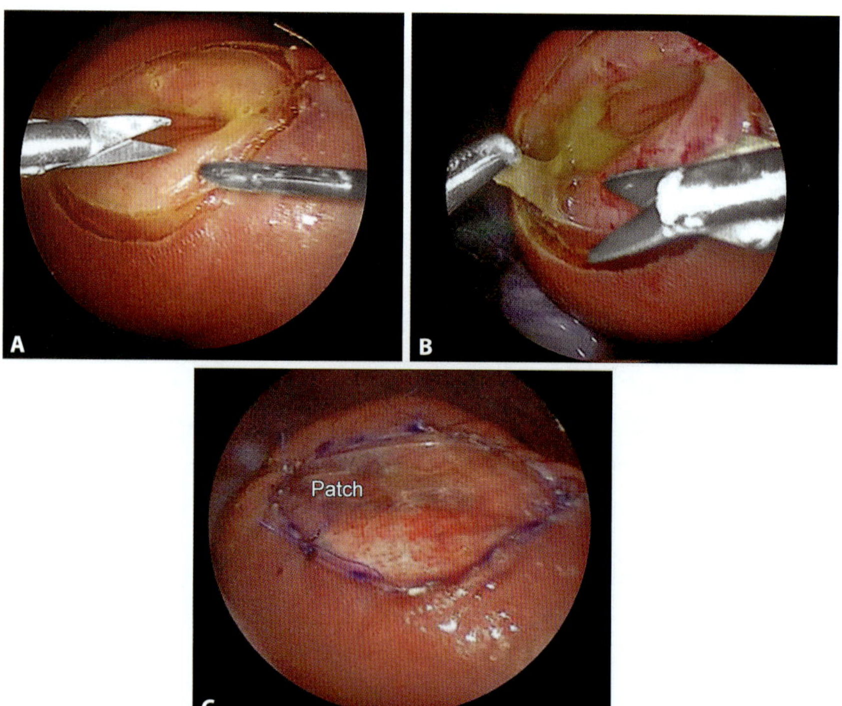


**Figs. 5A to C:** Foetoscopic repair of meningomyelocoele. (A) Lesion circumcised; (B) Meticulous dissection of neural tissue; (C) Closed with water-tight patch ***(Chapter 18)***.

# Plate 17

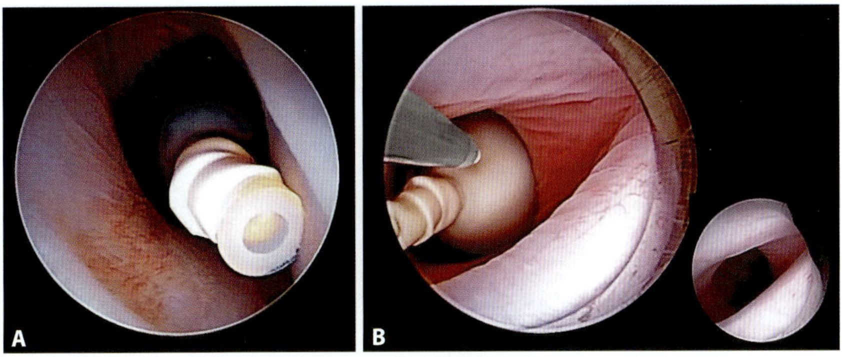

**Figs. 6A and B:** (A) Insertion of tracheal balloon; (B) Balloon puncture and removal ***(Chapter 18)***.

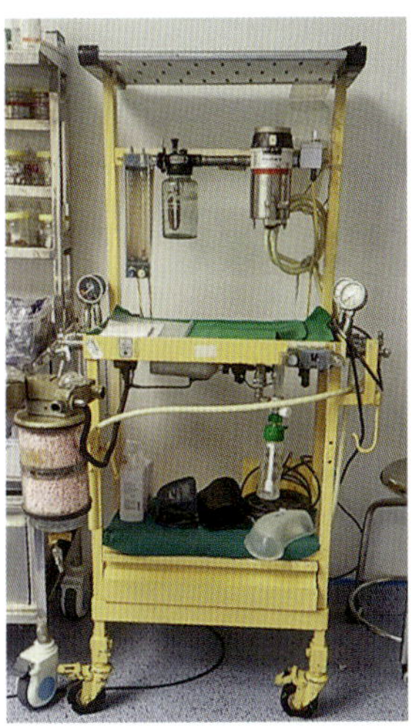

**Fig. 1:** Boyle's machine with sevoflurane vaporiser ***(Chapter 20)***.

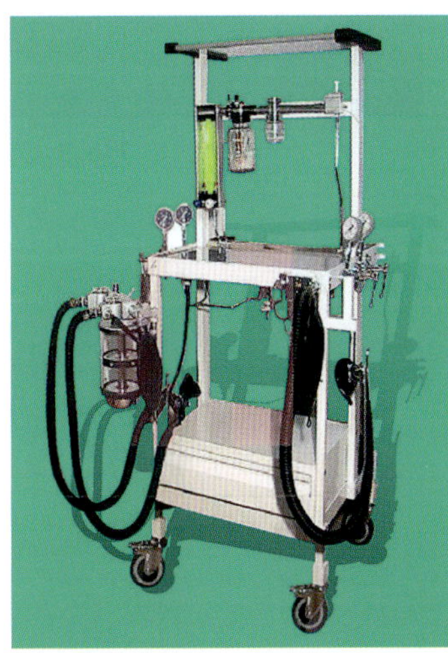

**Fig. 2:** Boyle's machine with halothane vaporiser ***(Chapter 20)***.

# Plate 18

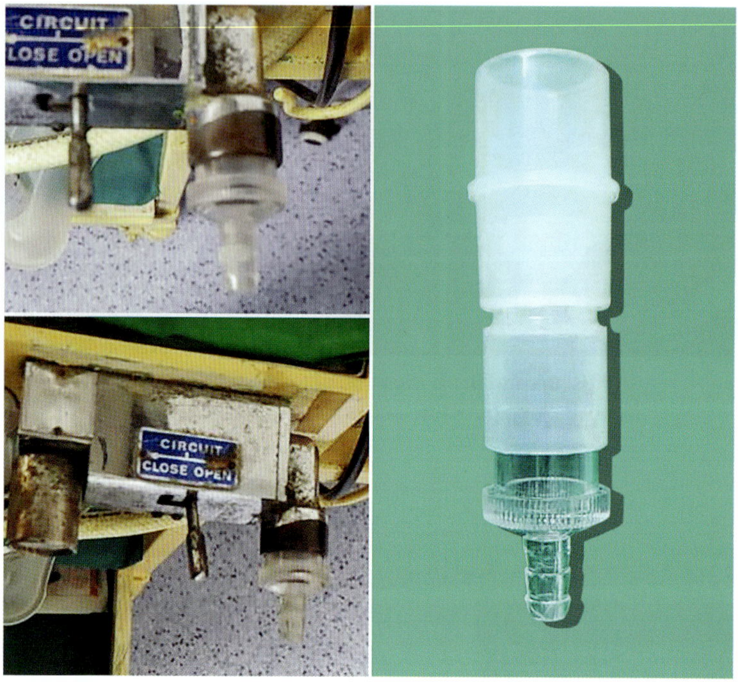


**Fig. 3:** Connectors *(Chapter 20)*.

CHAPTER 1

# Recent Advances in Molecular Pharmacology in Paediatric Anaesthesia: Stay Ahead of the Curve and Provide the Best Care!

*Sripriya R, Vanita Ahuja, Amrita Rath, Bhavna Gupta, Sukhminder Jit Singh Bajwa*

## ABSTRACT

The perioperative period requires the administration of multiple anaesthetic drugs, necessitating precise titration and careful management to ensure effective patient recovery. In paediatric patients, understanding pharmacokinetic and pharmacodynamic differences is crucial for optimising drug dosing and anaesthetic care. Advanced drug delivery systems, such as target-controlled infusion for intravenous drugs, have been developed based on paediatric-specific pharmacokinetic models. Additionally, pharmacodynamic variations and individual genetic differences significantly influence drug effects, emphasising the importance of personalising anaesthesia care. This chapter examines the pharmacokinetic differences in paediatric populations, recent innovations in pharmacogenomics, and advancements in drug delivery systems. It also explores the long-term effects of anaesthetic exposure during pregnancy and early childhood on neurodevelopment and neurocognition. Despite the challenges in conducting research in this vulnerable population, continued studies are crucial. Pharmacogenomics holds transformative potential for revolutionising the selection and dosing of anaesthetic drugs, paving the way for safer, more effective and individualised perioperative care.

***Keywords:*** Anaesthetic, Drugs, Neonates, Paediatrics, Pharmacogenetics, Pharmacogenomics, Titration.

## INTRODUCTION

Molecular pharmacology in paediatrics aims to enhance drug safety and efficacy by understanding molecular mechanisms of drug action, metabolism and interactions in children. Children cannot be regarded as 'small adults,' due to significant pharmacokinetic and pharmacodynamic differences. The pharmacokinetic and pharmacodynamic responses also vary among children of different ages. Pharmacogenetics and pharmacogenomics further influence the pharmacology of drugs in children.[1,2] Unlike the traditional 'one-size-fits-all' medicine, paediatric precision medicine can personalise medical care, based on an individual's genetic makeup, family history and environmental exposures, thereby ensuring that children receive the most appropriate care based on their unique genetic and biological characteristics.[1]

## PHARMACOLOGY IN PAEDIATRICS

### Pharmacokinetics

Pharmacokinetics encompasses four key processes: absorption, distribution, metabolism and clearance. Pharmacology in the paediatric age group depends on post-conceptual age or postmenstrual age, rather than post-natal age. Most neonatal drug dosing is weight-based (mg/kg or μg/kg), but increasing evidence confirms that there are many factors and variables beyond size that can be taken into consideration to optimise precision drug dosing in neonates. These variables include age, distribution (including plasma protein binding), route of elimination, isoenzyme maturation, renal development and transporter biology.[3,4] Ontogeny, age-related and development-related differences and changes in body size, composition, organ function, organ maturation and body chemistry, including enzyme activity and pharmacogenomics amongst children, can contribute to the variability in pharmacokinetics and pharmacodynamics. Changes in drug disposition at the level of tissues and cells with respect to drug transporter expression and function can affect drug efficacy and safety. Throughout childhood, from the time of birth to late adolescence, there is a 50-fold difference in drug disposition, most pronounced in the first year of life.[5]

Model-informed precision dosing (MIPD) is a novel and powerful tool to translate this updated knowledge of drug pharmacokinetics into dosing changes at the bedside.[6] It includes the use of pharmacokinetic models to tailor dosing to an individual patient's needs. It integrates mathematical models of drugs and diseases combined with individual patient characteristics such as genotype, anthropometric factors and organ function. This helps in attaining the therapeutic drug exposure targets and thereby improves the efficacy of the drug and reduces adverse events. It is used for drugs such as vancomycin in critically ill children.[7]

#### *Absorption*

In neonates, the pH in the stomach is neutral, which can affect the solubility and absorption of orally administered drugs. Additionally, gastric emptying and intestinal motility are slower, potentially prolonging drug absorption. By around 2 years of age, gastric pH, emptying time and motility generally approach adult levels, leading to more predictable absorption patterns. Rectal administration of drugs results in higher bioavailability due to avoidance of first-pass metabolism.[8]

The skin of neonates and infants is thinner and more hydrated, leading to higher absorption of topical medications. Blood flow to muscles and subcutaneous tissue can be erratic in neonates and infants, making absorption of intramuscular drugs unpredictable. Additionally, the lower muscle mass in young children can impact both the volume of distribution and the absorption rate.[9]

### *Distribution*

Neonates have a higher total body water content (~75–90%) compared to adults (~60%), resulting in a larger volume of distribution for hydrophilic drugs compared to lipophilic drugs, necessitating higher weight-based dosing. Body fat increases from 3% in premature neonates to about 10% at birth and approximately 20% by the end of infancy. This affects the distribution of lipophilic drugs. For example, propofol exhibits lower distribution in infants than in adults.[9,10]

At birth, the plasma albumin and α-1-acid glycoprotein are 75–80% and 50% of adult levels, respectively. This may result in a high free fraction of drugs, enhancing pharmacological effects and increasing the risk of toxicity. For instance, the unbound concentration of diazepam is four times higher in neonates compared to adults, reaching adult levels by 1–3 years of age.[8-11] In premature neonates, the blood-brain barrier is immature, leading to increased drug transfer into the central nervous system.[12]

### *Metabolism*

Neonates have immature liver enzyme systems, including cytochrome P450 enzymes, resulting in slower drug metabolism. Both phase I (oxidation, reduction and hydrolysis) and phase II (conjugation) reactions are affected, though they mature at different rates. The metabolism of drugs like thiopentone is dependent on phase I oxidative reactions.[8,9] Opioids, including morphine, fentanyl and other drugs such as amide local anaesthetics (LAs) and ketamine, are dependent on N-dealkylation of phase I metabolism. For phase II conjugation reactions, the main mechanism is glucuronamide reaction for morphine, fentanyl and naloxone. Cytochrome P450, family 3, subfamily A (CYP3A) has an effect in catalysing drug metabolism and increasing clearance with an increase in age. For example, hepatic extraction of midazolam is only 0.04 in neonates, as compared to 0.38 in adults. Other drugs affected by cytochrome P2D6 are selective serotonin reuptake inhibitors, morphine derivatives and prodrugs like tramadol. Cytochrome maturation occurs during the first months to years of life; however, esterase levels remain the same from neonates to adults. For example, remifentanil shows similar clearance in children aged 1 month to 9 years.[13]

### *Clearance*

*Renal clearance:* Renal development starts at 5–9 weeks of gestation and is completed around 36 weeks. The glomerular filtration rate (GFR) is 5 ml/min in full-term neonates. In preterm neonates, it may be as low as one-fifth of that. GFR functions are non-linear with a maximum value at 48 weeks of postmenstrual age. On average, GFR is 30% of adult GFR at 8–12 weeks of age. Renal function continues to mature over the first year, approaching adult levels by around 6–12 months. The kidney eliminates water-soluble drugs and metabolites. Age-dependent renal clearance, therefore, controls the drug dosing. Maturation of the kidney is independent of post-natal age and, hence, is a reliable method of clearance of a water-soluble drug.[1,5,8]

*Hepatic clearance:* Neonates also have immature biliary function, affecting both the binding and transport of bile salts, which limits the absorption of lipophilic drugs.[8,9,14] Intestinal enzyme cytochrome P450 family 3 subfamily A member 4 (CYP3A4) is present at lower levels in children compared to adults. In preterm infants, cytochrome P3A activity is also reduced, leading to decreased first-pass metabolism and increased bioavailability of certain drugs.[7,8]

The majority of the drugs used in anaesthesia, i.e. sedatives, hypnotics, benzodiazepines, opioids and neuromuscular blockers, are dependent on hepatic clearance. For drugs with a high extraction ratio, e.g. lignocaine, fentanyl, sufentanil and propofol, hepatic clearance is dependent on hepatic blood flow. For low-extraction drugs, e.g. diazepam and alfentanil, hepatic clearance is independent of hepatic blood flow and depends on intrinsic clearance for metabolism.[2,8]

## Mechanism of Action of Drugs Used in Paediatric Anaesthesia

### *Intravenous Induction Agents and Sedatives*

*Propofol:* The induction dose of propofol is 2.5–3.5 mg/kg in children aged > 3 years and 2 mg/kg in children aged 3–7 years. The dose is thus high compared to the dose of 2–2.5 mg/kg in adults. The intravenous infusion dose is 125–150 μg/kg/min for sedation and 1–3 mg/kg for emergence delirium. Propofol has rapid redistribution, short duration of action, large steady-state volume of distribution, slow elimination half-life and rapid clearance. Clearance of propofol exceeds liver blood supply, indicating that extra-hepatic sites such as lungs and intestines are involved in its metabolism. The loss of eyelash reflex is at 2 mg/kg in obese children as compared to 3.2 mg/kg in non-obese patients aged 3–17 years. Clearance attains mature adult values within 6 months of life. Context-sensitive half-life is 10.4 minutes for 1 hour's propofol infusion, and 19.6 minutes for 4 hours' infusion as compared to 6.7 and 9.5 minutes, respectively, in adults. Propofol reduces intraocular pressure and reduces emesis. Side effects of propofol include tolerance, pain on injection (more in infants, 50% and in children, 18%), spontaneous excitatory movements, anaphylactic reactions and propofol infusion syndrome (PRIS).[15]

*Thiopentone sodium:* Thiopentone sodium, an ultra-short-acting barbiturate, has an increased requirement in infants and children as compared to adults. There is a reduced requirement of thiopentone in premature neonates due to lower plasma protein binding, greater penetration of the brain or increased sensitivity of receptors. The induction dose in neonates is 3–4 mg/kg; in infants: 5–8 mg/kg; in 1–12 years: 5–6 mg/kg; and in >12 years: 3–5 mg/kg.[16]

*Etomidate:* Etomidate is a potent, short-acting, non-barbiturate sedative-hypnotic agent used due to its cardiac stable function. The induction dose is 0.2–0.4 mg/kg for anaesthesia. Etomidate 0.4 mg/kg does not impair systemic or regional cerebral blood flow in neonates or infants with congenital heart disease. The onset of action is rapid, within 5–15 seconds, with peak effect at 60 seconds and a short duration of 3–5 minutes. Clearance is highly variable and is reduced in neonates and infants having cardiac disease. It has both anticonvulsant and pro-convulsant quantities. Myoclonic movements occur in 30–75% of patients at induction. Pain on injection is a common side effect due to etomidate being a fat emulsion of medium and long-chain triglycerides. Etomidate reduces cortisol levels during and at 24 hours following surgery and hence should be avoided in patients with adrenal-suppressed states.[17]

*Ketamine:* Intravenous ketamine has rapid distribution and onset of anaesthesia within 30 seconds. In infants <3 months old, the volume of distribution is similar, the elimination half-life is prolonged, and there is reduced clearance due to reduced metabolism and renal excretion as compared to older infants. Ketamine can be administered orally (3–10 mg/kg), intramuscularly (3–7 mg/kg) or intranasally (6–9 mg/kg) for premedication.[18,19]

The intravenous sedation dose of ketamine is 0.5–2 mg/kg, the analgesic dose is 0.1 mg/kg, and the analgesic infusion dose is 0.1–0.3 mg/kg/h. Propofol or midazolam can be combined with ketamine 0.5 mg/kg during cardiac catheterisation, anaesthesia induction and sedation procedures. A ratio of 1:5 of ketamine: propofol for 30-minute anaesthesia and 1:6.7 for 90 minutes of anaesthesia is suggested.[20] Ketamine causes an increase in intracranial pressure, intraocular pressure and nystagmus. Ketamine can cause hallucinations and vivid dreams, with an incidence of 5–10% in prepubescent children. This occurs due to depression of the inferior colliculus and medial geniculate nucleus, leading to misinterpretation of auditory-visual signals and musculoskeletal gravity perception.[20] Repeated uses of ketamine in neonates causes γ-aminobutyric acid type A ($GABA_A$) R-mediated excitation of neuronal tissue of immature brains. Studies done on animal models and a few preclinical studies have demonstrated that ketamine may cause neuroapoptosis, especially in the forebrain, anterior cingulate cortex and hippocampus. These effects may cause neurodegenerative changes, learning deficits and memory impairment due to synaptic plasticity later in life. These changes are of concern in children <3 years and anaesthetic and sedation duration of >3 hours or longer.[21,22]

*Midazolam:* Benzodiazepines act via gamma-aminobutyric acid (GABA) receptors. GABA is an inhibitory neurotransmitter in the brain, amygdala, limbic system and spinal internuncial neurons and produces sedation and hypnosis. In preterm infants, midazolam has a lower clearance rate due to the developmental immaturity of CYP3A4 metabolism as compared to older children and adults. Premedication dose of midazolam via oral route is 0.25–0.5 mg/kg, intranasal 0.2–0.3 mg/kg, and 0.05 mg/kg intravenously. Sedation dose of midazolam is 0.2–0.3 mg/kg via intranasal route, 0.1–0.15 mg/kg via intramuscular route, 0.05–0.1 mg/kg intravenously at 6 months to 5 years, and 0.025–0.05 mg/kg intravenously for the age group of 5–12 years. The sedation dose is 1 mg/kg per rectal. Intranasal administration is irritating to the nasal mucosa and has poorer acceptance than the sublingual route.[23]

*Dexmedetomidine:* Dexmedetomidine acts via hyperpolarisation of non-adrenergic neurons in the locus coeruleus, inducing sedation like natural sleep. Dexmedetomidine 0.3 μg/kg/hour has the longest context-sensitive half-life in neonates, followed by infants at 3 months, 6 months, 1 year and then reaches adult level at 10 years. Dexmedetomidine has a bioavailability of 80% by the transmucosal route and 73% with the intramuscular route. The elimination half-life of dexmedetomidine is 2 hours, and the distribution half-life is 6 minutes. Preterm neonates have lower clearance; larger volume of distribution and longer elimination time as compared to full-term neonates and older children.[1,9,17]

Dexmedetomidine has a neuroprotective effect. It is more useful during magnetic resonance imaging (MRI) than midazolam with an intravenous loading dose of 1–2 μg/kg over 10 minutes, followed by an infusion of 0.5–1 μg/kg/hour. The premedication dose of dexmedetomidine is 2 μg/kg intranasally, 0.5 μg/kg intravenously and 1–2 μg/kg intramuscularly. For emergence delirium and shivering, it can be administered intravenously at a dose of 0.3–0.5 μg/kg.

## Inhalational Agents

The minimum alveolar concentration (MAC) of inhalational agents changes with age. MAC steadily increases until 2–3 months of age, but after 3 months, MAC starts declining with a slight increase during puberty. Uptake and elimination of inhalational agents are quicker in paediatric patients as compared to adults. This difference is seen as there is an increased respiratory rate and cardiac index in the paediatric population, with a greater distribution of cardiac output to vessel-rich organs. Changes in ventilation and cardiac output affect soluble inhalational agents more than less soluble anaesthetic agents, such as sevoflurane and desflurane.[8,9] Sevoflurane is widely used for induction during anaesthesia due to its low blood solubility and quick equilibration of alveolar and inspired concentrations.[1,24] Desflurane is pungent and may trigger upper airway reflexes such as breath-holding and laryngospasm during induction in children. 1 MAC of desflurane is 9.16% in neonates, 9.42% in 1-6 months, 9.92% in 6–12 months, 8.72% in 1-3 years, 8.62% in 3–5 years and 7.98% in 5–12 years age-group as compared to 7% in an adult.[16,23]

## *Opioids*

*Remifentanil*: Remifentanil is an ultra-fast-acting titratable opioid with a half-life of 3.2 minutes even after 3 hours of continuous intravenous infusion. Remifentanil has a strong affinity for mu receptors and less for kappa and delta-opioid receptors. The dose of remifentanil infusion is 0.05–0.1mg/kg/min with up to 0.5 mg/kg/min as mentioned in a recent study. It has predictable pharmacokinetics and an allometric exponent of 0.76. It has clinical application in short painful procedures due to its stable, haemodynamic and superior control of surgical stress response as compared to other opioids. Remifentanil can be combined with propofol with a clinical combination of 2.5, 5 and 10 mg of remifentanil combined per millilitre of propofol. Remifentanil has adverse effects of short duration. No dose adjustment is required in mild to moderate liver or renal disease.[25,26]

*Fentanyl:* Fentanyl is 50–100 times more potent than morphine. In premature infants, the half-life of fentanyl is 6–32 hours. The clearance of fentanyl is reduced in preterm neonates, resulting in respiratory depression. Fentanyl dosage via intravenous route is 1–2 μg/kg, continuous infusion 1–3 μg/kg/h, intranasal 1–2 μg/kg and oral transmucosal 5–15 μg/kg. Fentanyl may show variable kinetics (up to 17-fold variation in clearance) in preterm neonates after bolus or continuous infusion.[9,25,26]

*Morphine:* Morphine is 30–35% protein bound, but in neonates, it is 18–22% bound. Morphine-6-glucuronide metabolite is more potent than morphine. Morphine has a high hepatic extraction coefficient and is dependent on hepatic blood flow. Morphine is metabolised by sulfation rather than glucuronidation. The mean clearance of morphine is 32–52 ml/min/kg in children as compared to 2–16 ml/min/kg in neonates. Larger inter-individual variation has been observed with intravenous morphine in critically ill neonates and infants. Intravenous dose of morphine is 50 μg/kg in neonates and 100 μg/kg in infants and children up to 12 years of age. The dose of morphine as a continuous infusion in neonates is 5-20 μg/kg/h, in infants is 10–30 μg/kg/h, and in children is 20–30 μg/kg/h. Inter-individual variation in critically ill patients can prolong hepatic and renal clearance of morphine and lead to altered pharmacokinetics of morphine.[27]

*Tramadol:* Tramadol is a weak opioid with weak affinity to μ-opioid receptor. Polymorphism of the cytochrome P450 2D6 (*CYP2D6)* gene results in less conversion of tramadol to its active forms. The use of tramadol for pain relief is contraindicated in children younger than 12 years, and for post-operative tonsil/adenoid surgery, it is contraindicated in children younger than 18 years as per the latest Food and Drug Administration (FDA) safety announcement. The dosage of intravenous tramadol is 1–2.5 mg/kg, and infusion is 0.1–0.25 mg/kg/h.[1,27] Breastfeeding mothers receiving tramadol for pain relief need to be warned regarding the occurrence of serious respiratory depression in neonates and infants.

## *Muscle Relaxants*

The foetal acetylcholine receptors (AChRs) have 2$\alpha$, $\beta$, $\gamma$ and $\delta$ subunits. During development into adulthood, the $\gamma$ subunit is replaced by $\varepsilon$ subunit. Infants younger than 2 months have a lower train-of-four ratio, and infants > 2 months of age have increased fade. The volume of distribution is greater in children with water-soluble neuromuscular blocking drugs. So, increased dosages are required. Neonates and young infants have a large volume of distribution, and this results in altered response to depolarising neuromuscular agents, with dosage based on body weight. Neonates are resistant to depolarising neuromuscular agents when the administered dose of muscle relaxant is calculated based on body weight. However, when the dose of succinylcholine is calculated based on body surface area (which correlates with extracellular fluid) in neonates and young infants, the resistance to neuromuscular effect is not observed. In neonates, there is increased sensitivity to non-depolarising muscle relaxants due to reduced release of acetylcholine from immature motor nerves, but this effect is countered by the large volume of distribution. Hence, the dose calculations of non-depolarising muscle relaxants are calculated based on body weight.[8,28]

*Succinylcholine:* The dose is usually calculated based on weight. The dose is 1–3 mg/kg for infants and 2 mg/kg for children, with onset of action 30–60 seconds and duration of action 3–12 minutes.[28] Effective dose 90% ($ED_{90}$) of succinyl choline in neonates is 0.517 mg/kg and 8.24 mg/m$^2$.

*Vecuronium:* Vecuronium is a long-acting neuromuscular agent for infants and children. The dose in infants and children is 0.05–0.1 mg/kg. Onset is rapid in infants, 0.6–0.8 times that of a child and duration is increased by 1.7–2.9 times that of a child.[23,28]

*Rocuronium:* Rocuronium has a rapid onset and is longer acting in infants than in children. Both succinylcholine and rocuronium are of possible use in rapid sequence induction after ruling out any contraindication. The dose of rocuronium in infants and children is 0.3–1.0 mg/kg. The volume of distribution is larger in infants as compared to children, but clearance is slower in infants as compared to children.[28]

*Cisatracurium:* The dose of cisatracurium is similar to adults, with increased potency and greater specificity of drug action. Onset of action with intravenous cisatracurium 0.15 mg/kg occurs at 2 min in infants and 3 min in children. For cisatracurium, $ED_{95}$ values are similar for infants, children and adults.[28]

## *Local Anaesthetics*

Premature infants and neonates have a higher sensitivity to LAs due to their immature nervous system and increased sensitivity of sodium channels. Hence, reduced concentration and dose of LA are used in premature infants and neonates.[29] The larger volumes of distribution of water-soluble LAs in neonates and infants, as compared with older children, decrease the risk of high plasma concentrations after a single injection. However, the risk of drug accumulation after a continuous infusion or several injections is increased.[30]

Amino amide LA is metabolised in the liver. However, neonatal liver function is immature, with the maturation of cytochrome P450 enzyme systems occurring at different rates. For example, CYP3A4 typically matures within the first 9 months of life, whilst CYP1A2 may not reach full maturity until around 8 years of age.[31] In contrast, ester-type LA is metabolised by plasma cholinesterase, and the concentration and activity of plasma cholinesterase at birth are similar to those in adults.[29] This causes a higher risk of toxicity in neonates and infants with amide LA as compared to ester LA.

Infants have lower levels of LA-binding proteins, leading to a higher fraction of unbound LA and increased risk of toxicity. This risk is even greater before the age of 6 months when the liver is immature, and especially when continuous infusion or repeated bolus doses are used.[29] Clearance of these drugs is reduced in infants under 3 months, with adult levels reached by 8 months, resulting in longer elimination half-lives in neonates and infants compared to adults. Also, neonates and infants are at a higher risk of cardiac toxicity because of their higher heart rates and prolonged depolarisation phase.

When LA is used in peripheral nerve blocks, the duration of action is extended as compared to term neonates, as the premature neonates metabolise LA more slowly. However, when used for neuraxial anaesthesia, the duration of spinal block is shorter in infants than in adults, due to the larger volume of cerebrospinal fluid coupled with proportionally greater blood flow to the spinal cord, with more rapid uptake of drugs from the subarachnoid space. These phenomena are most pronounced in preterm infants compared with full-term infants.

Whilst using LA in fascial plane blocks, paediatric patients are at a higher risk of LA toxicity compared to adults due to the high vascularity of targeted tissue planes and the large volumes of anaesthetic required for effective spread in fascial planes.[32] Additionally, children's higher cardiac output and local blood flow elevate the likelihood of high plasma concentrations. To minimise risks, it is essential to adhere to dosing guidelines based on lean body weight, use dilute anaesthetic solutions, add epinephrine to reduce systemic absorption, select less cardiotoxic agents and monitor patients closely for 30–45 minutes after the block to observe peak plasma levels.

Furthermore, the concentration of LA used should be carefully selected, especially in children receiving general anaesthesia, where the block primarily provides analgesia. Lower concentrations (e.g., 0.125% levobupivacaine) are preferable for neonates to reduce the toxicity risk and to minimise complications such as masking compartment syndrome or delaying ambulation. However, higher concentrations (e.g., 0.5% levobupivacaine) are appropriate when a strong motor block is needed, such as in tendon transfer surgery for cerebral palsy. LA doses in children are calculated based on milligrams per kilogram, and not on volume as in adults. The recommended dosage of various LA drugs and adjuvants in paediatric patients is summarised in **Tables 1 and 2.**[33]

Synthetic opioids, such as fentanyl, lack evidence of efficacy as adjuvants in paediatric caudal blocks and do not enhance the effects of bupivacaine or ropivacaine.[33]

**TABLE 1:** Dosage of various local anaesthetic drugs in paediatrics.

| *Variables* | *Bupivacaine* | *Ropivacaine* | *Levobupivacaine* | *Lignocaine with adrenaline* |
|---|---|---|---|---|
| Allowable dose (mg/kg) | 2.5 | 2 | 2.5 | 7 |
| Bolus for upper and lower extremity blocks(mg/kg) | 0.5–1.5 | 0.5–1.5 | 0.5–1.5 | — |
| Bolus for fascial plane blocks (mg/kg) | 0.25–0.75 | 0.25–0.75 | 0.25–0.75 | — |
| Concentration for infusions (%) | 0.25 | 0.2 | 0.25 | — |
| Allowable infusion dose in mg/kg/h | 0.2 | 0.2 | 0.2 | — |

**TABLE 2:** Dosage of various local anaesthetic drug adjuvants in paediatrics.

| *Drug* | *Intrathecal dose* | *Caudal epidural doses* | *Peripheral nerve block* | *Side effects* |
|---|---|---|---|---|
| Morphine | 3 µg/kg | 30–90 µg/kg | | Nausea, vomiting and respiratory depression |
| Dexmedetomidine | 0.5–1 µg/kg | 1–2 µg/kg | 0.25–0.75 µg/kg | Sedation, bradycardia and hypotension |
| Clonidine | 0.5–1 µg/kg | 1–2 µg/kg | | Sedation, bradycardia and hypotension |

## EFFECT OF ANAESTHETIC EXPOSURE DURING CHILDHOOD ON THE DEVELOPING BRAIN

Animal studies suggest that anaesthetic exposure can harm the developing brain, leading to cognitive and functional impairments. Not only general anaesthetics but also hyperoxia can affect the developing brain. Hyperoxia is a well-known cause of cerebral white matter injury in preterm infants, with the male gender being an independent and critical risk factor for poor neurodevelopmental outcomes. Gender is therefore widely considered as one of the major decisive factors for the prognosis and treatment of these infants. Hyperoxia is a powerful trigger for the widespread apoptotic neuronal death and degeneration in the white matter tracts and periventricular regions in the developing brain. However, the molecular mechanisms and details regarding this still need to be uncovered.[34]

Recent research highlights the significant role of long non-coding ribonucleic acids (lncRNAs) in brain injury induced by hyperoxia.[35-37] For instance, the lncRNA metastasis-associated lung adenocarcinoma transcript 1 (MALAT1) has been identified as promoting neuroprotection during hypoxic/ischaemic injury. Additionally, studies have demonstrated that inhibiting lncRNA H19 can aid in the recovery from traumatic brain injury by activating the nuclear factor erythroid 2-related factor 2/heme oxygenase 1 (Nrf2/HO-1) pathway, facilitating both neuropathological and functional improvements.[36]

## MECHANISMS OF NEUROTOXICITY

### Inflammation and Immature Vascularisation

Systemic inflammation, potentially triggered by surgical stress or prenatal conditions, combined with hypoxia-ischaemia, activates microglia, releasing cytokines and free radicals and can lead to impaired cerebral flow. This leads to excitotoxicity, damaging pre-oligodendrocytes and resulting in hypomyelination. Prolonged exposure to anaesthetics such as sevoflurane and propofol can cause mitochondrial injury, increasing reactive oxygen species (ROS) production and brain damage.[38] Isoflurane disrupts astrocyte development, further affecting brain maturation.[39]

### Binding of Anaesthetics to N-Methyl-D-Aspartate and Gamma-Aminobutyric Acid Receptors

This binding disturbs intracellular calcium levels and mitochondrial function, thereby disrupting synaptic transmission and the excitatory-inhibitory balance essential for brain development.

Contrarily, sub-toxic doses of anaesthetics have been shown to confer neuroprotection. Isoflurane and sevoflurane preconditioning have been shown to improve outcomes in animal models through mechanisms such as protein kinase B activation, ROS release, and modulation of various signalling pathways.[40,41]

## LONG-TERM NEUROCOGNITIVE OUTCOMES

### Cognitive Deficits

Some studies suggest a risk of cognitive deficits, especially in language and abstract reasoning. However, the General Anaesthesia compared to Spinal anaesthesia (GAS) study found no increased neurocognitive impairment at 5 years.[42]

### Behavioural Problems

Early anaesthesia exposure may be linked to behavioural issues, such as hyperactivity.[43] The GAS study found no increased risk of autism spectrum disorder or attention deficit hyperactivity disorder, though these conditions are typically diagnosed in older children.[42]

## PRENATAL EXPOSURE TO ANAESTHETIC DRUGS AND EFFECTS ON THE FOETUS

Advanced medical and surgical technology has led to more frequent interventions during pregnancy. The mid-trimester of pregnancy is considered a safe period for surgery, but it is still a delicate phase for the foetus, as during this time, the central nervous system undergoes significant maturation, making it particularly susceptible to the anaesthetic drugs.

Understanding the anaesthetic transfer between the maternal and foetal systems is therefore crucial for minimising adverse effects. Although the placenta serves as a barrier to regulate the transfer of substances from the mother to the foetus, it is not completely effective in preventing the passage of certain drugs. Most inhalational anaesthetic agents, due to their fat-soluble nature, are capable of crossing the placental barrier with relative ease and attaining significant concentrations in the foetal brain. Muscle relaxants generally have minimal effects on the foetus due to their limited placental penetration.[44,45]

## Factors Influencing the Effect of Anaesthetic Drugs on the Foetus

### *The Duration of Anaesthesia*

Short-term (1–2 hours) exposure to about 1 MAC anaesthetic concentration can enhance neural stem cell proliferation, whereas prolonged exposure (6 hours) can reduce self-renewal capacity, leading to increased apoptosis and inhibited proliferation. For example, 6 hours of exposure to 2.5% concentrations of sevoflurane resulted in cell cycle arrest and learning deficits in the offspring.[44,45]

### *Repeated Exposure to Anaesthesia*

Whilst some studies suggest that single exposures do not significantly affect long-term behavioural outcomes or synaptic plasticity, others report detrimental effects from multiple exposures.

### *The Concentration of Anaesthetics*

High concentrations of inhalational anaesthetics during pregnancy have been associated with neurodegenerative changes and learning disorders in the offspring.[46]

### *The Trimester of Pregnancy*

During pregnancy, the foetal brain undergoes significant development, especially in the second trimester. Research suggests that during this trimester, the foetal brain may be more vulnerable to the potential adverse effects of inhalational anaesthetics compared to other trimesters. This vulnerability is due to the ongoing critical stages of brain development during this period.[46,47]

## Impact of Anaesthesia on Foetal Neurodevelopment

Animal studies have shown that exposure to certain anaesthetic agents during critical developmental periods can lead to cognitive impairments and alterations in motor coordination and reflexes. Studies in rodents have shown that exposure to isoflurane during stages of critical development can lead to memory and learning deficits. The underlying mechanisms involve neuroinflammation, apoptosis and disrupted synaptic plasticity, crucial for learning and memory processes. Sevoflurane has been shown to have neurotoxic effects when administered during pregnancy in rodent models, when exposed to high concentrations, linked to persistent cognitive deficits in the offspring. The impairments include difficulties in acquiring new information, slower processing speeds, and memory retention issues.[38,39]

Human studies are more complex due to ethical considerations and variability in exposure. However, observational studies have suggested potential associations between prenatal exposure to anaesthetics and neurodevelopmental disorders, increased risk of autism spectrum disorders, attention-deficit/hyperactivity disorder (ADHD) and developmental delays, such as speech and motor skills.[45,46] Prenatal exposures to general anaesthesia is associated with a 31% increased risk for a subsequent diagnosis of a disruptive or internalising behavioural disorder in children.[47]

Exposure to surgery and anaesthesia in early childhood has also been linked to an increased risk of behavioural deficits. These concerns have prompted the United States Food and Drug Administration (FDA) to issue warnings about prenatal exposure to general anaesthetics and sedative drugs, particularly in late pregnancy (risks associated with repeated or prolonged exposure) and in children under 3 years (potential impact on neurodevelopment with repeated or extended use).

The potential for increased behavioural problems in the offspring must be balanced against the immediate health needs of the mother and foetus. One should emphasise minimising exposure to anaesthetic agents during pregnancy and employing the lowest effective doses for the shortest duration necessary. Clinicians should develop strategies to address potential developmental concerns in children prenatally exposed to anaesthesia.

Not only the prenatal exposure, but Martynyuk et al. also describe the adverse effects of GABAergic general anaesthetic agents, such as sevoflurane, on germ cells. They highlight potential epigenetic changes and intergenerational effects resulting from exposure to these agents. These anaesthetics have been associated with two distinct types of long-term adverse outcomes: somatic neuroendocrine alterations and epigenetic programming of germ cells. The process of epigenetic reprogramming in germ cells during development involves deoxyribonucleic acid (DNA) methylation, histone modifications, and non-coding RNA expression, which are crucial for proper gene expression and cellular function. Exposure to anaesthetic agents during key stages of germ cell development can disrupt this reprogramming process. Germ cells appear to be more susceptible to the disruptive effects of anaesthetics compared to somatic cells, potentially leading to intergenerational consequences, where the offspring of exposed parents may also be affected.[23]

## EMERGING TRENDS IN PAEDIATRIC MOLECULAR PHARMACOLOGY

### Pharmacogenetics and Pharmacogenomics

Pharmacogenetics and pharmacogenomics are two related fields that explore how genetic variations influence an individual's response to drugs.[1] Both fields have the potential to play a critical role in paediatric anaesthesia by improving the safety and efficacy of anaesthetic drugs for children.

Pharmacogenetics is the study of genetic variations in specific genes and their impact on an individual's response to drugs.[2] In paediatric anaesthesia, it helps identify genetic factors that may affect how children metabolise or respond to anaesthetic agents. This field plays a crucial role in personalised drug selection and dosing by detecting variations in drug-metabolising enzymes, such as cytochrome P450, thereby enabling the adjustment of drug dosages to prevent both underdosing and overdosing. Genetic factors can also influence the risk of anaesthesia-related side effects, such as malignant hyperthermia in children with mutations in the *RYR1* gene.

Pharmacogenomics is a broader field that involves studying the entire genome and how it affects an individual's overall response to drugs. This includes understanding how variations in multiple genes and gene-environment interactions contribute to drug metabolism, efficacy, and side effects. Genome sequencing is an important component of precision medicine.[2] Pharmacogenomics allows for selecting anaesthetic drugs and doses that align with a child's genetic makeup, enhancing both efficacy and safety.

### Advances in Anaesthetic Drug Delivery Systems

Targeted drug delivery for anaesthetic drugs focuses on delivering medications directly to specific sites of action, minimising systemic exposure, and reducing side effects. This approach is particularly beneficial in children, who are more sensitive to drug toxicity and may have difficulty in tolerating systemic side effects. Key strategies for targeted anaesthetic drug delivery in paediatrics include microneedles, nanoparticles, liposomal carriers, hydrogels and transdermal patches for localised and controlled drug release, as well as ultrasound-guided precision injections and prodrug formulations for site-specific action.[48,49] LA drugs, fentanyl and dexmedetomidine, have been explored for targeted drug delivery.[50,51]

#### *Transmucosal Drug Delivery System*

There are two transmucosal routes: (1) Intranasal and (2) buccal. The intranasal route is convenient for premedication, as it is painless and offers high drug bioavailability. Intranasal formulations of dexmedetomidine and midazolam are commonly used for this purpose, with absorption occurring within 3–5 minutes. Buccal mucosal drug delivery bypasses first-pass metabolism. Fentanyl lozenges are available for delivery via this route.

### *Intranasal Drug Delivery System*

Intranasal administration is a non-invasive route that is well accepted by children and has a rapid onset with high bioavailability of drugs. It can be administered by drops or a mucosal atomiser device. Fentanyl (1.5 μg/kg), dexmedetomidine (0.5–4 μg/kg), ketamine (0.5–4 mg/kg) and midazolam (0.2–0.5 mg/kg) are commonly used intranasal drugs.

Nebulised drugs are absorbed through the nasal, buccal, and respiratory mucosa. Dexmedetomidine (2 μg/kg), ketamine (2 mg/kg), and midazolam (0.2 mg/kg) are some drugs that are administered via nebulisation.[52]

### *Transdermal Drug Delivery System*

The skin acts as the primary barrier to drug delivery via the topical route. It comprises of three main layers: (1) The outermost stratum corneum, (2) the middle epidermis and the thickest layer and (3) the dermis. The stratum corneum serves as the main barrier, permitting only specific molecules, such as lipophilic and low molecular-weight drugs, to penetrate. In the case of a transdermal patch, the drug must pass the stratum corneum barrier. Thus, it shows less bioavailability. It, however, has the advantage of bypassing first-pass metabolism. In neonates, the thin stratum corneum may increase drug absorption and toxicity, so transdermal delivery is best avoided. The topical creams spread only on the skin surface, with only 10–20% of the total drug permeating the skin.

Eutectic mixture of local anaesthetics (EMLA) (2.5% lignocaine and prilocaine) and Ametop (4% amethocaine gel) are used for topical anaesthesia for intravenous cannulation. Transdermal fentanyl patches designed to deliver approximately 12, 25, 50, 75 and 100 μg/h of fentanyl to the systemic circulation are available. The patches can be left in place for 72 hours. After application, fentanyl is absorbed by the skin, creating a depot in the upper skin layers. Plasma fentanyl concentrations gradually increase, maintaining constant drug levels. The release continues for 13–22 hours after removing the patch.

The addition of a permeation enhancer in the transdermal patch can improve the drug permeation, but up to a very limited extent. Techniques such as controlled heat, iontophoresis, and electroporation can promote the transfer of less lipid-soluble drugs but fail for large molecules.[52-55] The hypodermic needle goes deep into the dermis and can deliver 90–100% of the loaded drug, but it is very painful.

Microneedles are now being studied for the transdermal delivery of hydrophilic high molecular weight compounds into the stratum corneum.

The device combines the benefits of hypodermic needles (without the major drawback of pain) and transdermal patches (without the limitation of requiring low molecular weight, lipophilic drugs), thereby addressing the shortcomings of both. The device consists of tiny needles, each micron-sized, arranged on a small patch.[49,50] Apart from being painless, the bioavailability with these devices is high, making them a promising innovation for the future. Lignocaine microneedles could completely replace EMLA if they become widely available.[56]

### *Target-controlled Infusion in Children*

Considering pharmacokinetic differences in paediatrics, TCI models have been developed to deliver larger induction boluses and lower maintenance infusion rates.[57-59] Two common paediatric TCI models for propofol-based total intravenous anaesthesia (TIVA) are Paedfusor and Kataria.[59] Paedfusor is suitable for ages 1–16 years and patients weighing 5–61 kg, whilst the Kataria model is suitable for ages 3–16 years and patients weighing 15–61 kg. These models predict plasma site concentration (Cp) rather than effect-site concentration (Ce), so adequate time must be allowed for Cp-Ce equilibration when adjusting target levels. The target steady-state Cp for propofol as a sole agent is 4–6 µg/ml and 3–4 µg/ml with adjuncts, such as remifentanil infusion. In the absence of TCI pumps, manual infusion models such as McFarlan can be used in children 3–11 years old, and the manual infusion scheme of Steur et al. can be used in children younger than 3 years.[60,61] Electroencephalogram (EEG) based bispectral index (BIS) and entropy algorithms, based on adult data, are inconsistent for children aged $< 1$ year, so clinical signs are the primary method for assessing anaesthesia depth. Syringe pumps may not reliably deliver drugs at rates $\leq 0.5$ ml/h, but preparing drugs in lower concentrations can help. Closed-loop TCI systems have also been described for paediatric patients.

The Minto TCI remifentanil model is suitable for paediatric patients $\geq 12$ years, weighing $\geq 30$ kg. No TCI remifentanil regimens exist for those $<12$ years.[62] Fixed dose infusion rates of 0.1–0.3 µg/kg/min provide adequate intraoperative analgesia and are used to supplement propofol TIVA.

Total intravenous anaesthesia is primarily indicated for children with a known susceptibility to malignant hyperthermia or a family history of the condition. Future research should focus on developing TCI models and EEG monitoring algorithms for neonates and infants.

## CHALLENGES IN PAEDIATRIC AND FOETAL PHARMACOLOGICAL RESEARCH

Paediatric pharmacology research is crucial for understanding how drugs affect children; however, it faces significant ethical and practical challenges.[63] Ethically, children are a vulnerable population, and research involving them requires careful consideration of consent, potential harm, and long-term effects. Since children cannot legally provide informed consent, parental consent is required for trials, along with assent from older children. Additionally, stricter regulatory requirements add complexity to the research process. Practically, the paediatric population is smaller and more diverse, spanning various developmental stages (neonates, infants, children and adolescents). The limited number of children available for trials makes it difficult to collect sufficient data for each age group, restricting the scope of paediatric research. These constraints often lead to data being extrapolated from adult studies, which have inherent risks and limitations.

Research through comprehensive long-term studies is essential to fully understand the effects of prenatal exposure to anaesthetic drugs and ensure maternal safety and efficacy whilst avoiding any harm to the foetus or disruption of the labour process. Efforts need to be directed towards developing anaesthetic agents with reduced neurotoxic potential and establishing protocols to minimise exposure during critical periods of foetal development. Whilst animal research links general anaesthetic exposure to neurodevelopmental impairments, translating these findings to humans is complex due to differences in brain development and clinical contexts.

Further, there is a significant disparity between developed and developing nations in terms of resources, funding, and infrastructure for drug discovery and research, particularly in paediatric pharmacology and pharmacogenomics. International collaboration is essential to bridge this gap, ensuring that pharmacogenomic advancements benefit all paediatric populations.

## FUTURE SCOPE OF PAEDIATRIC MOLECULAR PHARMACOLOGY

Although the integration of pharmacogenomics into routine pre-anaesthetic evaluations is promising, it remains underutilised even in many developed countries. Its adoption in developing nations may take considerable time due to resource and infrastructure constraints. Continued research in this field will not only enable the personalisation of anaesthetic drug regimens for individual patients but also deepen our understanding of pharmacogenomic variations influenced by factors such as age, ethnicity, and developmental stage. The widespread application of pharmacogenomics could facilitate the creation of robust pharmacogenomic databases and predictive models. Furthermore, advancements in pharmacogenomics have the potential to drive innovation in research and the creation of novel anaesthetic agents. Point-of-care genetic testing may also become a viable option in the future. Therefore, the potential of pharmacogenomics in paediatric anaesthesia is both vast and transformative.

The role of professional societies such as the Indian Society of Anaesthesiologists (ISA) in advancing paediatric pharmacological research by facilitating collaboration among researchers, clinicians, and pharmaceutical companies, advocating for more resources and attention to the unique needs of the paediatric population in this direction will prove very useful. Their efforts can be critical in shaping the future of paediatric care and ensuring that research translates into better outcomes for children worldwide.

## CONCLUSION

In summary, whilst molecular pharmacology holds great promise for improving paediatric drug therapy, significant gaps in knowledge remain. Further research is essential to address developmental differences, genetic variations, and other paediatric-specific considerations to ensure safe and effective drug use in children.

## REFERENCES

1. Kaye AD, Mahakian T, Kaye AJ, Pham AA, Hart BM, Gennuso S, et al. Pharmacogenomics, precision medicine, and implications for anesthesia care. Best Pract Res Clin Anaesthesiol. 2018;32(2):61-81.
2. Behrooz A. Pharmacogenetics and anaesthetic drugs: Implications for perioperative practice. Ann Med Surg (Lond). 2015;4(4):470-4.
3. Hu TM. A general biphasic bodyweight model for scaling basal metabolic rate, glomerular filtration rate, and drug clearance from birth to adulthood. AAPS J. 2022;24(3):67.
4. Van Rongen A, Krekels EH, Calvier EA, de Wildt SN, Vermeulen A, Knibbe CA. An update on the use of allometric and other scaling methods to scale drug clearance in children: Towards decision tables. Expert Opin Drug Metab Toxicol. 2022;18(2):99-113.
5. Chapron BD, Chapron A, Leeder JS. Recent advances in the ontogeny of drug disposition. Br J Clin Pharmacol. 2022;88(10):4267-84.
6. Euteneuer JC, Kamatkar S, Fukuda T, Vinks AA, Akinbi HT. Suggestions for model-informed precision dosing to optimize neonatal drug therapy. J Clin Pharmacol. 2019;59(2):168-76.
7. Hughes JH, Tong DMH, Lucas SS, Faldasz JD, Goswami S, Keizer RJ. Continuous learning in model-informed precision dosing: A case study in pediatric dosing of vancomycin. Clin Pharmacol Ther. 2021;109(1):233-42.
8. Batchelor HK, Marriott JF. Paediatric pharmacokinetics: key considerations. Br J Clin Pharmacol. 2015;79(3):395-404.
9. O'Hara K. Paediatric pharmacokinetics and drug doses. Aust Prescr. 2016;39(6):208-10.
10. Sethi PK, White CA, Cummings BS, Hines RN, Muralidhara S, Bruckner JV. Ontogeny of plasma proteins, albumin and binding of diazepam, cyclosporine, and deltamethrin. Pediatr Res. 2016;79(3):409-15.
11. Stutman HR, Parker KM, Marks MI. Potential of moxalactam and other new antimicrobial agents for bilirubin-albumin displacement in neonates. Pediatrics. 1985;75(2):294-8.

12. Sullins AK, Abdel-Rahman SM. Pharmacokinetics of antibacterial agents in the CSF of children and adolescents. Paediatr Drugs. 2013;15(2):93-117.
13. Ladumor MK, Bhatt DK, Gaedigk A, Sharma S, Thakur A, Pearce RE, et al. Ontogeny of hepatic sulfotransferases and prediction of age-dependent fractional contribution of sulfation in acetaminophen metabolism. Drug Metab Dispos. 2019;47(8):818-31.
14. Hines RN. The ontogeny of drug metabolism enzymes and implications for adverse drug events. Pharmacol Ther. 2008;118(2):250-67.
15. Filho EM, Riechelmann MB. Propofol use in newborns and children: is it safe? A systematic review. J Pediatr (Rio J). 2020;96(3):289-309.
16. Sneyd JR. Thiopental to desflurane - an anaesthetic journey. Where are we going next? Br J Anaesth. 2017;119(Suppl 1):i44-i52.
17. Mellon RD, Simone AF, Rappaport BA. Use of anesthetic agents in neonates and young children. Anesth Analg. 2007;104(3):509-20.
18. Bhutta AT. Ketamine: a controversial drug for neonates. Semin Perinatol. 2007;31(5):303-8.
19. Poonai N, Canton K, Ali S, Hendrikx S, Shah A, Miller M, et al. Intranasal ketamine for procedural sedation and analgesia in children: A systematic review. PLoS One. 2017;12(3):e0173253.
20. Iqbal AU, Shuster ME, Baum CR. Ketofol for Procedural Sedation and Analgesia in the Pediatric Population. Pediatr Emerg Care. 2022;38(1):28-33.
21. Wang R, Lin Q. Prolonged ketamine exposure induces enhanced excitatory GABAergic synaptic activity in the anterior cingulate cortex of neonatal rats. Neurosci Lett. 2021;745:135647.
22. Yan J, Jiang H. Dual effects of ketamine: neurotoxicity versus neuroprotection in anesthesia for the developing brain. J Neurosurg Anesthesiol. 2014;26(2): 155-60.
23. Allegaert K, Van de Velde M, Van den Anker J. Neonatal clinical pharmacology. Paediatr Anaesth. 2014;24(1):30-8.
24. Martynyuk AE, Ju LS, Morey TE, Zhang JQ. Neuroendocrine, epigenetic, and intergenerational effects of general anesthetics. World J Psychiatry. 2020;10(5):81-94.
25. Suwa K, Takahashi K, Iizuka Y, Lefor AK. High-dose remifentanil anesthesia with minimal sedation in neonates: A single-center retrospective study. Cureus. 2024;16(8):e67801.
26. Ziesenitz VC, Vaughns JD, Koch G, Mikus G, van den Anker JN. Pharmacokinetics of fentanyl and its derivatives in children: A comprehensive review. Clin Pharmacokinet. 2018;57(2):125-49. Erratum in: Clin Pharmacokinet. 2018;57:393-417.
27. Thigpen JC, Odle BL, Harirforoosh S. Opioids: A review of pharmacokinetics and pharmacodynamics in neonates, infants, and children. Eur J Drug Metab Pharmacokinet. 2019;44(5):591-609.
28. Gronert BJ, Brandom BW. Neuromuscular blocking drugs in infants and children. Pediatr Clin North Am. 1994;41(1):73-91.
29. El-Boghdadly K, Pawa A, Chin KJ. Local anesthetic systemic toxicity: current perspectives. Local Reg Anesth. 2018;11:35-44.
30. Mazoit JX, Dalens BJ. Pharmacokinetics of local anaesthetics in infants and children. Clin Pharmacokinet. 2004;43(1):17-32.

31. O'Hara K, Wright IM, Schneider JJ, Jones AL, Martin JH. Pharmacokinetics in neonatal prescribing: evidence base, paradigms and the future. Br J Clin Pharmacol. 2015;80(6):1281-8.
32. Lönnqvist PA. Fascial plane blocks in children-Scientifically supported or not? Paediatr Anaesth 2024;34:13-18.
33. Suresh S, Ecoffey C, Bosenberg A, Lonnqvist PA, de Oliveira GS Jr, de Leon Casasola O, et al. The European Society of Regional Anaesthesia and Pain Therapy/American Society of Regional Anesthesia and Pain Medicine Recommendations on Local Anesthetics and Adjuvants Dosage in Pediatric Regional Anesthesia. Reg Anesth Pain Med. 2018;43(2):211-6.
34. Felderhoff-Mueser U, Bittigau P, Sifringer M, Jarosz B, Korobowicz E, Mahler L, et al. Oxygen causes cell death in the developing brain. Neurobiol Dis. 2004;17(2):273-82.
35. Wang L, Li S, Stone SS, Liu N, Gong K, Ren C, et al. The role of the lncRNA MALAT1 in neuroprotection against hypoxic/ischemic injury. Biomolecules. 2022;12(1):146.
36. Chen Q, Wu B, Shi Z, Wang Y, Yuan Y, Chen X, et al. LncRNA H19 knockdown promotes neuropathologic and functional recovery via the Nrf2/HO-1 axis after traumatic brain injury. CNS Neurosci Ther. 2024;30(7):e14870.
37. Wu J, Zhang G, Xiong H, Zhang Y, Ding G, Ge J. miR-181c-5p mediates apoptosis of vascular endothelial cells induced by hyperoxemia via ceRNA crosstalk. Sci Rep. 2021;11(1):16582.
38. Boscolo A, Starr JA, Sanchez V, Lunardi N, DiGruccio MR, Ori C, et al. The abolishment of anesthesia-induced cognitive impairment by timely protection of mitochondria in the developing rat brain: The importance of free oxygen radicals and mitochondrial integrity. Neurobiol Dis. 2012;45(3): 1031-41.
39. Ryu YK, Khan S, Smith SC, Mintz CD. Isoflurane impairs the capacity of astrocytes to support neuronal development in a mouse dissociated co-culture model. J Neurosurg Anesthesiol. 2014;26(4):363-8.
40. Kitano H, Kirsch JR, Hurn PD, Murphy SJ. Inhalational anesthetics as neuroprotectants or chemical preconditioning agents in ischemic brain. J Cereb Blood Flow Metab. 2007;27(6):1108-28.
41. Zuo Z, Wang Y, Huang Y. Isoflurane preconditioning protects human neuroblastoma SH-SY5Y cells against in vitro simulated ischemia-reperfusion through the activation of extracellular signal-regulated kinases pathway. Eur J Pharmacol. 2006;542(1-3):84-91.
42. McCann ME, de Graaff JC, Dorris L, Disma N, Withington D, Bell G, et al. Neurodevelopmental outcome at 5 years of age after general anaesthesia or awake-regional anaesthesia in infancy (GAS): an international, multicentre, randomised, controlled equivalence trial. Lancet. 2019;393(10172):664-77.
43. Ing C, Ma X, Sun M, Lu Y, Wall MM, Olfson M, et al. Exposure to surgery and anesthesia in early childhood and subsequent use of attention deficit hyperactivity disorder medications. Anesth Analg. 2020;131(3):723-33.
44. Balinskaite V, Bottle A, Sodhi V, Rivers A, Bennett PR, Brett SJ, et al. The risk of adverse pregnancy outcomes following nonobstetric surgery during pregnancy: estimates from a retrospective cohort study of 6.5 million pregnancies. Ann Surg. 2017;266(2):260-6.

45. Cheek TG, Baird E. Anesthesia for nonobstetric surgery: maternal and fetal considerations. Clin Obstet Gynecol. 2009;52(4):535-45.
46. De Tina A, Palanisamy A. General anesthesia during the third trimester: any link to neurocognitive outcomes? Anesthesiol Clin. 2017;35(1):69-80.
47. Ing C, Silber JH, Lackraj D, Olfson M, Miles C, Reiter JG, Jain S, et al. Behavioural disorders after prenatal exposure to anaesthesia for maternal surgery. Br J Anaesth. 2024;132:899-910.
48. Prausnitz MR, Langer R. Transdermal drug delivery. Nat Biotechnol 2008;26(11):1261-8.
49. Sharma D. Microneedles: an approach in transdermal drug delivery: a Review. PharmaTutor. 2018;26:7-15.
50. Waghule T, Singhvi G, Dubey SK, Pandey MM, Gupta G, Singh M, et al. Microneedles: A smart approach and increasing potential for transdermal drug delivery system. Biomed Pharmacother. 2019;109:1249-58.
51. Baek SH, Shin JH, Kim YC. Drug-coated microneedles for rapid and painless local anesthesia. Biomed Microdevices. 2017;19(1):2.
52. Dave NM. Premedication and induction of anaesthesia in paediatric patients. Indian J Anaesth. 2019;63(9):713-20.
53. Eberhart L. The safety and tolerability of the fentanyl HCl iontophoretic transdermal system: An alternative to currently available analgesic modalities. J Opioid Manag. 2007;3(5):249-56.
54. Kinoshita M, Yamamoto R, Kominami K. In-vitro and in-vivo transdermal iontophoretic delivery of tramadol, a centrally acting analgesic. J Pharm Pharmacol. 2011;63(11):1437-45.
55. Polat BE, Blankschtein D, Langer R. Low-frequency sonophoresis: Application to the transdermal delivery of macromolecules and hydrophilic drugs. Expert Opin Drug Deliv. 2010;7(12):1415-32.
56. Zhang Y, Brown K, Siebenaler K, Determan A, Dohmeier D, Hansen K. Development of lidocaine-coated microneedle product for rapid, safe, and prolonged local analgesic action. Pharm Res. 2012;29(1):170-7.
57. Eleveld DJ, Colin P, Absalom AR, Struys MMRF. Pharmacokinetic-pharmacodynamic model for propofol for broad application in anaesthesia and sedation. Br J Anaesth. 2018;120(5):942-59.
58. West N, Dumont GA, van Heusden K, Petersen CL, Khosravi S, Soltesz K, et al. Robust closed-loop control of induction and maintenance of propofol anesthesia in children. Paediatr Anaesth. 2013;23(8):712-9.
59. Kataria BK, Ved SA, Nicodemus HF, Hoy GR, Lea D, Dubois MY, et al. The pharmacokinetics of propofol in children using three different data analysis approaches. Anesthesiology. 1994;80(1):104-22.
60. McFarlan CS, Anderson BJ, Short TG. The use of propofol infusions in paediatric anaesthesia: a practical guide. Pediatr Anesth. 1999;9(3):209-16.
61. Steur RJ, Perez RS, DeLange JJ. Dosage scheme for propofol in children under 3 years of age. Pediatr Anesth. 2004;14(6):462-7.
62. Minto CF, Schnider TW, Egan TD, Youngs E, Lemmens HJM, Gambus PL, et al. Influence of age and gender on the pharmacokinetics and pharmacodynamics of remifentanil. I. Model development. Anesthesiology. 1997;86(1):10-23.
63. Barker CIS, Standing JF, Kelly LE, Faught LH, Needham AC, Rieder MJ, et al. Pharmacokinetic studies in children: recommendations for practice and search. Arch Dis Child. 2018;103(7):695-702.

CHAPTER 2

# Role of Soft Skills and Consent in Paediatric Anaesthesia: Enhance Your Communication Skills and Provide the Best Care

*Sujata Chaudhary, Sangeeta Khanna, Vibhavari Naik, Priya Rudingwa*

## ABSTRACT

Soft skills can be defined as qualities and attributes of a person which enable him or her to interact effectively with others as a well-rounded professional. Dealing with children as patients requires paediatric anaesthesiologists to enhance these skills for a pleasant outcome. To understand the importance of soft skills and informed consent in paediatric anaesthesia, one must slip into the parent's shoes and see the world through the child's perspective. The operating room environment, fear of needles and the prospect of anaesthesia causes a lot of stress and anxiety to both the parents and the child. On the day of surgery, prolonged fasting, parental separation, a busy preoperative room and paperwork cause a lot of discomfort and anxiety. To add to this, their fear and anxiety is aggravated if the attending anaesthesiologist appears very busy and indifferent. Hence, it is imperative for the anaesthesiologist to hone the necessary soft skills as he sedates the child and wheels him to the operating room and back into the postoperative room to reunite him with his parents. As anaesthesiologists, we need to ensure that it is a smooth and pleasant experience.

This article is all about how to improve the experience and build memories—not nightmares. Our soft skills go a long way in making the patients and relatives understand the need for and benefits of the procedure, the mode of anaesthesia, the risks involved, alternative options available and opportunity to ask questions if any.

***Keywords:*** Adolescents, Child, Communication, Consent, Parents, Skills.

## INTRODUCTION

Non-technical skills (NTS) in anaesthesia are broadly divided into (1) cognitive and mental skills: these are important at the individual level. (2) Social and interpersonal skills: these are important at team level.[1]

'Soft skills' are NTS and individual interpersonal qualities that we utilise in clinical anaesthesia practice. We all encounter common situations such as the anxiety of surgery, the stress of separating a child from the parents, the mental trauma that parents undergo during the perioperative period, etc. Effective communication along with compassionate care goes a long way in alleviating this apprehension. Development of soft skills such as interpersonal skill, emotional intelligence, communication, empathy and compassion toward the patient, collaboration and negotiation skills are important attributes that help in trust building and fostering adherence to long-term patient care. Through improving the communication with families, anaesthesiologists can impact patient and family experiences of care and decision-making. These are associated with greater satisfaction, improved adherence to treatment and more favourable health outcomes.[2] Special attention is required when talking to children as our patients. The idea is to provide information in a precise way which is easy to understand, both for the child as well as the parents.[3] Open and frank communication is an art which should be developed and inculcated from the beginning of the medical career. A relation of trust and cooperation needs to be developed. Each phase of paediatric anaesthesia starting from pre-anaesthetic evaluation, periprocedural management and postoperative care presents with unique opportunities for effective communication. When discussing the 'humanistic' dimension of patient care, rushing through the operation room list should not be the sole aim. Our patients, especially children, need our time, attention, loving and compassionate care. Spending time with the child and family, talking and even playing with the child helps us to enter his or her zone.

The development of different aspects of soft skills in anaesthesia is derived from the aviation industry where this was first introduced as both domains involve attention to minute details and performance in high pressure situations.[4]

Soft skills go a long way in making the patients and caregivers understand the need for and benefits of the procedure, mode of anaesthesia, the risks involved, alternative options available and gives them an opportunity to ask questions if any. Ultimately, the child should be convinced that whatever treatment options are being offered are in his or her best interest. This is essential for having a shared and informed decision-making. Nevertheless, before embarking on any treatment, obtaining a written and informed consent is a must. With children as patients, this must be obtained from parents or legal guardians. This should be a voluntary consent, explained in the language which the patient understands, not given under any external pressures or coercion with a reasonable background information and understanding.[5]

## COMMUNICATION SKILLS FOR THE PAEDIATRIC ANAESTHESIOLOGISTS

'Communication' is the ability to proficiently convey and receive information, thoughts, emotions and concepts. This encompasses, but is not limited to, the ability to convey ideas effectively to others, to attentively listen during conversations, to provide and receive constructive feedback and to deliver public speech. Effective verbal communication should involve delivery of clear messages in a language which is easy to understand for the child and parents, accept their different realities like the opinion/beliefs, actively listen to their queries and suggest the best treatment modality. Hence forming a flexible, child-centric and age-appropriate approach should be the goal. Communication is not just about using words, which form the verbal component of communication, but the tone, pitch and speed of our communication. These provide a lot of information and constitute paraverbal communication, which is equally important. And lastly, non-verbal communication is all about what can be heard or understood without being said.[6] Maintaining eye-to-eye contact, adaptability, empathy, gestures, ensuring privacy, facial expressions, encouraging smiles and affirming nods, body language and postures are some of the key aspects of non-verbal communication. These cues can significantly influence perceptions and can enhance communication effectiveness.[7] The stark absence of formal training in this area highlights a need to include communication skills in the paediatric anaesthesia fellowship curriculum and formulated structured course for training fellows.[8]

## COMMUNICATION SKILLS WITH THE CHILD

The perioperative experience of a child is indeed a critical period where poor experiences can lead to distress and psychological trauma with potential long-term effects.[9] Effective communication with the child begins with establishing good rapport. One of the ways to establish rapport is LAURS (*L*: Listening to concerns; *A*: Acceptance of child's perceptions; *U*: Utilisation of child's thought process; *R*: Reframing positive connotations; *S*: Supportive suggestion) technique, a structured approach described by Cyna AM **(Table 1)**.[10] Communication can be initiated over a topic of relevance depending on the child's age. Some tips to improve child engagement involve sitting down at the level of the child, making eye contact, using a language appropriate for the child, and sharing simple factual information based on the comprehension of the child. Involvement of the child in an age-appropriate activity that simulates the components of the perioperative period can also be useful. Some examples include giving them a virtual reality experience to reduce anxiety of unfamiliar surroundings, making them watch their favourite video to allow venous access placement, giving them a cycle to ride to allow parental separation and making them blow a balloon to help in inhalational induction. Negative communication can play as nocebo (negative subconscious thought process affecting the outcome negatively), having the potential to cause harm and should be avoided.[11] Socioeconomic background and cultural differences have a major impact on the decision-making process. Understanding these through patient-driven interactions not only improves satisfaction but also reduces the incidence of malpractice suits.

**TABLE 1:** Elucidation of LAURS technique to establish rapport with the child.

| | *Situation* | *Anaesthesiologist's response* |
|---|---|---|
| *L*—Listening to concerns | Anaesthesiologist is about to begin inhalational induction and child refuses face mask. Child says—I do not want this | Anaesthesiologist has full attention and eye contact with the child and asks—tell me why do you not want this? |
| *A*—Acceptance of child's perceptions | Child narrates a story from his previous experience and then says—I am very scared of injections | Anaesthesiologist accepts and reassures—its okay to be scared of injections, many children are. But, we will not be giving you any |
| *U*—Utilisation of child's thought process | Child continues to have concerns around breathing through mask, feeling of choking through it and says—'But, what if I hate the smell during breathing through the mask?' | Anaesthesiologist smells the mask and says—Wow! This is specially made for you with your favourite strawberry shake flavour. Here, hold my hand and breathe. If you dislike the smell, press my hand so that I can add more strawberries to it |
| *R*—Reframing positive connotations | Child agrees to breathe through the mask but has negative thoughts like — Do I have to keep breathing through this for a very long time? | Anaesthesiologist reframes child's connotations about breathing through mask and says—'Every time you blow through this, it will make this balloon big. And bigger the balloon, sooner it will take you to your mummy' |
| *S*—Supportive suggestion | Child while breathing says—I think I am feeling sleepy | Anaesthesiologist supports the feeling by saying—Yes, you will now sleep and have lovely dreams of drinking strawberry shake made by your mummy |

## COMMUNICATION SKILLS WITH THE PARENTS

Paediatric anaesthesiologists need to master communication skills not just with the patient but also with the anxious and nervous parents. Establishing a rapport with the child relieves the parent anxiety and improves parent satisfaction scores.[12] Counselling is a vital component of communication with parents. Counselling differs from advice in that the former allows autonomy for decisions. Elements of counselling may be remembered by the acronym GATHER **(Box 1)**.[11]

**BOX 1:** Constituents of the acronym GATHER.

- *G*reet the parents
- *A*scertain need for coming
- *T*ell the choices available
- *H*elp parents make a voluntary choice
- *E*xplain the procedure
- *R*eturn with something more interesting

Occasionally, we have a situation where the parents need to be informed about the poor health and morbid condition of their child. Breaking bad news is the most challenging communication for the paediatric anaesthesiologist. The Society of Paediatric Anaesthesia (SPA) recommends the use of SPIKES, a well-established protocol for breaking bad news to the family.[13] This includes *S*etting up the interview, Assessing the patient family's *P*erception, obtaining the family's *I*nvitation, giving *K*nowledge and more information, and addressing *E*motions with empathy, strategy and summary. Empathy towards children and their parents can help to build trust and rapport, easing anxiety and fear. Nonetheless, the language should be simple and easy to understand without use of medical jargon.

## COMMUNICATION SKILLS WITH THE SURGEON AND THE TEAM

The perioperative care of children may be associated with a higher potential for conflict due to shared decision-making responsibilities and may be aggravated during times of crisis. Good camaraderie between surgeons and anaesthesiologists; both, the pillars of the operating room team help to avoid conflicts.[14] Team briefing performed before starting an anticipated difficult case helps to address specific concerns and reduce errors.[15] Crisis situations should be followed by 'debrief.' Effective communication among healthcare team members is widely acknowledged as a crucial factor in providing top-notch care. The World Health Organization (WHO) checklist provides an opportunity for the team to discuss pertinent issues related to the case and has been shown to improve communication, reduce complications and enhance provider and patient outcomes.[16] The European Society for Paediatric Anaesthesiology has suggested paediatric-specific checklist with additional components specific to children such as fasting status, venous access check, patient positioning, X-ray and electrocautery protection.[17] Parental involvement in the checklist is adopted by many paediatric surgical units and has shown to reduce child anxiety and improve parental satisfaction.[18]

## INFORMED CONSENT AND ASSENT

One of the important areas for the anaesthesiologist where communication and soft skills are of utmost importance is during the consent-taking process which reflects a person's right to make his choices, have views, and act according to his values and beliefs. The essential components of informed consent including voluntariness (willingness of the patient to undergo treatment), capacity (ability to understand the type of treatment) and knowledge (adequate information about the treatment and alternative treatment options) should be disclosed to the patient by the treating anaesthesiologist.

In paediatric patients, where competency is not fulfilled and the decision-making capacity is limited, parents or legal guardians provide informed consent. This surrogate decision-making process is based on the belief that parents or guardian will act in the best interest of the child.[19] The process of informed consent in children is challenging for anaesthesiologists, and they must consider various ethical, legal and medical issues involved in that process. The informed consent in children includes obtaining informed assent from paediatric patients whenever possible and obtaining parental permission. The term 'informed permission' is used when the parent provides legal consent for the child to emphasise that the consent is not by the patient. Though a child may be unable to make legally binding decisions, his status as a minor does not preclude him from decision-making.[20] The process of informed refusal is equally important as informed consent and needs the anaesthesiologist to explain in detail to the children and their guardians about the risk and benefits while respecting refusal to assent and avoiding coercion.[21] The American Academy of Paediatrics recommends that minors should be involved in decision-making as per their developmental capacity and the medical issues involved.[22]

## INFORMED ASSENT IN CHILDREN

Assent is the child's agreement to a medical procedure when it is not legally authorised or lacks an understanding of consent completely. Children over 12 years have decision-making capacity and can provide informed assent for the procedure. To enable informed assent, children must be made aware of the condition and what to expect during the procedure, and the patient's understanding of the situation should be assessed before soliciting their approval for the planned care. In Western countries, emancipated minors are legally eligible for informed consent, but in India, 18 years is the legal age for giving valid consent for treatment as per the Indian Majority Act, Guardian and Wards Act and Indian Contract Act. Different jurisdictions have varying guidelines about the age at which children should be involved in the consent process and be able to provide assent and there is no universally accepted standard. For an assent to be reliable and valid it is essential to determine whether a child fully understands the information provided and is capable of providing meaningful assent.

## CONTENTS AND GOAL OF INFORMED CONSENT

An informed consent form includes a description of the proposed plan, information on alternative options, risks and benefits involved, the discussion of uncertainties, comprehension of the information, and solicitation of a voluntary preference or decision. The information provided in informed consent varies greatly, including excessive details about the technical aspects of care. The parent's understanding of risks, benefits and other therapeutic options is also unsatisfactory.[23] From the anaesthesiologist's perspective, there is reduced emphasis on shared decision-making and elicitation of patients' concerns.

The primary goal of informed consent in the paediatric context is to empower parents or legal guardians to make a well-informed decision that is in the best interest of their child.[24] The secondary purpose is to reduce anxiety by addressing concerns and by reassurance. To achieve these goals, it is essential to provide information that meets the patients' needs and comprehension ability in simple vernacular language with minimal medical jargon.[25] A few studies have found improved knowledge, patient satisfaction and anxiety reduction with the usage of written information leaflets.

### Recent Advances in Informed Consent in Paediatric Anaesthesia

In recent times, technological advancements have become a part of consent-taking in children. Virtual reality usage to simulate the surgical environment and the anaesthesia process reduces anxiety and improves understanding among paediatric patients and their parents.[26] This reduction in anxiety can facilitate the consent-taking process. Usage of multimedia in the form of interactive consent forms that include interactive elements such as videos, animations and quizzes can help parents and children to better understand the procedure, risks and benefits. These tools can be customised to the child's developmental level and medical literacy. Usage of mobile apps designed to guide families through the consent process can provide information in an engaging and easily accessible format.

Providing a copy of the consent form to the parents so that it can be read at home and clarifications can be made in the next visit is a helpful step in this process. This approach allows autonomy of the patient and family, enables legal safety for healthcare providers and encourages a shared understanding of the treatment plan.[27]

Shared decision-making is the need of hour. It emphasises a collaborative approach where healthcare providers and families work together to make decisions. This includes discussing the child's values and preferences and involving them in the decision-making process as much as possible.

## SPECIAL CONSIDERATIONS

### Confidentiality for Adolescents

Adolescents may not want to share personal information with their parents or relatives. Anaesthesiologists, like all healthcare providers, must navigate the delicate balance between respecting the adolescent's confidentiality and the need to involve parents in their care when appropriate.[28] Social workers may be involved if required to facilitate effective communication. Anaesthesiologists should not breach confidentiality unless there is a chance of harm to self or society.

### Pregnant Adolescent

Adolescents may present with a positive pregnancy test on preoperative anaesthesia workup. The dilemma to inform parents should not be clouded by personal experiences and emotions. The adolescent may not want to inform the parent about the same and hence to convince parents for postponement of an elective surgery may require tact and skill.[29] Moreover, professional guidelines often advocate for respecting minors' autonomy, particularly in reproductive health matters, while also considering the role of parents in the adolescents' healthcare decisions.[30] Use of vague unremarkable reasons without scaring the parents may sometimes be useful. The legal counsel, surgical team and social worker should be taken into confidence before talking to the parent.

### Children of Jehovah's Witnesses

Jehovah's Witnesses are patients who refuse transfusion of blood/blood products due to biblical reasons. Moreover, the refusal of blood transfusions by Jehovah's Witnesses raises ethical and legal debates, particularly when it involves the treatment of children or when the refusal contradicts the medical standard of care.[31] Anaesthesiologists should obtain written permission from parents on what fluids can be transfused to their children. The other interventions/options that are available should be discussed as transfusion therapy is deemed a 'matter of conscience.'[32]

## CONCLUSION

Conventional training in anaesthesia has involved teaching technical skills to the trainees. However, along with this technical dexterity, emphasis should be placed on other strategies or NTS like care with empathy and compassion, teamwork, clear communication, planning, resource management, stress management and decision-making for better patient care. Effective communication plays a pivotal role in ensuring positive outcomes and enhancing the overall experience of children and their families in the perioperative period by fostering trust, addressing concerns and facilitating informed consent.

## REFERENCES

1. Radhakrishnan B, Katikar MD, Myatra SN, Gautam PL, Vinayagam S, Saroa R. Importance of non-technical skills in anaesthesia education. Indian J Anaesth. 2022;66(1):64-9.
2. Claus LE, Links AR, Amos J, DiCarlo H, Jelin E, Koka R, et al. Parent Experience of Communication about Children's Surgery: A Qualitative Analysis. Pediatric Quality and Safety. 2021; 6(3): e403.
3. Carlyle AV, Ching PC, Cyna AM. Communication during Induction of Paediatric Anaesthesia: An Observational Study. Anaesth Intensive Care. 2008;1;36(2):180-4.
4. Ghodki P. Soft Skills for successful Anaesthesia Practice. J Anaesth Crit Care Case Rep. 2017;3(1):3-4.
5. McCombe K, Bogod DG. Consent and capacity: issues for paediatric anaesthesia. BJA Educ. 2020;20(11):377-81.
6. Ranjan P, Kumari A, Chakrawarty A. How can doctors improve their communication skills? J Clin Diagn Res. 2015;9(3):JE01-4.
7. Azhar F. The role of nonverbal communication in enhancing effective leadership in organizational contexts. Gema Wiralodra. 2024;15(1): 324-33.
8. Mann CM, Kennedy C. Identifying the core attributes of pediatric communication techniques to be taught to anesthetic trainees. Paediatr Anaesth. 2020;30(5):614-23.
9. Brown EA, De Young A, Kimble R, Kenardy J. Review of a parent's influence on pediatric procedural distress and recovery. Clin Child Fam Psychol Rev. 2018;21(2):224-5.
10. Cyna AM, Andrew MI, Tan SG. Communication skills for the anaesthetist. Anaesthesia. 2009;64(6):658-65.
11. Cyna AM. Little words BIG impact: Perioperative communication for children with burns. Anaesth Intensive Care. 2020;48(2):123-8.
12. Ehwerhemuepha L, Feaster W, Kain Z. Impact of anesthesiologists on parental perioperative satisfaction scores. Paediatr Anaesth. 2017;27(9):949-54.
13. Society of Pediatric Anesthesia. (2021). How to break bad news to families. [online] Available from https://pedsanesthesia.org/wp-content/uploads/2021/03/How-to-Break-Bad-News-to-Families.pdf [Last accessed May, 2025].
14. Sinskey JL, Chang JM, Shibata GS, Infosino AJ, Rouine-Rapp K. Applying conflict management strategies to the pediatric operating room. Anesth Analg. 2019;129(4):1109-1.
15. Keil O, Brunsmann K, Boethig D, Dennhardt N, Eismann H, Girke S, et al. Incidence and characteristics of errors detected by a short team briefing in pediatric anesthesia. Paediatr Anaesth 2022;32(10):1144-50.
16. Armstrong BA, Dutescu IA, Nemoy L, Bhavsar E, Carter DN, Ng KD, et al. Effect of the surgical safety checklist on provider and patient outcomes: a systematic review. BMJ Qual Saf 2022;31(6):463-78.
17. European Society for Paediatric Anaesthesiology. (2024). WHO surgical checklist. [online] Available from https://www.euroespa.com/science-education/

specialized-sections/espa-guidelines/safety/who-surgical-checklist/ [Last accessed May, 2025].

18. Lagoo J, Lopushinsky SR, Haynes AB, Bain P, Flageole H, Skarsgard ED, et al. Effectiveness and meaningful use of paediatric surgical safety checklists and their implementation strategies: a systematic review with narrative synthesis. BMJ Open. 2017;7(10):e016298.
19. Hickey K. Minors' rights in medical decision making. JONAS Healthc Law Ethics Regul. 2007;9(3):100-6.
20. Feinstein MM, Pannunzio AE, Lobell S, Kodish E. Informed Consent in Pediatric Anesthesia: A Narrative Review. Anesth Analg. 2018;127(6):1398-405.
21. Shah M, Waisel D, Lalwani K. Ethics in pediatric anesthesiology. In: Lalwani K, Cohen IT, Choi EY, Raman VT (Eds). Pediatric Anesthesia: A Problem-based Learning Approach. New York: Oxford Academic; 2018. pp. 601-21.
22. Katz AL, Webb SA; COMMITTEE ON BIOETHICS. Informed Consent in Decision-Making in Pediatric Practice. Pediatrics. 2016;138(2):e20161485.
23. Pianosi K, Gorodzinsky AY, Chorney JM, Corsten G, Johnson LB, Hong P. Informed consent in pediatric otolaryngology: what risks and benefits do parents recall? Otolaryngol Head Neck Surg. 2016;155:332-9.
24. Rezvani S, Fadavi M, Bazmi S. Study of obtaining informed consent in pediatric wards from the viewpoint of physicians and children's parents. Arch Pediatr Infect Dis. 2021;10(1):e111168.
25. Rai E, Chen RYY, Noi CS, Hee HI. Evaluation of anesthesia informed consent in pediatric practice—An observation cohort study. J Anaesthesiol Clin Pharmacol. 2019;35(4):515-21.
26. Tas FQ, van Eijk CAM, Staals LM, Legerstee JS, Dierckx B. Virtual reality in pediatrics, effects on pain and anxiety: A systematic review and meta-analysis update. Paediatr Anaesth. 2022;32(12):1292-304.
27. Fitriana D. The role of informed consent as legal protection for doctors in conducting medical procedures. Sinergi Int J Law. 2023;1(3):235-45.
28. Crawford K, Low JK, Le Page AK, Mulley W, Masterson R, Kausman J, et al. Transition from a renal paediatric clinic to an adult clinic: Perspectives of adolescents and young adults, parents and health professionals. J Child Health Care. 2022;26(4):531-47.
29. Waisel DB. Ethical issues in pediatric anesthesiology. In: Cote CJ, Lerma J, Anderson BJ (Eds). A Practice of Anesthesia for Infants and Children, 6th edition. USA: Elsevier; 2019. pp. 327-76.
30. Blumling A, McGowan M, Prows C, Childers-Buschle K, Martin L, Lynch J, et al. Engaging Adolescents and Young Adults in Decisions About Return of Genomic Research Results: a mixed-methods longitudinal clinical trial protocol. Res Sq [Preprint]. 2023:rs.3.rs-2819191. Update in: BMC Med Inform Decis Mak. 2024;24(1):391.
31. Néill CO. Jehovah's Witnesses and Blood Transfusions: An Analysis of the Legal Protections Afforded to Adults and Children in European/English Human Rights Contexts. Eur J Health Law. 2017;24(4):368-89.
32. Waisel DB. Ethical considerations. In: Gregory GA, Andropoulos DB (Eds). Gregory's Pediatric Anesthesia, 5th edition. USA: Wiley-Blackwell; 2012. pp. 1-14.

CHAPTER 3

# Paediatric Airway Management: Stay Updated on the Latest Techniques and Strategies!

*Indu M Sen, Pradnya Sawant, Richa Saroa, Anudeep Jafra, Mridul Dua*

## ABSTRACT

Paediatric airway management requires vigilance, knowledge and expertise to practise updated management strategies in view of the functional and physiological differences as compared to adults. Since this population is predisposed to more perioperative complications due to immature systems, thorough preoperative evaluation and review of records are essential for the safe conduct of anaesthesia. The introduction of perioperative risk stratification tools for children has led to a better understanding of the overall risk by integrating comorbidities and the risk associated directly with surgery and anaesthesia. Advancements in the use of perioperative monitoring devices, use of point of care ultrasonography (POCUS), para-oxygenation and hybrid airway management techniques have revolutionised airway management in the paediatric population. Newer ventilation strategies, multimodal analgesic regimens and planned extubation have paved the path to improved outcomes in paediatric surgical interventions. Amidst the technological advancements, artificial intelligence has significantly contributed to patient safety by virtual airway examination that helps in formulating a management plan and prevent catastrophic adverse events. With rapid developments in the field of paediatric anaesthesia, it is imperative to impart education to the anaesthesia trainees early in the residency programmes to imbibe the concept of teamwork and protocolised management. However, airway management in the paediatric patient needs to be tailored based upon the case scenario, availability of airway gadgets and technical expertise. Continuous surveillance of existing setups and critical evaluation of untoward perioperative outcomes further serve to make future safety recommendations.

***Keywords:*** Airway, Assessment, Devices, Management, Paediatrics, Risk.

## INTRODUCTION

The paediatric population is fraught with perioperative challenges and requires expertise, vigilance and updated management strategies in view of anatomical and physiological differences as compared to adults. The field of paediatric anaesthesia has made tremendous progress in the last decade in patient care and safety. The incorporation of guidelines and checklists helps in predicting difficulties in airway management and also focuses on normalising vital parameters.[1-3] This chapter will re-emphasise upon the need for thorough patient evaluation and meticulous planning while utilising the available modalities. Airway-related challenging case scenarios have also been discussed where hybrid techniques facilitated successful airway management.

# PREOPERATIVE EVALUATION AND RISK STRATIFICATION

## Airway Assessment in the Paediatric Population

A thorough evaluation is recommended within 2 weeks for patients undergoing major elective surgical procedures. Though telecommunication or questionnaire-based preoperative assessment approach has recently been introduced to facilitate evaluation in remote areas or to minimise preoperative hospital visits, it still mandates physical examination before the scheduled operative procedure by a trained anaesthesiologist.[4] It is of paramount importance to detect alarming symptoms such as history of difficulty in breathing, apnoeic spells, audible wheeze, cyanosis, history of obstructive sleep apnoea (OSA) or failure to thrive. The presence of predictors of a difficult airway, e.g. facial asymmetry, micrognathia, retrognathia, prognathies, fixed cervical spine, oral or neck mass, temporomandibular joint (TMJ) ankylosis and syndromes such as the Crouzon, Pierre Robin, Pfeiffer and Treacher Collins warrants a detailed airway examination using a 'line of sight' approach. Estimation of room air oxygen saturation ($SpO_2$) and preoperative optimisation should be done wherever feasible.[2]

Systematic assessment is challenging in infants due to immature behaviour and difficulty in obeying commands. There is no validated data and there are no parameters to assess difficult intubation and laryngoscopy in neonates. In a study conducted by Aparna D et al. in 2020[5] to determine the relationship between various anthropometric parameters in neonates with difficult laryngoscopy and intubation, no single parameter could provide a high index of sensitivity and specificity to predict difficult airway. A combination of parameters which included body weight, thyromental distance, sternomental distance and frontal plane to chin distance divided by weight ratio could predict the difficulty but needed validation.[5,6]

Another score used is the Colorado Paediatric Airway Score (COPUR).[7] This is a composite of five parameters wherein each parameter is scored from 1 to 4. A composite score of >12 suggests difficulty in intubation [(Cormack-Lehane (CL) grades 3 and 4]. These parameters are C: chin (side profile), O: Opening (mouth opening-interdental distance), P: history of previous intubations and history of OSA, U: Uvula (percentage of uvula visible) and R: range of neck movement.

## Perioperative Risk Stratification

Tools which integrate the underlying comorbidity and risk associated with surgical and anaesthetic exposure have been utilised for better understanding of the overall risk. The American Society of Anesthesiologists physical status tool has traditionally been utilised for risk stratification, and it reliably predicts the incidence of perioperative respiratory events.[3]

**TABLE 1:** COLDS score.

| *Parameter* | *Grading (1, 2 and 5)* |
|---|---|
| C: *Current* signs and symptoms of upper respiratory tract infection | • None (1)<br>• Mild symptoms (2)<br>• Moderate-to-severe symptoms (5) |
| O: Timing of *Onset* of symptoms | • 4 weeks (1)<br>• 2–4 weeks ago (2)<br>• <2 week ago (5) |
| L: Presence of *Lung* disease | • None (1)<br>• Mild (2)<br>• Moderate to severe (5) |
| D: Airway *Device* to be used (mask/supraglottic airway device/ endotracheal tube) | • None/face mask (1)<br>• Supraglottic device (2)<br>• Endotracheal tube (5) |
| S: Type of *Surgery* (airway/non-airway/ major or minor surgery) | • Other (1)<br>• Minor airway (2)<br>• Major airway (5) |

COLDS score is a validated preoperative screening tool that is widely employed to quantify the risk of increased perioperative respiratory adverse events (PRAEs) airway reactivity and need for medication **(Table 1)**.[8] The total score ranges from 5 to 25 with each category being assigned a score of 1, 2 or 5 and an increasing score is associated with increased PRAEs.

Similarly, the American College of Surgeons National Surgical Quality Improvement Program-Pediatric (ACS NSQIP-Pediatric) online calculator is a risk prediction model with 18 fixed difficulty predictors. It has predefined cut-off values as derived from the clinical data and algorithmically predicts the surgical outcomes and 30-day mortality in the paediatric population based on machine learning.[9,10]

Despite the availability of the predictive models, non-modifiable risk factors such as prematurity (post-conceptual age <44 weeks), type of surgery, otolaryngological procedures, emergency airway surgeries and non-operating room anaesthesia (NORA) contribute significantly to PRAEs and postoperative outcomes. National Audit Project 7 (NAP7, 2024) has reported that the incidence of PRAEs is highest in otolaryngological procedures (23%), out of which 14% of the total are solely attributed to airway-related issues.[11]

## Utility of Ultrasonography in Paediatrics

Ultrasonography (USG) has gained widespread popularity in paediatrics during the perioperative period and has distinct advantages, especially being non-invasive and the ease of making repeated assessments at the bedside. POCUS can facilitate decision-making in the perioperative period and outside the operating room locations.[12,13] Preoperative POCUS has been reliably utilised to estimate the preoperative hydration status, screen for cardiac anomalies, residual gastric contents and diagnose underlying lung conditions such as pneumothorax (lung point sign) or pneumonia (lung hepatisation).[11] Preoperative sonographic airway assessment has been established to predict difficult laryngoscopy by measuring various indices that include tongue thickness, palatine tonsils, epiglottis, vocal cord pathologies/movement abnormalities and hyo-mental distance ratio. Selection of the appropriate endotracheal tube size has also been made by measurement of the subglottic diameter.[14] USG can also aid in the detection of oesophageal/endobronchial intubation. Post-operatively, it can be used for the diagnosis of laryngomalacia, i.e. dynamic collapsibility of airway structures signalling difficult or delayed extubation.[15]

The use of USG in anticipated difficult airway is recommended for scenarios where front-of-neck access (FONA) may have to be resorted to and thereby implement strategies to identify landmarks for quick FONA. USG is primarily used to precisely delineate the cricothyroid membrane in an anticipated difficult airway. This may be accomplished using two methods. The first involves obtaining the 'string of pearls' appearance in the sagittal plane and the other is the TACA (thyroid cartilage-airline interface-cricoid cartilage-airline interface) method in transverse plane. Both methods help in identification of the cricothyroid membrane for FONA to the airway in emergency situations.[16] One must remember that in patients <8 years of age, surgical tracheostomy should be done by an experienced person. Moreover, the use of USG is limited by availability of the device, probes or technical expertise, especially in resource-limited countries. Therefore, regular training programmes for residents involving hands-on workshops should be conducted to improve their competency.

## CONDUCT OF ANAESTHESIA: MONITORING, EQUIPMENT AND TECHNIQUES

Paediatric anaesthesia has advanced tremendously owing to the development of monitoring techniques, thereby allowing surgical interventions with complex physiological derangements. The quest for continuous perioperative, non-invasive monitoring is still evolving.

### Preoxygenation

Children have higher metabolic rates, higher oxygen consumption, lower functional residual capacity and higher closing volumes, making them prone to oxyhaemoglobin desaturation. Hence, preoxygenation using 5 L/min flow of nasal oxygen before the conduct of anaesthesia as well as para-oxygenation during apnoea has been found to be beneficial during endotracheal intubation or during other airway interventions by increasing the apnoea time.[17]

The oxygen reserve index (Ori™) is a non-invasive continuous parameter that provides insight into the reserve of patients receiving supplemental oxygen. It can predict hypoxaemia before changes in the pulse oximeter readings owing to its capability to detect the changes in arterial partial pressure of oxygen in the range of 80–200 mm Hg.[18]

The Kids Transnasal Humidified Rapid Insufflation Ventilatory Exchange (THRIVE) trial is a multicentre, international, randomised controlled trial to determine whether THRIVE can reduce hypoxaemia episodes, increase first-attempt success rate compared with standard practice in paediatric emergent endotracheal intubations and reduce respiratory adverse events.[19]

## Newer Devices for Paediatric Airway Management

The introduction of modern anaesthesia workstations with various modes of ventilation and the development of newer monitoring devices has facilitated surgical interventions in children with complex physiologically difficult airways with improved patient safety. However, there are concerns regarding the availability of age- and size-appropriate monitoring systems and the validation of certain monitored parameters in the paediatric population.[20]

## Monitoring

Minimal mandatory monitoring guidelines are already established while the need to strengthen anaesthesia delivery systems and surgical facilities in resource-constrained settings has been highlighted.[21-23] Novel wireless and flexible sensors using blue tooth to accurately measure physiological parameters have been employed. Continuous non-invasive arterial pressure monitors can provide beat-to-beat variation of blood pressure as well as cardiac output measurements using finger cuffs.[24]

Non-invasive and wearable optical sensors for fast and accurate measurement of transcutaneous oxygen and carbon dioxide monitoring are being used in place of invasive arterial catheters for arterial blood gas analysis.[25]

There has been a paradigm shift towards cerebral perfusion pressure monitoring along with respiratory and haemodynamic monitoring as all these variables are susceptible to rapid changes under anaesthesia, especially in neonates and young children undergoing complex surgical procedures.[26] Intraoperative neuromonitoring including motor and sensory evoked potentials and depth of anaesthesia monitors have been employed to titrate optimal anaesthetic drug delivery and for early detection of complications so that rapid corrective measures can be taken. However, these devices require further refinement to circumvent the underlying issues related to prolonged placement and accuracy of monitoring in children of different age groups.

## Short-acting Fast Emergence Medications

With recent concerns over the effect of anaesthetics on a developing brain, a balanced anaesthetic technique, using short-acting fast emergence (SAFE) agents along with non-depolarising muscle relaxants and $\alpha$-2 agonist drugs, has been proposed. These agents provide optimum sedation-analgesia and also reduce the requirement of anaesthetic agents.[27] In addition to various non-pharmacological methods, ultra-short-acting agents such as remifentanil and remimazolam infusions have been introduced. Different routes of administration and drug dosages are being tried based on the bioavailability of the drugs.[28,29] In an effort to reduce dosing errors, the Paediatric Anaesthetic Emergency Drug Solution (PAEDS) approach which combines a colour-coded chart with medication box colours has been suggested to prevent medication errors. The utility of this approach has been tested in a simulated environment.[28]

## Newer Supraglottic Airway Devices

Newer supraglottic airway devices with gastric channels, intubating laryngeal mask airways, videolaryngoscopes (VLs) and microcuff endotracheal tubes have revolutionised airway management. Angulated, hyperangulated and channelled VLs have been shown to improve first attempt intubation success in anticipated as well as unanticipated difficult airway by providing better glottic view in children with anatomical complexities. Therefore, the VLs have been incorporated into the difficult airway management algorithm in paediatrics.[30,31] Video-assisted direct laryngoscopy has an advantage of confirmation of successful endotracheal tube placement while serving as a good teaching aid at the same time. Ultrasound visualisation of saline-filled cuff tracheal rapid ultrasound saline test (TRUST) can accurately detect endotracheal versus endobronchial intubation in children.[32]

## Hybrid Techniques

This involves the simultaneous use of two different techniques to capitalise upon the strength of one while overcoming the limitations of the other to secure and maintain the airway. These include non-angulated rigid VL with the use of ventilating bougies and lighted stylets, hyperangulated rigid bronchoscopy with flexible video laryngotracheobronchoscopy and intubation and extubation through supraglottic airway devices while maintaining continuous oxygenation and ventilation. For the management of challenging airways, hybrid techniques along with three-dimensional printing and machine learning are being proposed.[33-35]

## Advanced Ventilation Modalities

Newer modes of ventilation like flow-controlled ventilation, using technology based on Bernoulli's principle to achieve active expiration, physiologically variable ventilation that mimics the spontaneous respiration by integrating breath-to-breath variations with respiratory rate and negative pressure ventilation are being used in paediatric patients with deranged haemodynamics. These modes provide better oxygenation, optimising oxygen delivery, decreasing physiological disruptions and are known to reduce the incidence of ventilator-induced lung injury.

Ventrain™ is a manual device designed for complete ventilatory failure conditions in paediatrics. This can be used with intravenous cannulas and has a unique ability for oxygenation as well as carbon dioxide removal by active expiration owing to the suction effect created on patient airflow and, thereby, reduces air trapping and barotrauma. However, there is still limited experience regarding this device in paediatric patients.[36]

## Extubation

An elective extubation in a paediatric patient warrants a careful planning and assessment, which includes patient readiness, adequate reversal of neuromuscular blockade and sufficient respiratory drive. The timing, location of extubation, appropriate equipment for reintubation and safe transfer of patients should be ensured. In cases of difficult extubation, monitoring should be continued for at least 24 hours for early detection of post-operative complications and prompt management.

## Practice Guidelines, Simulation and Artificial Intelligence

Practice guidelines/algorithms are useful tools if appropriately used along with judgement and vigilance by the attending team. Recently published guidelines on airway management in neonates and infants in European Journal of Anesthesiology emphasise that experts from different paediatric specialties can collaborate to form an universal algorithm.[37] The need of the hour is to keep ourselves updated by practising various airway management techniques, first on the manikins and then on normal patients, to successfully manage the challenging airway.

Airway training in a simulated environment provides opportunities for practice, recording and debriefing without harming patients. Artificial intelligence uses data from electronic health records, databases, stored images for pattern recognition and computer modelling analysis to provide a continuum of perioperative care. These modalities may prove to be useful in paediatric population.[38,39]

## CHALLENGING AIRWAY CASE SCENARIOS

*Prerequisites:* Para-oxygenation, haemodynamic and respiratory monitoring, optimum positioning, back-up planning, post-extubation care and record keeping.

### Case 1: Vallecular Cyst (Left) Compressing Epiglottis and Type 3 Laryngomalacia (Fig. 1)

This is a rare disorder with progressive stridor, respiratory distress and life-threatening laryngomalacia warranting urgent supraglottoplasty and epiglottopexy.[40]

A 3-month-old 3 kg baby boy diagnosed with a large cystic lesion over the epiglottis after a flexible fibreoptic bronchoscopy was scheduled to undergo excision of the same under general anaesthesia. Since the vocal cords were not visible by conventional Miller's laryngoscope, the fluid in the cyst was aspirated with an 18 G needle by an otorhinologist using zero-degree rigid bronchoscopy under propofol sedation. Spontaneous respiration using intravenous anaesthesia and high-flow nasal oxygen (STRIVE-Hi) technique and 1% lignocaine topicalisation of the glottic structures. Subsequently, the child underwent cyst marsupialisation, epiglottopexy and supraglottoplasty. Intravenous propofol and dexmedetomidine infusion was administered to secure the airway using VL with size 1 Miller's blade and uncuffed endotracheal tube. Intravenous atracurium was given after confirmation of endotracheal tube placement. After the completion of surgery, the patient

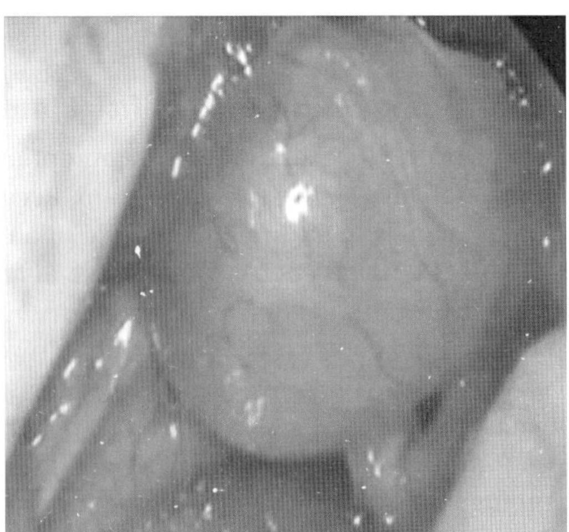

**Fig. 1:** Vallecular cyst. *(For color version, see Plate 1)*

was extubated once fully awake and shifted to the post-anaesthesia care unit (PACU) for post-operative monitoring/escalation of care. *This case highlights the need for prompt surgical intervention and post-operative monitoring for favourable patient outcomes.*

## Case 2: Congenital Anterior Glottic Web for Emergent Tracheostomy (Fig. 2)

A 10-month-old 5 kg baby girl was admitted with progressive stridor and failure to thrive. Airway assessment revealed a congenital anterior glottic web.

A 2 mm fibreoptic bronchoscope could not be negotiated through the laryngeal opening and hence, a supraglottic airway (I-gel™; 1.5) was placed under sevoflurane anaesthesia. However, ventilation through the I-gel was also inadequate even in the extended neck position required for tracheostomy. The I-gel was therefore removed, and tracheostomy was performed under mask anaesthesia with sevoflurane and local anaesthetic infiltration, supplemented by intravenous ketamine and glycopyrrolate. The entire intraoperative course was uneventful and the child was shifted to the paediatric intensive care unit after successful tracheostomy. *This case highlights the need for quick airway assessment to establish a diagnosis, minimum handling and early decision for tracheostomy, preferably by an otorhinolaryngology surgeon.*[41]

## Case 3: Submental Teratoma (Fig. 3)

A 9-day-old female neonate weighing 1.8 kg with a submental mass developed respiratory arrest while in the computed tomography suite. She

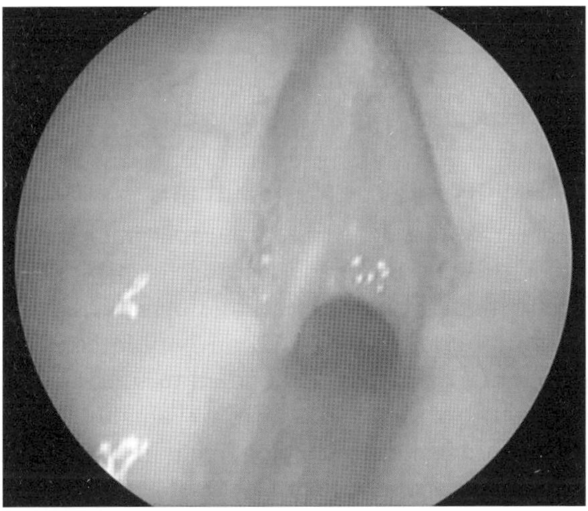

**Fig. 2:** Laryngeal web. *(For color version, see Plate 1)*

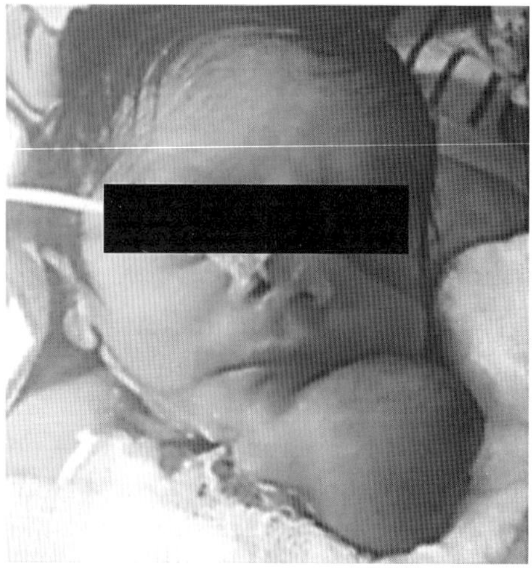

**Fig. 3:** Submental mass.

was shifted to operating room for securing the airway after multiple failed attempts in ventilation and intubation. As face mask ventilation too was difficult, I-gel was inserted and subsequently, anaesthesia was induced with fentanyl, ketamine and atracurium. A 3.0 mm uncuffed endotracheal tube was inserted using a size zero Miller blade of C-MAC video laryngoscope. Two-dimensional echocardiography revealed a double outlet right ventricle with a large subpulmonic ventricular septal defect (VSD) and a patent ductus arteriosus. Computerised tomography was suggestive of teratoma. She required ventilatory and ionotropic support in the intensive care unit before and after the surgery.

*This case highlights the importance of the anaesthesiologist in NORA and complex syndromic neonatal interventions that help in prompt rescue in cases of airway emergencies. It is safer to secure the airway in a well-equipped setup. Written informed consent must be taken after explaining all the complications and the need for mechanical ventilatory support.*

## Case 4. Cystic Hygroma of the Neck (Figs. 4A to C)

A 2-day-old female neonate delivered by lower segment caesarean section presented with airway compromise leading to inspiratory stridor and suprasternal retractions because of a large mass in the neck. She was maintaining a peripheral $SpO_2$ of 75% on bubble continuous positive airway pressure. The patient was scheduled to undergo cyst aspiration and bleomycin injection. Meticulous airway evaluation, case-appropriate preparation and use of advanced technology including VL and USG facilitated the safe management of the difficult airway. Para-oxygenation, quick aspiration of the cyst by the surgeon followed by manual displacement of mass

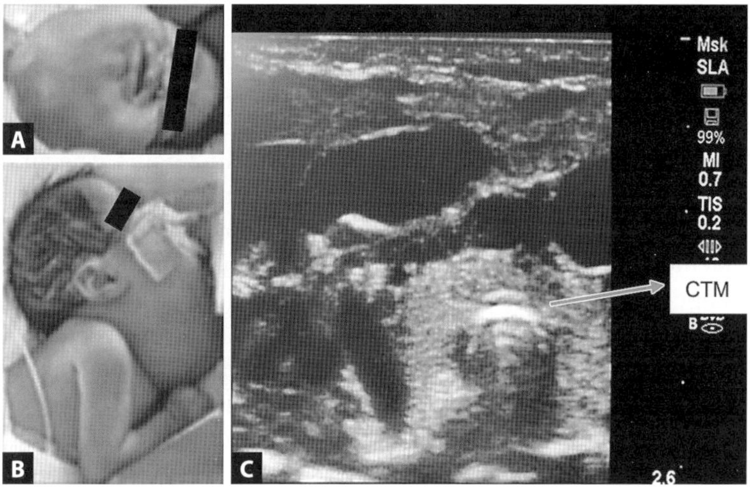


**Figs. 4A to C:** Cystic hygroma. *(For color version, see Plate 2)*

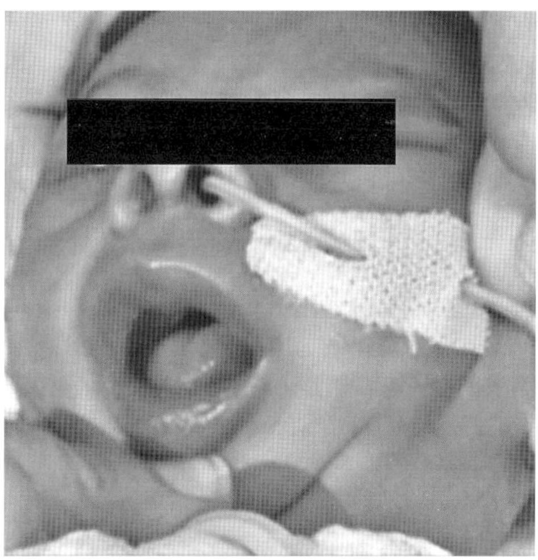

**Fig. 5:** Multiple birth defects. *(For color version, see Plate 2)*

facilitated endotracheal tube insertion in the lateral position. Subsequently, planned extubation was done in the neonatal intensive care unit 1 week post-sclerotherapy. *This case highlights the use of POCUS along with other airway gadgets in emergency scenarios and post-procedural intensive care unit care for a favourable outcome.*[42]

## Case 5. Airway Issues in a Neonate with Multiple Birth Defects (Fig. 5)

A 2-day-old full-term 3.5 kg male with cleft palate grade III, VSD, atrial septal aneurysm, short limbs and neonatal jaundice was referred with obstructed inguinal hernia. He had cyanotic spells, a seizure episode and required emergency endotracheal intubation (3.0 mm uncuffed endotracheal tube fixed at 7 cm). In the operating room, the tube was repositioned over a stylet using video laryngoscopy (C-MAC), after which the $SpO_2$ improved from 85 to 97%. The surgery was completed uneventfully in 2 hours. The air entry was not adequate while shifting on an artificial manual breathing unit. Igel™ was inserted followed by endotracheal tube removal (Bailey manoeuvre). The haemodynamics and ventilation temporarily improved. A neonatal fibrescope was not available. Blind endotracheal tube insertion through I-gel and reintubation using video laryngoscopy was unsuccessful since the large tongue completely obstructed the glottic view. Pulling the tongue with a Magill's forceps did not help. In this scenario, the surgeon applied a silk suture for pulling the tongue. The glottic view improved to CL grade 2A. A microcuff endotracheal tube (3 mm) was placed. This simple manoeuvre averted invasive cricothyrotomy or nasal intubation in this syndromic baby. *This case highlights that extubation and shifting should be carefully monitored and one should be prepared for the worst possible scenario.*

## Case 6: Temporomandibular Joint Ankylosis (Fig. 6)

A 4-year-old 12 kg boy was admitted for staged TMJ arthrotomy and mandibular distraction in view of post-traumatic TMJ ankylosis. Mouth opening was <2 cm. Flexible fibreoptic intubation was planned under sedation. The patient was premedicated with oral midazolam and oral atropine. 2% of lignocaine and adrenaline nebulisation was administered. The nose was packed with adrenaline-soaked gauze pieces, and xylometazoline nasal drops were instilled. As the child did not have an

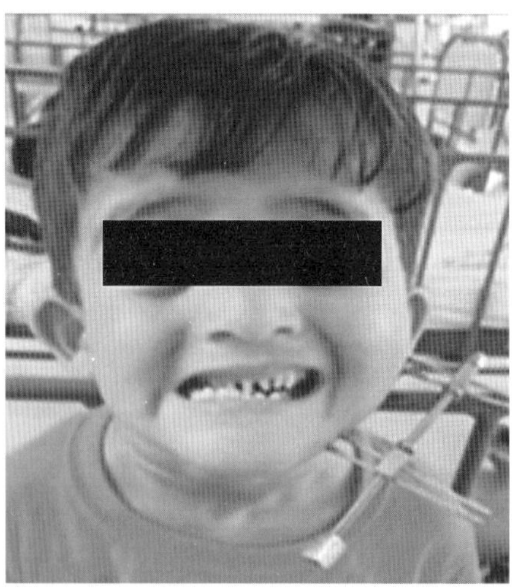

**Fig. 6:** Temporomandibular joint ankylosis.

intravenous line preoperatively, anaesthesia was induced using sevoflurane in an air-oxygen mixture. Intravenous ketamine 1 mg/kg was given, and a dexmedetomidine infusion was started at 1 µg/kg/hour. Fibreoptic nasal bronchoscopy was done using a 2.2 mm bronchoscope with a preloaded 5 mm (internal diameter) uncuffed endotracheal tube. Left-sided TMJ arthrotomy was done uneventfully. The child was extubated on meeting the criteria for extubation and monitored in the PACU. The right side was operated uneventfully 1 month later using the same airway management technique. *This case highlights that thorough preparation and expertise are needed to manage difficult TMJ ankylosis in children with no mouth opening. Opioid-sparing intravenous anaesthesia techniques are the preferred choice for the conduct of anaesthesia.*[43]

## CONCLUSION

Difficult airway management demands thorough preoperative evaluation, essential radiological imaging, meticulous planning, an experienced team, a well-equipped setup and a multidisciplinary approach. Practice guidelines/algorithms are helpful; but in actual situations, judgement and vigilance of the attending team plays a vital role. The need of the hour is to keep ourselves updated by practising various airway management techniques, first on the mannequins and then on normal patients to successfully manage the challenging airway. Continuous surveillance of existing setups and critical evaluation of untoward perioperative outcomes further serves as a guide to prepare for future safety recommendations.

## REFERENCES


1. Pazderka PA, Mastenbrook J, Billian J, Caulfield R, Khan F, Ekblad G, et al. Quality evaluation of a checklist for intubation preparation in graduate medical education. Cureus 2022;14(6):e25830.
2. Kumar R, Kumar S, Misra A, Kumar NG, Gupta A, Kumar P, et al. A new approach to airway assessment-"Line of Sight" and more. Recommendations of the task force of airway management foundation (AMF). J Anaesthesiol Clin Pharmacol. 2020;36:303-15.
3. Lynne F, Izabela L, Steven JS, Jay B. The Pediatric specific american society of anesthesiologists physical status score: A multicenter study. Anesth Analg. 2021;132:807-17.
4. Lesher AP, Shah SR. Telemedicine in the perioperative experience. Semin Pediatr Surg. 2018;27:102-6.
5. Aparna D, Jafra A, Bhardwaj N, Jain D, Luthra A, Malik MA. Evaluation of various anthropometric airway parameters as predictors of difficult airway in neonates: A prospective observational study. Int J Pediatr Otorhinolaryngol. 2020;138:110387.
6. Petrov I, Stankovic Z, Soldatovic I, Tomic A, Simic D, Milenovic M, et al. Difficult airway prediction in infants with apparently normal face and neck features. J Clin Med. 2024;13(15):4294.

7. Raj D, Luginbuehl I. Managing the difficult airway in the syndromic child. Contin Educ Anaesth Crit Care Pain. 2015;15:7-13.
8. Lee LK, Bernardo MKL, Grogan TR, Elashoff DA, Ren WHP. Perioperative respiratory adverse event risk assessment in children with upper respiratory tract infection: Validation of the COLDS score. Paediatr Anaesth. 2018;28:1007-14.
9. Saito JM, Barnhart DC, Grant C, Brighton BK, Raval MV, Campbell BT, et al. The past, present and future of ACS NSQIP-Pediatric: Evolution from a quality registry to a comparative quality performance platform. Semin Pediatr Surg. 2023;32(2):151275.
10. Bertsimas D, Li M, Zhang N, Estrada C, Scott Wang HH. High-performance pediatric surgical risk calculator: A novel algorithm based on machine learning and pediatric NSQIP data. Am J Surg. 2023;226:115-21.
11. Oglesby FC, Scholefield BR, Cook TM, Smith JH, Pappachan VJ, Kane AD, et al. Peri-operative cardiac arrest in children as reported to the 7th National Audit Project of the Royal College of Anaesthetists. Anaesthesia. 2024;79:583-92.
12. Burton L, Bhargava V. A Scoping review of ultrasonographic techniques in the evaluation of the pediatric airway. J Ultrasound Med. 2023;42:2463-79.
13. Guimarães Ferreira Fonseca L, Bertolizio G, Engelhardt T, Karlsson J. Pediatric point of care airway ultrasound (POCUS): Current evidence and future practice. Anaesthesiologie. 2024. English. Epub ahead of print.
14. Ariff S, Ali KQ, Tessaro MO, Ansari U, Morris S, Soofi SB, et al. Diagnostic accuracy of point-of-care ultrasound compared to standard-of-care methods for endotracheal tube placement in neonates. Pediatr Pulmonol. 2022;57:1744-50.
15. Hamilton CE, Su E, Tawfik D, Fernandez E, Veten A, Conlon T, et al. Assessment of vocal cord motion using laryngeal ultrasound in children: a systematic review and meta-analysis. Pediatr Crit Care Med. 2021;22:e532-9.
16. Kristensen MS, Teoh WH. Ultrasound identification of the cricothyroid membrane: the new standard in preparing for front-of-neck airway access. Br J Anaesth. 2021;126:22-7.
17. Fuchs A, Koepp G, Huber M, Aebli J, Afshari A, Bonfiglio R, et al. Apnoeic oxygenation during pediatric tracheal intubation: a systematic review and meta-analysis. Br J Anaesth. 2024;132:392-406.
18. Vos JJ, Willems CH, van Amsterdam K, van den Berg JP, Spanjersberg R, Struys MMRF, et al. Oxygen reserve index: validation of a new variable. Anesth Analg. 2019;129:409-15.
19. George S, Gibbons K, Williams T, Humphreys S, Gelbart B, Le Marsney R, et al; Kids THRIVE Investigators; Paediatric Research in Emergency Departments International Collaborative (PREDICT); Australia, New Zealand Intensive Care Society Paediatric Study Group (ANZICS PSG). Transnasal humidified rapid insufflation ventilatory exchange in children requiring emergent intubation (Kids THRIVE): a statistical analysis plan for a randomised controlled trial. Trials 2023; 24(1):369.
20. Van Wijk JJ, Weber F, Stolker RJ, Staals LM. Current state of non-invasive, continuous monitoring modalities in pediatric anesthesiology. Curr Opin. 2022;33:781-7.
21. Gelb AW, Morriss WW, Johnson W, Merry AF. International Standards for a Safe Practice of Anesthesia Workgroup. World Health Organization-World Federation

of Societies of Anaesthesiologists (WHO-WFSA) international standards for a safe practice of anesthesia. Can J Anaesth. 2018;65:698-708.
22. Rai E, Bhardwaj N. (2016). Guidelines for minimal mandatory monitoring for paediatric anaesthesia. [online] Available from https://www.iapaindia.com/images/downloads/iapa-monitoring-guidelines-2016.pdf [Last accessed May, 2025].
23. Shahbaz S, Howard N. Anaesthesia delivery systems in low and lower-middle-income asian countries: A scoping review of capacity and effectiveness. PLOS Glob Public Health. 2024;4(3):e0001953.
24. Chen H, Soetikno A, Xu S, Suresh S. Advanced wireless monitoring for children in cardiac perioperative setting. Paediatric Anesthesia. 2023;33:670-2.
25. Bernasconi S, Angelucci A, De Cesari A, Masotti A, Pandocchi M, Vacca F, et al. Recent technologies for transcutaneous oxygen and carbon dioxide monitoring. Diagnostics (Basel). 2024;14(8):785.
26. Pichler G, Höller N, Baik-Schneditz N, Schwaberger B, Mileder L, Stadler J, et al. Avoiding arterial hypotension in preterm neonates (AHIP)-A single center randomised controlled study investigating simultaneous near infrared spectroscopy measurements of cerebral and peripheral regional tissue oxygenation and dedicated interventions. Front Pediatr. 2018;6:15.
27. Bisesi SA, Stauber SD, Hutchinson DJ, Acquisto NM. Current practices and safety of medication use during pediatric rapid sequence intubation. J Pediatr Pharmacol Ther. 2024;29:66-75.
28. Sequera-Ramos L, Laverriere EK, Garcia-Marcinkiewicz AG, Zhang B, Kovatsis PG, Fiadjoe JE; PeDI Collaborative. Sedation versus general anesthesia for tracheal intubation in children with difficult airways: a cohort study from the pediatric difficult intubation registry. Anesthesiology. 2022;137:418-33.
29. Neches SK, DeMartino C, Shay R. Pharmacologic adjuncts for neonatal tracheal intubation: the evidence behind premedication. Neoreviews. 2023;24(12):e783-e796.
30. Goodier R, Partyka C, Moore N, Middleton P, Abdullah Q. Mixed-methods pilot study exploring the influence of the novel paediatric anaesthetic drug solution tool on clinician cognitive load during simulated paediatric rapid sequence intubation in the emergency department. J Paediatr Child Health. 2023;59:808-13.
31. Lingappan K, Neveln N, Arnold JL, Fernandes CJ, Pammi M. Videolaryngoscopy versus direct laryngoscopy for tracheal intubation in neonates. Cochrane Database Syst Rev. 2023;5:CD009975.
32. Stein ML, Park RS, Kovatsis PG. Emerging trends, techniques and equipment for airway management in paediatrics. Paediatr Anaesth. 2020;30:269-79.
33. Tessaro MO, Salant EP, Arroyo AC, Haines LE, Dickman E. Tracheal rapid ultrasound saline test (T.R.U.S.T.) for confirming correct endotracheal tube depth in children. Resuscitation. 2015;89:8-12.
34. Stein ML, Park RS, Kiss EE, Adams HD, Burjek NE, Peyton J; PeDI Collaborative Investigators. Efficacy of a hybrid technique of simultaneous videolaryngoscopy with flexible bronchoscopy in children with difficult direct laryngoscopy in the Pediatric Difficult Intubation Registry. Anaesthesia. 2023;78:1093-101.
35. Stein ML, Sarmiento Argüello LA, Staffa SJ, Heunis J, Egbuta C, Flynn SG, et al; PeDI Collaborative Investigators. Airway management in the paediatric difficult

intubation registry: a propensity score matched analysis of outcomes over time. EClinicalMedicine. 2024;69:102461.
36. Dos Santos Rocha A, Habre W, Albu G. Novel ventilation techniques in children. Paediatr Anaesth. 2022;32:286-94.
37. Disma N, Asai T, Cools E, Cronin A, Engelhardt T, Fiadjoe J, et al; and airway guidelines groups of the European Society of Anaesthesiology and Intensive Care (ESAIC) and the British Journal of Anaesthesia (BJA). Airway management in neonates and infants: European Society of Anaesthesiology and Intensive Care and British Journal of Anaesthesia joint guidelines. Eur J Anaesthesiol. 2024;41:3-23.
38. Kim JH, Choi JW, Kwon YS, Kang SS. Predictive model for difficult laryngoscopy using machine learning: retrospective cohort study. Braz J Anesthesiol. 2022;72:622-8.
39. Duffy CC, Bass GA, Yi W, Rouhi A, Kaplan LJ, O Sullivan E. Teaching airway, management using virtual reality: A scoping review. Anesth Analg. 2024;138:782-93.
40. Tsai YT, Lee LA, Fang TJ, Li HY. Treatment of vallecular cysts in infants with and without coexisting laryngomalacia using endoscopic laser marsupialization: fifteen-year experience at a single-center. Int J Pediatr Otorhinolaryngol. 2013;77:424-8.
41. Gosavi K, Dey P, Swami S, Salunke A. Anesthesia management for a case of laryngeal keel placement. Saudi J Anaesth. 2017;11:486-9.
42. Puri S, Jafra A, Dogra N, Sen IM, Solanki S. Anesthetic management of a massive cystic hygroma of the neck in a neonate. J Indian Assoc Pediatr Surg. 2024;29:183-5.
43. Bhalotra AR, Balyan R, Manchanda G, Singh S. Opioid-free anaesthesia in children with severe mandibular hypoplasia and TMJ ankylosis with sleep apnoea for mandibular distraction osteogenesis. Indian J Anaesth. 2019;63:412-4.

CHAPTER 4

# Updates and Concerns in Perioperative Fluid Management

*Madhuri Kurdi, Anil Kumar MR, Ridhima Sharma, Mayank Kumar, Shilpa Goyal*

## ABSTRACT

The perioperative fluid management in children has always been challenging in all three phases: (1) The pre-operative, (2) intraoperative, and (3) post-operative phases. The strategies, including the type of intravenous (IV) fluid to be infused and calculations for the volume and rate of infusion of the chosen fluid, need to be selected keeping in mind the fluid losses, the paediatric physiology and the type of surgery. Our understanding of the physiological basis of fluid management in children is growing day by day. It is now clear that the period of pre-operative fasting has an impact on post-operative outcomes. Various formulae and guidelines for perioperative fluid management in children have been devised, and the practitioner who administers paediatric anaesthesia should be well adept with these developments. The objective prior to surgery should be to minimise the duration of fasting and, when possible, provide clear oral fluids until 1 hour prior to the procedure. Fluid deficits and maintenance fluids should be determined using the Holliday–Segar formula. The evidence supporting the use of balanced crystalloid solutions in paediatric patients is growing. Isotonic fluids are the mainstay of maintenance fluids. Glucose supplementation is usually not necessary for healthy children undergoing surgery beyond the neonatal period. 1–2% dextrose may be added if there is a possibility of hypoglycaemia. The correct strategies to replace blood loss with fluids, blood and alternatives need to be utilised. Post-operatively, it is best to restart enteral feeding early. If IV fluids need to be continued, isotonic fluids are preferred.

Nevertheless, the current modalities in paediatric perioperative fluid and blood loss management, including formulae for replacement, choice of IV fluid, upcoming methods for monitoring fluid therapy, goal-directed fluid therapy and fluid protocols in the enhanced recovery after surgery pathway are discussed in this chapter.

***Keywords:*** Balanced salt solutions, Blood loss, Colloids, Crystalloids, Fasting, Fluid, Guidelines, Intravenous, Paediatric, Perioperative.

## INTRODUCTION

The topic of perioperative fluid management, especially the type, composition and quantity of fluid to be infused, has always been of interest to the anaesthesiologist managing the paediatric surgical patient. This chapter focuses upon the latest trends in perioperative fluid management in children, including (1) minimisation of the pre-operative fasting period, (2) risk of hyponatraemia and importance of glucose in fluid management, (3) the choice between different balanced crystalloids and between crystalloids and colloids, (4) formulae and guidelines for intraoperative fluid management, (5) management of the bleeding surgical child, (6) newer strategies in fluid management such as goal-directed fluid therapy, upcoming technology-based monitoring of fluid therapy, and (7) post-operative fluid management.

## PHYSIOLOGICAL BASIS OF FLUID MANAGEMENT IN CHILDREN

Though the fluid management strategy in children has always been a topic of frequent discussion, our knowledge of paediatric physiology has remained the same, and there are not many new developments in this field. There are specific differences between adult and infant/child physiology that can influence the perioperative fluid management strategy.

The total body water and the extracellular fluid compartment in children represent a higher proportion of the body weight compared to that of adults. The extracellular fluid accounts for 1/3rd of the total body water in children. Sodium is the primary cation, and chloride is the primary anion in the plasma.[1] Potassium, magnesium, proteins and organic/inorganic phosphate are components of the intracellular compartment. The fluid losses in children are extensive, mainly due to their higher metabolic rate, larger surface area to weight ratio and faster respiration. Hence, their fluid requirement is higher.[2]

The cardiovascular system plays an important role in perioperative fluid dynamics. The infant myocardium has reduced compliance and reduced contractile force compared to that of the adult. Infant cardiac output is mainly dependent on the heart rate. The heart rate is the most sensitive guide to fluid replacement and changes in intravascular volume in children, and it progressively increases with increasing fluid loss. The blood pressure is maintained until more than 10% of the body water is lost.[3]

The immaturity of the renal system limits fluid and electrolyte balance in children. Low systemic arterial pressure, high renal vascular resistance and decreased capillary surface area for filtration lead to low glomerular filtration rate (GFR) in a full-term neonate.[4] The GFR is 15–30% of normal adult values in the first few weeks of life, and it reaches adult values by approximately 1 year. The kidneys achieve rapid maturation by the 5th day of life and reach 80–90% of adult capacity by 1 year of life. The newborns are obligatory salt losers and unable to concentrate the urine maximally during the first few weeks of life. Hence, newborns poorly tolerate sodium loads and water deprivation.[3] They will become hyponatraemic early, and in spite of hyponatraemia, the urinary sodium loss will continue. This obligatory sodium loss proportionally increases the water turnover. The limited urine concentrating ability adds to this and makes the infant prone to develop dehydration when fluid intake is restricted or when fluid losses occur, e.g. during prolonged pre-operative fasting. Nevertheless, perioperative fluid deficits in children can also occur due to renal/cutaneous/gastrointestinal and third space losses. The estimated blood volume and deficit differ with age. Hence, whenever fluid administration is needed, it has to be based on calculations adjusted on age and weight.

Neonates, young infants (<2 months of age), and premature neonates have decreased hepatic glycogen stores, making them more prone for hypoglycaemia. The oxygen consumption, metabolic rate and cardiac index of the neonates are approximately double that of an adult, which can predispose them to hypoglycaemia.[3]

## IMPACT OF PRE-OPERATIVE FASTING ON PERIOPERATIVE FLUID MANAGEMENT AND POST-OPERATIVE PERIOD

Pre-operative fasting is mandatory in the paediatric patient needing any type of anaesthesia. Prolonged pre-operative fasting can lead to dehydration, catabolism, neurohormonal changes and ketosis.[5-7] In a study, children <36 months of age had shown higher concentration of plasma ketone bodies and lower mean arterial pressure (MAP) immediately after anaesthetic induction following prolonged duration of fasting. However, there was no significant difference in the plasma glucose concentrations.[8] Nonetheless, it should be kept in mind that children, especially neonates and small infants, are prone to intraoperative hypoglycaemia resulting from prolonged fasting and the liver metabolism not being fully developed.

Different societies have given their guidelines for pre-operative fasting in children. The recommended period of pre-operative fasting in the past was 2 hours for clear fluids.[9] This was reduced to 1 hour for clear fluids by paediatric anaesthesia societies such as the Association of Paediatric Anaesthetists of Great Britain and Ireland (APA), Australian and New Zealand College of Anaesthetists, European Society of Anaesthesiology and Intensive Care, European Society for Paediatric Anaesthesiology and L'Association des Anesthésistes Réanimateurs Pédiatriques d'Expression Française.[6] The Practice Guidelines of the Indian Society of Anaesthesiologists also strongly recommend that consumption of water, up to 3 ml/kg, should be allowed until 1 hour prior to the administration of anaesthesia. Consumption of clear liquids other than water, up to 3 ml/kg until 2 hours prior to the administration of anaesthesia, has got a weak recommendation.[10]

Reducing the pre-operative fasting times will improve the fluid dynamics in a child posted for surgery and avoid post-operative complications.[6] It will help in the following ways:

- Reduction in the need for perioperative intravenous (IV) fluid supplementation, avoiding the complications pertaining to fluid overload in various major surgeries.

- Positive impact on the physiological and psychological well-being of the child.[11]
- Reduction in pre-operative parent separation anxiety, which is most common in the age group of 1–6 years.[6]
- Reduction in pre-operative parent/caregiver anxiety scores; Studies have proven that high anxiety scores among children are correlated with higher anxiety scores amongst parents/caregivers.[6,12]
- Reduction in post-operative emergence delirium and nausea, more so in the 1–6 years age group.[6,8]
- Playing an important role in enhanced recovery after surgery (ERAS).

## PERIOPERATIVE CHOICE OF INTRAVENOUS FLUID

The tonicity (primarily determined by the sodium concentration), chloride (which buffers the fluid and makes it balanced) and glucose content of IV fluid play an important role in paediatric perioperative fluid management. These factors and their relation to the development of acid-base imbalance, hyponatraemia, hypoglycaemia and hyperglycaemia and ketoacidosis in surgical neonates have been extensively researched upon.

Studies have reported an approximately 11–13% incidence of hospital-acquired hyponatraemia in healthy children after surgery. The hyponatraemia is due to the release of anti-diuretic hormone (ADH) in the post-operative period. Studies have shown that perioperative infusion of hypotonic IV fluids is associated with hyponatraemia.[4]

The dilemma between perioperative crystalloids versus colloids in the operating room has been going on since decades. The choice of crystalloid is frequently debated. The choice of crystalloids has to be made between isotonic balanced crystalloid solutions (BCSs), such as Plasma-Lyte and Ringer's lactate and isotonic fluids, such as 0.9% sodium chloride. A BCS contains electrolytes in concentrations similar to those found in human plasma and is physiologically more similar to human plasma than the 0.9% saline solution. A BCS contains lactate, acetate, or malate as a bicarbonate precursor to prevent hyperchloraemic and dilutional metabolic acidosis, which is observed after 0.9% saline infusions. It has long been known that a 0.9% saline solution is neither 'normal' nor 'physiological.' The elevated chloride concentration in 0.9% sodium chloride solution (154 mmol/L compared to the physiological level of 103 mmol/L) can lead to several adverse effects. These include renal vasoconstriction, decreased renal blood flow and GFR, diuresis, and suppression of the renin-aldosterone system.[5] In critically ill children, hyperchloraemia can result in poor outcomes and has been associated with a higher death rate.[13,14]

In randomised controlled trials (RCTs) and meta-analyses, the use of BCSs resulted in a smaller increase in post-operative chloride levels, less decrease in base excess, and a lower frequency of hyperchloraemic acidosis compared to 0.9% saline solution. These findings indicate that BCSs are more effective in maintaining homeostasis during the perioperative period.

In a study by Lima et al., Plasma-Lyte and normal saline were compared for perioperative IV fluid therapy in children undergoing craniotomy for brain tumour removal; saline infusions resulted in higher variability in serum chloride levels pre- and post-surgery. The incidence of hyperchloraemic acidosis was substantially greater in the saline group than in the balanced salt solution (BSS)group.[15] Conversely, BCS infusions provide a more stable electrolyte and acid-base balance, making them a safer substitute for regular saline.

Plasma-Lyte contains sodium acetate and sodium gluconate instead of sodium lactate, which is a component of Ringer's lactate. Priyanka et al. compared the use of Ringer's lactate and Plasma-Lyte in children undergoing intra-abdominal surgery. Patients who received Plasma-Lyte had an acid-base status similar to those who received Ringer's lactate but had lower levels of hyponatraemia and hyperlactatemia.[16] Plasma-Lyte is associated with other advantages too; as compared with lactate, metabolisation of acetate in Plasmalyte is significantly faster, more independent of hepatic function, with a lower increase in oxygen consumption and no interference with the diagnostic use of lactate as a marker of low tissue perfusion.

A meta-analysis comparing isotonic and hypotonic IV maintenance fluid therapy in hospitalised children found that isotonic fluids significantly reduced the risk of mild hyponatraemia, especially for longer fluid therapy durations. Isotonic fluids also decreased the risk of moderate and severe hyponatremia over 24 hours.[17]

Physiological factors, scientific data and guidelines of various paediatric societies favour BSS as the most accepted perioperative fluid, mainly because of its superior safety and efficacy.[6]

Nevertheless, the administration of IV fluids for intraoperative maintenance in children has shifted from the historical practice of using hypotonic 5% dextrose solution to the current preference of isotonic BSS combined with 1–2% dextrose.[4] The recommended type of fluid to be administered in an infant <1 year of age is 1–2.5% dextrose with BSS.[6] But, neonates of age <48 hours should be supplemented with 10% dextrose to avoid incidences of hypoglycaemia.[9] Hypoglycaemia can adversely affect the central nervous system, especially in neonates. It can provoke counterregulatory stress response and alteration of cerebral metabolism, leading to permanent neural damage. On the other hand, hyperglycaemia can also worsen neural outcomes after an ischaemic/hypoxic event. It can reduce phagocytic function and delay gastric emptying. It can induce severe osmotic diuresis and lead to dehydration.[4] Glucose concentrations >150 mg/dl are associated with glycosuria and osmotic diuresis. It has been suggested that capillary blood sugar levels should be assessed in children, especially neonates, posted for surgery. This will help to decide the type of fluid to be given perioperatively.

Glucose supplementation is usually not necessary for healthy children undergoing surgery, beyond the neonatal period.[6] However, in lengthy surgical procedures where glucose is not administered, it is important to closely monitor blood sugar levels. Introducing 1–2.5% glucose may aid in avoiding disruption of glucose and endocrine homeostasis. A 1% glucose solution can be made by mixing 2 ml of 50% glucose with 100 ml of water or by combining 10 ml of 50% glucose with 500 ml of water. There is an increasing agreement that intraoperative dextrose should only be given to children who are at the highest risk for hypoglycaemia (malnutrition, hypermetabolism, liver failure, hypothermia, mitochondrial disorders, beta-blocker therapy or critical illness). APA consensus guidelines and European consensus statement guidelines recommend intraoperative use of low dextrose (1–2.5%) containing isotonic fluids, which have been shown to maintain acceptable blood glucose levels and prevent electrolyte imbalances during surgery.[9,18] Association of the Scientific Medical Societies in Germany recommends a balanced isotonic electrolyte solution containing 1–2.5% glucose to be used for the background infusion. The initial infusion rate can begin at 10 ml/kg/h and should be adjusted according to the patient's needs over time to maintain a normal extracellular fluid volume.[17]

Colloids are non-crystalline homogeneous particles suspended in either isotonic saline or BSS. They have the property of remaining in the intravascular space for a longer period. They increase the oncotic pressure in the intravascular space and expand the plasma volume. They are either derived from blood in the form of albumin or prepared commercially, such as dextrans and hydroxyethyl starch (HES).[19] There are various studies regarding the preferred colloids in adults, but the recommendations are not very clear in children.[19]

In adults, different studies have highlighted the side effects of various colloids. Dextran can cause anaphylaxis or coagulopathy. Gelatin can induce allergic reactions. HES can lead to renal failure. All these side effects of commercially available colloids or albumin have not been proven in children.[6,18] Albumin is the most commonly available plasma protein and the main determinant of plasma oncotic pressure.[6,20] It binds to acidic drugs. It is commercially available in different concentrations, such as 4%, 5%, 20%, and 25%. It can lead to side effects like nausea, flushing and anaphylactic reactions, although it has less allergenic potential as compared to HES and is costly to produce and store.[6] Caution must be exercised in those with fluid overload, heart or kidney failure. Although the role of albumin as a resuscitative fluid in children with burns >15% and within 8–12 hours of burn injury has been proven in a study,[21] its role in healthy children with hypoalbuminaemia and burns has not been proven.[22] In a study conducted in children aged 2–12 years, undergoing surgery for congenital heart disease, it was found that haemodynamic changes with need for inotropic and vasopressor support, blood loss, need for blood transfusion and renal impairment were comparable with albumin and HES.[22]

Nonetheless, since there are very few robust RCTs on the perioperative use of colloids and their safety in children, the evidence is weak, and it is recommended that, intraoperatively, colloids can be used in children for non-cardiac surgery only when inadequate volume correction is achieved with crystalloids.[23]

## FORMULAE AND GUIDELINES FOR INTRAOPERATIVE FLUID MANAGEMENT IN CHILDREN

The objectives of intraoperative fluid management are to maintain tissue perfusion, intravascular volume, electrolyte balance, and stable acid–base and hormonal levels throughout the procedure.[5] Effective fluid management for a particular patient relies on the coexisting medical condition and the type of surgical procedure the child undergoes. The intraoperative fluid replacement in paediatric surgery is commonly done using formulae based on the child's body weight to replace fasting requirements, maintenance fluid and additional third space loss. Intraoperative fluid needs can occur to replenish volume lost before surgery (resuscitative volume) or to address the deficit caused by fasting. Maintenance fluids are necessary to cover physiological losses from respiration, perspiration, and urine output over a 24-hour period, as well as replacement fluids to offset ongoing surgical blood or fluid losses.[4]

In order to reach the above objectives in infants and children beyond 4 weeks of age, the National Institute for Health and Care Excellence (NICE) guidelines[6] and APA[9] recommend using the Holliday and Segar[24] equation to calculate the deficit and basal daily fluid requirements **(Table 1)**.

The equation (4-2-1 rule) provides a solid foundation for prescribing fluids during surgery, and is recommended for intraoperative fluid management, but modifications must be made to account for the additional

**TABLE 1:** The 4-2-1 rule.[24]

| *Weight (kg)* | *Hourly fluid requirement (ml/h)* | *Fluids per day* |
|---|---|---|
| <10 | 4 × body weight (BW) | 100 ml/kg/day |
| 10–20 | 40 + 2 × (BW-10) | 1,000 ml/day + 50 ml/kg/day for each kg > 10 kg |
| >20 | 60 + 1 × (BW-20) | 1,500 ml/ day + 20 ml/ kg/ day for each kg >20 kg |

obligatory fluid losses associated with the procedure. Such losses can arise from factors such as evaporation during open-cavity operations, burns, fever, sepsis, gastrointestinal fluid losses, and bleeding. For superficial surgical procedures, insensible losses are generally around 1–2 ml/kg/h and usually do not necessitate specific replacement. In the case of thoracotomy, insensible losses range from 4 to 7 ml/kg/h, while during open abdominal surgeries, they rise to between 5 and 10 ml/kg/h.[6,25] For instance, a 25 kg child undergoing peripheral superficial surgery will need 65 ml of maintenance fluid per hour. Conversely, the same child undergoing open abdominal surgery might require 65 ml/h for maintenance along with an extra 125–250 ml/h to account for insensible losses, reaching a total of 190–315 ml/h.

Furman and colleagues suggested determining the pre-operative deficit by taking the Holliday–Segar hourly rate and multiplying it by the number of hours the patient was not allowed to eat or drink. During the initial hour of surgery, half of this calculated amount is replaced, and the remaining half is administered over the following two hours.[26] Later, Berry et al. suggested that children 3 years and younger should receive 25 ml/kg, whereas children 4 years and older should receive 15 ml/kg of basic salt solution over the first hour of surgery.[27] German guidelines recommend administration of balanced electrolyte solution with 1–2.5% dextrose at the rate of 10 ml/kg/h as an initial infusion, followed by adjustment in rate based on requirement. This method generally supplies the required maintenance fluid and accounts for the replacement of insensible losses in a single calculation.[19]

Nevertheless, the pre-operative deficit should be assessed individually for each case. The duration of fasting related to volume deficits impacts intraoperative fluid management. Due to an improved comprehension of paediatric physiology, which encompasses organ maturation, perioperative fluid and electrolyte needs, as well as the recent paediatric pre-operative fasting recommendations (fasting of 1–2 hours for clear liquids), the intraoperative fluid needs are lessened and can be determined using the "2-1-0.5" rule **(Table 2)**.[5] This 2-1-0.5 rule is followed for intraoperative fluid maintenance in long-duration surgeries and those involving major fluid shifts, where the surgical stress response and the resultant release of ADH will be high. The anaesthesiologist, following this rule, looks for clinical signs of dehydration and gives additional fluid as required. In a survey conducted amongst 202 anaesthesiologists of the department of anaesthesiology in

**TABLE 2:** 2-1-0.5 rule.[5]

| *Weight (kg)* | *Hourly fluid requirement using the "2-1-0.5" rule (ml/h)* |
|---|---|
| <10 | 2 × body weight (BW) |
| 10–20 | 20 + 1 × (BW-10) |
| >20 | 30 + 0.5 × (BW-20) |

**TABLE 3:** Assessment of dehydration in children.[1,29]

| *Dehydration (%)* | *Signs (two or more of these should be present)* |
|---|---|
| <5 (No signs of dehydration) | Alert, normal HR/breathing/BP/skin colour, normal eyes, not thirsty, skin turgor instant recoil, and CCRT normal |
| 5–10 (Dehydration present) | Restless, irritable, normal HR/mild tachycardia, tachypnoea, normal BP/skin colour/peripheral pulses, sunken eyes, thirsty, skin turgor mildly decreased, CCRT prolonged |
| >10 (Severe) | Lethargic/unconscious, tachycardia, tachypnoea, acidotic breathing, hypotension, pale skin, weak peripheral pulses, cold extremities, sunken eyes, skin turgor decreased |

HR: heart rate; BP: blood pressure; CCRT: central capillary refill time

an institute in Johannesburg, it was found that registrars with 3–5 years of experience used the 2-1-0.5 rule much more readily than the registrars with 1–2 years of experience, who preferred to use the 4-2-1 rule for intraoperative fluid maintenance.[28]

If pre-operative and post-operative fasting times are as per fasting guidelines, perioperative IV fluid therapy is not required in children beyond neonatal age who undergo short procedures less than one hour with IV access in place. If the child is fasting for >6 hours, an appropriate volume of fluid can be administered based on the degree of dehydration **(Table 3)**. (1% dehydration = 10 ml/kg fluid loss).[1,29]

For fluid resuscitation, it is advised to give a crystalloid solution without glucose that contains sodium (within a range of 131–154 mmol/L) as a bolus of 20 ml/kg over a duration of 10 minutes in children, with a maximum total of 40–60 ml/kg, assuming there is no prior cardiac or renal disease.[18]

## MANAGEMENT OF INTRAOPERATIVE BLEEDING IN CHILDREN

The two most common causes of intraoperative bleeding are failure to control blood vessel bleeding at the surgical site or surgery done in highly vascularised tissues. The second cause is non-surgical or haemostatic bleeding secondary to a pre-existing undiagnosed coagulation disorder prior to surgery or coexistence of established underlying pathologies (such as chronic renal disease, liver disease, and malignancies), the use of drugs, and alteration of haemostasis related to the surgical procedure as in the case of cardiopulmonary bypass or liver transplantation.[30]

The principles of paediatric intraoperative bleeding management include identifying patients who are at risk of bleeding, addressing surgery-related haemostatic changes, adequately replacing blood losses, preventing and treating complications from massive transfusions, and pharmacological therapies, including topical agents to control excessive perioperative bleeding.[30] The goal during the treatment of intraoperative bleeding should be to preserve normovolaemia and be vigilant for hypervolaemia and dilutional coagulopathy, especially while using crystalloids. The prevention and early recognition of coagulopathy due to acidosis, haemodilution, and hypothermia—the so-called lethal triad and subsequent blood losses is important.[5]

## Adequately Replacing Blood Losses with Fluids

The continuous blood and fluid loss needs to be closely monitored and compensated for with the use of a BCS free of glucose.[5] When there is bleeding, a 1:2 ratio of colloids to crystalloids is utilised for the initial transfusion volume. After bleeding has reached 20% of the blood volume, the ideal crystalloid-to-colloid ratio is 1:1.[1] The replacement of intraoperative blood losses with isotonic solution or blood depends on the patient's haematocrit.[1] Furthermore, an additional 2 ml/kg/h of isotonic solution for superficial surgery, 4–7 ml/kg/h for thoracotomy, and 5–10 ml/kg/h for abdominal surgery are required.[1] Sümpelmann et al. recommend that in patients with circulatory instability, balanced isotonic electrolyte solutions without glucose can be administered as repeat dosage infusions of 10–20 ml/kg until the desired effect is achieved.[18] If the volume of crystalloids exceeds, colloids are used as repeat dose infusions to prevent interstitial fluid excess, which causes haemodilution and a decrease in oxygen delivery. A third-generation HES in a balanced solution with a molecular weight of 1,30,000 Da (HES 130) is the preferred synthetic colloid in children. It should be administered in boluses of 5–10 ml/kg if clinically needed, and a moderate total dose of 10–20 ml/kg should be aimed for (maximum 30 ml/kg).[23]

### *Fluid Responsiveness*

Autotransfusion manoeuvres are the most reliable way to predict fluid responsiveness. These include passive leg raise test (in children over 5 years old), Trendelenburg positioning, and external hepatic compression. Autotransfusion dynamically changes central volume and cardiac preload, mimicking the impact of an IV fluid bolus. Positioning and draping the patient frequently prevent these tests from being conducted; thus, fluid responsiveness is more often determined through a dynamic clinical assessment based on treatment response. Judicious IV "fluid challenges" (10–20 ml/kg balanced isotonic crystalloid or 5–10 ml/kg colloid solution) are given while monitoring for positive trends in physiological endpoints (blood pressure, heart rate, urine output, and skin perfusion) and point-of-care testing [pH, base excess, lactate, haemoglobin (Hb), and echocardiography].[6]

## Replacing Blood Losses with Blood

The need for blood transfusion is determined by factors such as age, preoperative Hb levels, type of surgery and maximum allowable blood loss (MABL). Neonates and newborns have more blood volume per weight, but they are less tolerant of blood loss. Additionally, their metabolic rate and basal oxygen demands are higher than adults.[31] MABL is computed as EBV × (H0-H1)/H0 (EBV = estimated blood volume; H0 = starting haematocrit; H1 = lowest allowable haematocrit). The Paediatric Critical Care Transfusion and Anaemia Expertise Initiative (TAXI) guidelines and the European Society of Anaesthesia and Intensive Care (ESAIC) guidelines recommend against transfusion if the child is haemodynamically stable intraoperatively with a Hb concentration of at least 7 g/dl (Grade 1B evidence). Once transfusion is initiated, recommendations are to avoid overtransfusion, with a post-transfusion Hb target of 9.5 g/dl in the haemodynamically stable child without active bleeding.[32] Current evidence for optimum Hb threshold in neonates is controversial and evolving (12 g/dl). High-risk groups, such as cyanotic children and neonates, might require higher thresholds. The needed volume of packed cells in ml is estimated by multiplying body weight (kg) by the desired Hb increase (g/dl) × 5. Massive blood loss is defined as losing one blood volume in 24 hours, 50% of one blood volume in 3 hours, losing over 1.5 ml/kg/min for 20 minutes, or receiving a transfusion of >40 ml/kg of red cells. Routine blood draws should be avoided; laboratory studies should be integrated, when possible, with low-volume extraction and closed-loop collecting methods.

### *Fibrinogen and Prothrombin Complex Concentrate*

Factor concentrates as alternatives to conventional haemostatic blood products (plasma and cryoprecipitate) offer potential advantages of targeted factor composition, small volume, decreased immunogenicity and infectious risks, and accessibility. Fibrinogen concentrate is recommended as an alternative to cryoprecipitate to be administered to children suffering from perioperative bleeding and hypofibrinogenemia.[33] Little to no research exists in the paediatric literature on the efficacy and safety of prothrombin complex concentrate for perioperative haemostatic management, and the use for this indication remains off-label.

## Use of Intraoperative Blood Conservation Modalities

Intraoperatively, blood conservation strategies can be used. These include (1) careful blood pressure and fluid management to avoid haemodilution, (2) restrictive transfusion strategy guided by physiological parameters, (3) goal-directed transfusion algorithms with point-of-care testing, (4) optimisation of haemostatic surgical technique, (5) anti-fibrinolytics such as tranexamic acid (TXA), epsilon aminocaproic acid and aprotinin, (6) topical haemostatic agents, (7) recombinant coagulation products, (8) autologous cell-salvage, (9) normovolaemic haemodilution, and (10) maintenance of normothermia.[34]

TXA can be considered an important modality, especially in those undergoing high blood loss surgery.[35] Optimal recommended dose of TXA in children is 10–30 mg/kg (maximum dose of 2 g) and an infusion of 5–10 mg kg/hour to maintain therapeutic and safe plasma concentrations during surgery. Restrictive transfusion strategies include optimal blood use, limiting blood transfusion by administering the right component, in the right dose, to the right patient, at the right time, for the right reason.[34] Hb concentrations and laboratory coagulation panel thresholds should be assessed in the context of the patient's end-organ function, oxygen delivery, haemostatic status, fluid status, haemodynamics, and the degree of cardiopulmonary reserve; with the goal of tolerating a lower number level if non-clinically significant anaemia, bleeding, or coagulopathy exist.[36]

## Monitoring and Use of Modern Technology in Guiding Perioperative Fluid Therapy in Children

The intraoperative fluid management in children demands close monitoring due to their limited reserve capacity. Ideally, plasma electrolytes, glucose and Hb (or haematocrit) should be measured regularly in any child receiving large volumes of IV fluid, or who remains on IV fluids for >24 hours.[37]

Reliable haemodynamic monitoring techniques are still lacking in paediatric anaesthesia. Many monitoring techniques used in adults have limited value in children. Monitoring techniques that can be used for guiding perioperative fluid therapy in children are as follows:

- For minor surgeries in a child with a normal pre-operative hydration status, standard monitoring techniques such as pulse oximetry, capnography, non-invasive blood pressure and electrocardiography will be sufficient. Additional information can be obtained from a capillary or venous blood gas analysis (base-excess, lactate and glucose).
- In major surgery, beat-by-beat blood pressure monitoring and serial blood gas analysis can be done by insertion of arterial or central venous lines. Pulmonary artery catheters and transpulmonary thermodilution can be used depending on comorbidities in the patient.
- The 2022 ESAIC guidelines recommend utilising viscoelastic haemostatic assay (VHA) guided interventions to help guide transfusion in neonates and children undergoing cardiac and non-cardiac surgery (Grade 2C evidence).[33] VHAs are increasingly available to guide rational and evidence-based haemostatic diagnosis and management, including the administration of blood products such as fresh frozen plasma, platelets, cryoprecipitate, coagulation factor concentrates, or fibrinogen.

Point-of-care viscoelastic testing (VET) allows the anaesthesia team to track haemostatic derangements in real time, guiding point-of-care and goal-directed management of coagulation decisions. The most relevant use of goal-directed bleeding management and transfusion algorithms is in the setting of massive haemorrhage.[34]

- Respiratory variation of aortic blood flow peak velocity (ΔVpeak) measured by pulsed wave Doppler with transthoracic or transoesophageal echocardiography has been reported to be the most consistent predictor of fluid responsiveness in mechanically ventilated children.[38] Flow measurements by ΔVpeak are not affected by arterial compliance or changes in peripheral perfusion. The technique requires a skilled echocardiographer, which may limit its use in everyday practice. Variants of the ΔVpeak technique include measurement using the suprasternal notch view instead of the usual apical 5-chamber view[39] and transfontanelle measurement of respiratory variation of carotid artery blood flow peak velocity (ΔVpeak_CA), which has been reported to be useful in cardiac surgery.[38]
- Continuous blood flow velocity measurement in the descending aorta with an oesophageal Doppler system (CardioQ™; Deltex Medical) showed promising results in a study by Weber et al.[40] A cutoff value of >135.5 cm/s was found to be an indicator of termination of further fluid challenges.
- Non-invasive cardiac output monitors based on thoracic electrical bioimpedance, also known as electrical cardiometry, can be used to reliably estimate the cardiac output and stroke volume variation. Relative phase shifts of either constant or oscillating electrical currents are analysed by these monitors when traversing the thorax. Variations in thoracic resistance are then registered due to changes in blood velocity throughout the cardiac cycle. Their clinical use in the operating room may be limited by interference from monopolar electrocautery and changes in intrathoracic impedance in clinical settings such as interstitial oedema, open thorax surgery, etc.[41]
- Emerging literature suggests that novel technologies such as cerebral and somatic near-infrared spectroscopy(NIRS), can better quantify and monitor oxygen consumption and delivery, especially when taken together with patient haemodynamic and laboratory markers indicative of sufficient perfusion (e.g. lactate, base deficit and pH).[42] NIRS is a technology that is easy to use and can provide helpful information about organ oxygenation and perfusion by measuring regional tissue oxygen saturation ($rSO_2$) with near-infrared light. Infants are ideal for NIRS monitoring as nearly all their vital organs lie near the skin surface which near-infrared light penetrates through. Measuring $rSO_2$ does not require a patient to have adequate pulsatile blood flow or good perfusion, as required when obtaining pulse oximetry measurements. There are

multiple anatomical sites where NIRS sensors can be placed. The most common sites used in children are the forehead [for caesium superoxide ($CrSO_2$)], the abdomen (for splanchnic $rSO_2$, $SrSO_2$), and the flank (for renal $rSO_2$, $RrSO_2$).[43]

Static variables such as heart rate, central venous pressure, pulmonary artery occlusion pressure, dynamic parameters generated from arterial pressure waveforms such as systolic pressure variation, pulse pressure variation and stroke volume variation, respiratory variations in inferior vena cava diameter (ΔIVC), pulse contour analysis monitors such as PiCCO™ (Pulsion), Vygon™ (Vytech) and Flotrac™ (Edwards Lifesciences) that analyse the arterial pressure waveform, dynamic parameters derived from plethysmography such as pulse oximeter plethysmograph amplitude variation (ΔPOP) and plethysmography variability index (PVI) have not shown reliable evidence/or have shown conflicting evidence in predicting fluid responsiveness in children because of higher chest/lung and vascular compliance, lower cardiac compliance and cardiac output in children.[44]

## Fluid Therapy Protocols in Enhanced Recovery after Surgery Pathway in Children

Prolonged pre-operative fasting is avoided in the ERAS pathway. The child is encouraged to drink clear liquids up to 1 hour prior to elective surgery, breast milk up to 4 hours, and formula, solids and non-human milk up to 6 hours prior to general anaesthesia for an elective procedure. Ingestion of a carbohydrate drink 2–3 hours prior to the elective procedure by the child has been shown to reduce post-operative insulin resistance, maintain glycogen reserves, decrease protein breakdown, improve muscular strength, provide a more stable metabolic state at induction, maintain intraoperative normothermia and probably reduce post-operative nausea and vomiting.[45,46]

One has to keep in mind that when the steps of ERAS, such as reduced fasting and avoidance of mechanical bowel preparation, are applied, the child will have less intravascular volume deficits and fluid needs and hence, the fluid administration needs to be adjusted accordingly. A neutral fluid balance is maintained intraoperatively to avoid complications such as pulmonary oedema and post-operative adynamic ileus.[45] Standardised anaesthetic protocols for IV fluids can be used to prevent fluid overload, e.g. IV fluids can be administered via a syringe pump at 2–5 ml/kg/h, less for laparoscopic surgery and more for open gastrointestinal surgery.[47] Nevertheless, there may be a few variations in the fluid management protocols depending on the type of surgery.

Goal-directed fluid therapy or the zero fluid balance model can be used to guide intraoperative and post-operative fluid management.[48] Restricted fluid intake and early enteral feeding in children is being encouraged post-operatively.[49]

### Goal-directed Fluid Therapy in Children

The response of every child to perioperative stress is different, and their perioperative fluid needs are different. Hence, it has been suggested that individualised goal-directed therapy using an appropriate amount of colloid and crystalloid in order to optimise certain selected objective goals of haemodynamic parameters is required, and this may reduce post-operative complications.[1] In goal-directed fluid therapy, one or more of static and/or dynamic haemodynamic parameters (variables) are used to guide fluid administration, with a goal of maximising tissue oxygen delivery and optimising tissue microperfusion without fluid overload. These parameters include PVI, stroke volume, stroke volume variation, cardiac output, mixed venous oxygen saturation, central venous pressure, pulmonary capillary wedge pressure and lactic acid. Transoesophageal echocardiography, pulmonary artery catheterisation, arterial waveform analysis, oesophageal Doppler and bioimpedance-based technologies have to be used to derive these parameters. Recent studies in children undergoing open bowel surgery and elective urological surgery concluded that intraoperative PVI-guided fluid therapy is superior to conventional fluid therapy and significantly reduces the volume of IV crystalloids administered.[50,51] In this technique, the maintenance IV fluid is started. PVI and MAP are used to guide further fluid administration. Fluid boluses are given if the PVI is too high or the MAP is too low. Repeat boluses are given until the PVI and MAP are corrected. In case the PVI and MAP are not corrected with these boluses, phenylephrine is administered.

## SOME UNIQUE PERIOPERATIVE FLUID MANAGEMENT CONSIDERATIONS IN SPECIAL SURGERIES

### Neurosurgery

- The child can have pre-operative fluid and electrolyte disturbances secondary to diuretic therapy, diabetes insipidus, vomiting, and poor fluid and food intake due to impaired consciousness. Preoperatively, enteral fluids may have to be withheld for a longer duration, and IV fluids should be started to maintain fluid balance in children with decreased levels of consciousness, loss of protective airway reflexes, delay in surgical timings or in the presence of vomiting.
- Administration of hypoosmolar fluids can result in the movement of water across the blood–brain barrier into brain tissue and cause cerebral oedema. Iso-osmolar fluids like 0.9% sodium chloride or BSSs such as Plasma-Lyte maintain the osmotic gradient across the blood–brain barrier and hence are preferred maintenance fluids.[52,53] Ringer's lactate solution, though used as an isotonic fluid, has slightly lower osmolality (275 mOsm/L) as compared to plasma and may increase brain oedema.

- Administration of human albumin 5% has been associated with a lesser degree of cerebral oedema than isotonic crystalloids following traumatic brain injury.[54] Albumin and HES 130/0.42 may produce a weaker clot in neurosurgical patients, and hence, monitoring of the coagulation during their use has been advocated.[55] These effects are clinically insignificant if the infused volume is <25% of the patient's blood volume.[56]
- Blood loss and cerebrospinal fluid loss are major contributors to intraoperative fluid loss. Blood loss up to 10–15% blood volume may be replaced with isotonic crystalloids, and additional blood loss should be replaced with packed red cells if the haematocrit falls below 25. Colloids such as tetrastarch and gelatine are used for volume replacement if blood products are not readily available.
- The majority of children may be given fluids without dextrose in the intraoperative period without risk of hypoglycaemia during neurosurgery.[57] However, blood glucose should be monitored, and hypoglycaemia should be avoided, especially in smaller children on long-term IV fluids, diabetic children, neonates and malnourished children. Hyperglycaemia can aggravate ischaemic brain injury, and blood glucose levels > 250 mg% should be avoided.
- Hyponatraemia (serum Na < 135 mmol/L) may occur during or following surgery, secondary to the syndrome of inappropriate anti-diuretic hormone secretion (SIADH), cerebral salt wasting and overzealous fluid resuscitation. Hypernatraemia (serum Na >150 mmol/L) commonly occurs following multiple doses of mannitol or hypertonic saline (3% sodium chloride).
- Craniofacial surgeries are often prolonged procedures involving large blood loss and are more commonly done in infants and small children. There can be extensive blood loss and third space fluid loss from the scalp and the cranium, and, therefore, at least two large indwelling cannulae should be secured, one for maintenance fluids and drugs and the other for rapid fluid and blood replacement.[58]

## Cardiac Surgery

- All infants and children can have clear fluids up to 2 hours pre-operatively. Infants with shunts and cyanotic infants and children (saturation ≤80%), especially with haematocrit >0.55, should be offered clear fluids up to 2 hours preoperatively, and IV fluids if pre-operative fasting duration is >4 hours.
- All children should have diuretics withheld on the day of surgery.[59] Common diuretics used in paediatric cardiology are frusemide, amiloride, spironolactone and bumetanide.[60]
- Patients undergoing congenital heart surgery with cardiopulmonary bypass frequently require the administration of IV fluids and blood

products due to haemodynamic instability. Excessive fluid administration and acute kidney injury may promote fluid overload.[61]

- The underlying cardiac disease and impaired cardiovascular reserve of patients should be taken into account for fluid management.
- There is a risk of fluid overload from cardiopulmonary bypass, which stimulates a significant 'stress' response (up to 72 hours post-operatively) particularly in neonates and infants, due to inflammation, release of ADH, and capillary leak. This results in fluid and salt retention by the kidneys. Unlike gastrointestinal surgery or sepsis, there are usually no ongoing losses and hence extra fluid input is not required; nonetheless, the fluid and salt need to be restricted. Fluid intake is usually limited to 50% of normal maintenance in the first 24 hours post-operatively for those requiring cardiopulmonary bypass and to 75% of normal maintenance for those not requiring cardiopulmonary bypass.[60]

## POSTOPERATIVE FLUID MANAGEMENT IN CHILDREN

Children should begin consuming liquids as soon as they can after anaesthesia, where no medical or surgical contraindications exist.[10] It has been observed that early post-operative oral hydration (within half an hour of arrival in the post-anaesthesia care unit) in preverbal and younger children undergoing elective surgery is efficacious in terms of patient and parent satisfaction and safe compared to delayed feed in the wards. However, forcing children to drink right after surgery can lead to a higher risk of vomiting. The timing should depend on the child's desire to drink. The child should be offered the drink in a conducive atmosphere with adequate analgesia so that the acceptance of the drink will be better.[62]

If early oral fluid intake is not feasible or is inadequate, IV fluid support is important to keep the blood volume normal. Managing IV fluids post-surgery includes two distinct components: continuous body fluid loss and the retention of free water triggered by the secretion of ADH due to surgical stress. Intravascular volume depletion is the most potent stimulus of ADH release. Free water retention can lead to hyponatraemia. Various factors such as pain, inflammation, surgical stress, hypoxia, hypercapnia, sepsis, organ dysfunction and medications can enhance the secretion of excessive amounts of ADH, resulting in the development of SIADH. It is therefore necessary to decrease the infusion rate of isotonic balanced solutions to prevent dilutional hyponatremia in the post-operative phase. If the hourly urine volume is less due to ADH, and IV fluid management is necessary, isotonic fluids should be administered as maintenance fluid with the rate reduced as per the 2-1-0.5 rule/reduced to 50–80% of the usual maintenance.[6] The rate can be increased after the urine volume normalises.[5]

Administering a hyponatraemic solution as a maintenance fluid after surgery carries a significant risk of causing iatrogenic hyponatraemia.

A meta-analysis of studies primarily involving surgical patients revealed an increased risk of hospital-acquired hyponatraemia associated with the use of hypotonic IV fluids.[4] Hence, it has been recommended that hypotonic fluids should not be used as post-operative maintenance fluids. Ringer's Lactate or BSS with added dextrose if needed are preferred fluids for maintenance in the post-operative phase.

Ongoing blood loss may need to be replaced by blood products. Other losses through surgical drains and nasogastric tube should be regularly measured and replaced with an isotonic fluid like 0.9% sodium chloride with or without potassium supplementation. The American Academy of Paediatrics (AAP) advises that patients aged 28 days to 18 years who need maintenance IV fluids should be administered isotonic solutions containing the right amounts of potassium chloride and dextrose, as this greatly reduces the likelihood of hyponatraemia.[63]

Continuous and thorough evaluation of fluid volume, losses, and electrolytes are essential, with the rate of fluid administration, the type of fluid, and any additives adjusted based on needs. The overall length of IV fluid therapy should be minimised, taking into account nutritional needs and the possible requirement for total parenteral nutrition if enteral feeding is not resumed within a few days after surgery.[6]

## CONCLUSION

The objective of fluid management before surgery should be to minimise the duration of fasting and, when possible, provide clear fluids until 1–2 hours prior to the surgical procedure. Volume replacement should be tailored to the individual. Fluid deficits and maintenance fluids should be determined using the Holliday–Segar formula. BCSs such as Plasma-Lyte or Ringer's Lactate, or BSSs, are the mainstay of maintenance fluids. Use of modern technology in haemodynamic monitoring can help in improving perioperative fluid therapy in children. Post-operatively, it is best to restart enteral feeding early. If IV fluids need to be continued, BSSs/BCSs are preferred.

Well-designed multicentric RCTs on the use of intraoperative IV fluids, especially BCSs in children, need to be conducted. Robust studies on the safety of colloids and large-scale studies on blood conservation and haemostatic blood product transfusion strategies in children are also needed. More studies on technology-based monitoring of perioperative fluid therapy and replacement are warranted.

## KEY POINTS

- The pre-operative fasting time should be as short as possible. Liberal clear fluid intake (e.g. water 3 ml/kg) until 1 hour prior to induction of anaesthesia improves patient and parent comfort, the child's metabolic and haemodynamic status after the induction of anaesthesia and enhances recovery.

- The choice of crystalloids has to be made between isotonic BCSs, such as Plasma-Lyte and Ringer's lactate, and isotonic fluids such as 0.9% sodium chloride. Balanced isotonic crystalloids (e.g. Plasma-Lyte) are the first-line fluids for intraoperative maintenance and volume replacement. Glucose 1–2% may be added if there is a risk of intraoperative hypoglycaemia. The recommended type of fluid to be administered in an infant < 1 year of age is 1–2.5% dextrose with balanced salt solution.
- The Holliday–Segar equation ("4-2-1" rule), along with additional fluid requirements based on the invasiveness of the surgical procedure (2 ml/kg/h for minor, 4 mg/kg/h for intermediate, and 6 ml/kg/h for major trauma) is still useful for calculating intraoperative maintenance in children.
- The 2-1-0.5 rule is followed for intraoperative fluid maintenance in long-duration surgeries and those involving major fluid shifts, where the surgical stress response and the resultant release of ADH will be high. The anaesthesiologist, following this rule, looks for clinical signs of dehydration and gives additional fluid as required.
- The evidence for the safe use of colloids in children is weak. Colloids can be used in children for non-cardiac surgery only when inadequate volume correction is achieved with crystalloids and to avoid fluid overload. Hetastarch (HES130) is the preferred synthetic colloid in children.
- Autotransfusion manoeuvres, such as the Passive Leg Raise test, are the most reliable way to predict fluid responsiveness.
- The need for blood transfusion is determined by factors such as age, pre-operative Hb levels, type of surgery and maximum allowable blood loss.
- If the child is haemodynamically stable intraoperatively with a Hb concentration of at least 7 g/dl, blood transfusion is not recommended. A post-transfusion Hb target of 9.5 g/dl in the haemodynamically stable child without active bleeding is recommended.
- VHA guided interventions are useful to help guide transfusion in neonates and children.
- Goal-directed fluid therapy with one or more static and/or dynamic haemodynamic variables can be used to guide fluid administration, with a goal of maximising tissue oxygen delivery and optimising tissue micro-perfusion without fluid overload.
- Novel technologies such as cerebral and somatic NIRS can better quantify and monitor oxygen consumption and delivery.
- Early post-operative oral hydration (within half an hour of arrival in the post-anaesthesia care unit) in preverbal and younger children is efficacious and safe. If a patient is at risk for water retention due to ADH secretion because of high levels of surgical stress, fluid intake is restricted

to 50%–80% of the usual maintenance. Hypotonic/hyponatremic fluids should not be used as post-operative maintenance fluids. Ringer's Lactate or balanced salt solution with added dextrose if needed are preferred fluids for maintenance in the post-operative phase.
- Fluid management forms an important part of the enhanced recovery after surgery pathway.

## REFERENCES


1. Mathew A, Rai E. Pediatric perioperative fluid management. Saudi J Anaesth. 2021;15(4):435-40.
2. Meyers RS. Pediatric fluid and electrolyte therapy. J Pediatr Pharmacol Ther. 2009;14(4):204-11.
3. Rasch DK, Carter B. Fluid balance in pediatric anesthesia. In: Rasch DK, Webster DE (Eds). Clinical manual of pediatric anesthesia. Singapore: McGraw-Hill Book Co;1994. pp.145-60.
4. Bhardwaj N. Perioperative fluid therapy and intraoperative blood loss in children. Indian J Anaesth. 2019;63(9):729-36.
5. Lee H, Kim JT. Pediatric perioperative fluid management. Korean J Anesthesiol. 2023;76(6):519-30.
6. Eaddy N, Watene C. Perioperative management of fluids and electrolytes in children. BJA Educ. 2023;23(7):273-8.
7. Dennhardt N, Beck C, Huber D, Nickel K, Sander B, Witt LH, et al. Impact of preoperative fasting times on blood glucose concentration, ketone bodies and acid-base balance in children younger than 36 months: A prospective observational study. Eur J Anaesthesiol. 2015;32(12):857-61.
8. Dennhardt N, Beck C, Huber D, Sander B, Boehne M, Boethig D, et al. Optimized preoperative fasting times decrease ketone body concentration and stabilize mean arterial blood pressure during induction of anesthesia in children younger than 36 months: a prospective observational cohort study. Paediatr Anaesth. 2016;26(8):838-43.
9. American Psychological Association. (2007). APA Consensus guideline on perioperative fluid management in children 2007. [Online] Available from https://www.apagbi.org.uk/sites/default/files/inline-files/Perioperative_Fluid_Management_2007.pdf [Last accessed June, 2025].
10. Dongare PA, Bhaskar SB, Harsoor SS, Garg R, Kannan S, Goneppanavar U, et al. Perioperative fasting and feeding in adults, obstetric, paediatric and bariatric population: Practice Guidelines from the Indian Society of Anaesthesiologists. Indian J Anaesth. 2020;64(7):556-84.
11. Zhang E, Hauser N, Sommerfield A, Sommerfield D, von Ungern-Sternberg BS. A review of pediatric fasting guidelines and strategies to help children manage preoperative fasting. Paediatr Anesth. 2023;33(12):1012-9.
12. Al-Robeye AM, Barnard AN, Bew S. Thirsty work: exploring children's experiences of preoperative fasting. Paediatr Anaesth. 2020;30(1):43-9.
13. Stenson EK, Cvijanovich NZ, Anas N, Allen GL, Thomas NJ, Bigham MT, et al. Hyperchloremia is associated with complicated course and mortality in pediatric patients with septic shock. Pediatr Crit Care Med. 2018;19(2): 155-60.

14. Zampieri FG, Cavalcanti AB, Di Tanna GL, Damiani LP, Hammond NE, Machado FR, et al. Balanced crystalloids versus saline for critically ill patients (BEST-Living): a systematic review and individual patient data meta-analysis. Lancet Respir Med. 2024;12(3):237-46.
15. Lima MF, Neville IS, Cavalheiro S, Bourguignon DC, Pelosi P, Malbouisson LMS. Balanced crystalloids versus saline for perioperative intravenous fluid administration in children undergoing neurosurgery: A randomized clinical trial. J Neurosurg Anesthesiol. 2019;31(1):30-5.
16. Priyanka A, Ganapathy U, Choudhary R, Arulprakasam S Sr, Krishna CMR, Calairadjane J. A comparative study of peri-operative fluid therapy with ringer lactate and plasmalyte in children undergoing intra-abdominal surgery: A randomized control trial. Cureus. 2023;15(5):e39124.
17. Amer BE, Abdelwahab OA, Abdelaziz A, Soliman Y, Amin AM, Mohamed MA, et al. Efficacy and safety of isotonic versus hypotonic intravenous maintenance fluids in hospitalized children: an updated systematic review and meta-analysis of randomized controlled trials. Pediatr Nephrol. 2024;39(1):57-84.
18. Sümpelmann R, Becke K, Zander R, Witt L. Perioperative fluid management in children: can we sum it all up now? Curr Opin Anaesthesiol. 2019;32(3): 384-91.
19. Sümpelmann R, Becke K, Brenner S, Breschan C, Eich C, Höhne C, et al. Perioperative intravenous fluid therapy in children: guidelines from the Association of the Scientific Medical Societies in Germany. Paediatr Anaesth. 2017;27(1):10-8.
20. Chen B, Hammo B, Barry J, Radhakrishnan K. Overview of Albumin Physiology and its Role in Pediatric Diseases. Curr Gastroenterol Rep. 2021;23(8):11.
21. Dittrich MHM, Brunow de Carvalho W, Lopes Lavado E. Evaluation of the "early" use of albumin in children with extensive burns: a randomized controlled trial. Pediatr Crit Care Med. 2016;17(6):e280-6.
22. Van der linden P, De Ville A, Hofer A, Heschl M, Gombotz H. Six percent hydroxyethyl starch 130/0.4 (Voluven®) versus 5% human serum albumin for volume replacement therapy during elective open-heart surgery in pediatric patients. Anesthesiology. 2013;119(6):1296-309.
23. Beels M, Stevens S, Saldien V. Perioperative fluid management in children: an updated review. Acta Anaesth Bel. 2022;73(3):179-89.
24. Holliday MA, Segar WE. The maintenance need for water in parenteral fluid therapy. Pediatrics. 1957;19(5):823-32.
25. https://www.nice.org.uk. Algorithms for IV fluid therapy in children and young people in hospital. [Online] Available from https://www.nice.org.uk/guidance/ng29/resources/algorithms-for-iv-fluid-therapy-in-children-and-young-people-in-hospital-set-of-6-pdf-2190274957 [Last accessed June, 2025].
26. Furman EB, Roman DG, Lemmer LA, Hairabet J, Jasinska M, Laver MB. Specific therapy in water, electrolyte and blood-volume replacement during pediatric surgery. Anesthesiology. 1975;42(2):187-93.
27. Berry F. Practical aspects of fluid and electrolyte therapy. In: Berry F (Ed). Anesthetic management of difficult and routine pediatric patients. New York: Churchill Livingstone; 1986. pp.107-35.
28. Bruckmann KI. (2018). Anaesthetists practice of intra-operative fluid management in the paediatric population in three academic hospitals. [Online]

Available from https://wiredspace.wits.ac.za/bitstreams/b44967fa-e8b2-404d-b0fa- 17214/download [Last accessed June, 2025].
29. The Royal Children's Hospital Melbourne. Clinical Practice Guidelines 2020. Available from https://www.rch.org.au/clinicalguide/guideline_index/dehydration/ [Last accessed June, 2025].
30. Giraldo MZ. Pediatric perioperative bleeding – Basic considerations. Colombian J Anesthesiol. 2013;41(1):44-9.
31. Lewis SR, Pritchard MW, Evans DJ, Butler AR, Alderson P, Smith AF, et al. Colloids versus crystalloids for fluid resuscitation in critically ill people. Cochrane Database Syst Rev. 2018;2018(8):CD000567.
32. Valentine SL, Bembea MM, Muszynski JA, Cholette JM, Doctor A, Spinella PC, et al. Consensus recommendations for RBC transfusion practice in critically ill children from the pediatric critical care transfusion and anemia expertise initiative. Pediatr Crit Care Med. 2018;19(9):884-98.
33. Kietaibl S, Ahmed A, Afshari A, Albaladejo P, Aldecoa C, Barauskas G, et al. Management of severe peri-operative bleeding: Guidelines from the European Society of Anaesthesiology and Intensive Care: Second update 2022. Eur J Anaesthesiol. 2023;40(4):226-304.
34. Goobie SM, Faraoni D. Perioperative paediatric patient blood management: a narrative review. Br J Anaesth. 2025;134(1):168-79.
35. Patel PA, Wyrobek JA, Alexander BJ, Pivalizza EG, Hare GMT, Mazer CD, et al. Update on applications and limitations of perioperative tranexamic acid. Anesthesia Analg. 2022;135(3):460-73.
36. Goobie SM, Haas T. Perioperative bleeding management in pediatric patients. Curr Opin Anaesthesiol. 2016;29(3):352-8.
37. Wilson CM, Walker IA. Perioperative fluids in children. Update Anaesth. 2005;19:36-8.
38. Lee JH, Kim EH, Jang YE, Kim HS and Kim JT. Fluid responsiveness in the pediatric population. Korean J Anesthesiol. 2019;72(5):429-440.
39. Desgranges FP, Desebbe O, Pereira de Souza Neto E, Raphael D, Chassard D. Respiratory variation in aortic blood flow peak velocity to predict fluid responsiveness in mechanically ventilated children: a systematic review and meta-analysis. Paediatr Anaesth. 2016;26(1):37-47.
40. Weber T, Wagner T, Neumann K, Deusch E. Low predictability of three different noninvasive methods to determine fluid responsiveness in critically ill children. Pediatr Crit Care Med. 2015;16(3):e89-94.
41. Sanders M, Servaas S, Slagt C. Accuracy and precision of non-invasive cardiac output monitoring by electrical cardiometry: a systematic review and meta-analysis. J Clin Monit Comput. 2020;34(3):433-60.
42. Liu L, Qiang Z, Zhang J, Ren Y, Zhao X, Fu W, et al. Effect of hemoglobin content on cerebral oxygen saturation during surgery for scoliosis in pediatric patients. BMC Anesthesiol. 2021;21(1):165.
43. Bailey SM, Prakash SS, Verma S, Desai P, Kazmi S, Mally PV. Near-infrared spectroscopy in the medical management of infants. Curr Probl Pediatr Adolesc Health Care. 2022;52(11):101291.
44. Gan H, Cannesson M, Chandler JR, Ansermino JM. Predicting fluid responsiveness in children: a systematic review. Anesth Analg. 2013;117(6):1380-92.

45. Rafeeqi T, Pearson EG. Enhanced recovery after surgery in children. Transl Gastroenterol Hepatol. 2021;6:46.
46. Laird A, Bramley L, Barnes R, Mount E, Nataraja RM, Pacilli M. Effects of a preoperative carbohydrate load on postoperative recovery in children: a randomised, double-blind, placebo-controlled trial. J Pediatr Surg. 2023;58(9):1824-31.
47. Phillips MR, Adamson WT, McLean SE, Hance L, Lupa MC, Pittenger SL, et al. Implementation of a pediatric enhanced recovery pathway decreases opioid utilization and shortens time to full feeding. J Pediatr Surg. 2020;55(1):101-5.
48. Roberts K, Brindle M, McLuckie D. Enhanced recovery after surgery in paediatrics: a review of the literature. BJA Educ. 2020;20(7):235-41.
49. Rove KO, Edney JC, Brockel MA. Enhanced recovery after surgery in children: promising, evidence-based multidisciplinary care. Paediatr Anaesth. 2018;28(6):482-92.
50. Mathew PJ, Sharma S, Bhardwaj N, Ashok V, Malik MA. Goal-directed fluid therapy guided by plethysmographic variability index (PVI) versus conventional liberal fluid administration in children during elective abdominal surgery: A randomized controlled trial. J Pediatr Surg. 2023;58(4):735-40.
51. Ankita D, Bhardwaj N, Abas MM, Mathew PJ. Plethysmography variability index guided fluid management is superior to conventional approach for elective urological surgery in children - a prospective randomised controlled trial. Europ J Anaesthesiol. 2024;41(12):932-4.
52. Allen CH, Goldman RD, Bhatt S, Simon HK, Gorelick MH, Spandorfer PR, et al. A randomized trial of Plasma-Lyte A and 0.9% sodium chloride in acute pediatric gastroenteritis. BMC Pediatr. 2016;16:117.
53. Houghton J, Wilton N. Choice of isotonic perioperative fluid in children. Anesth Analg. 2011;112(1):246-7.
54. Singh P. Intravenous fluid considerations in the resuscitation of a head injured patient. Indian J Neurotrauma 2005;2:87-90.
55. Nilsson CU, Strandberg K, Engström M, Reinstrup P. Coagulation during elective neurosurgery with hydroxyethyl starch fluid therapy: An observational study with thromboelastometry, fibrinogen and factor XIII. Perioper Med (Lond). 2016;5:20.
56. Arya VK. Basics of fluid and blood transfusion therapy in paediatric surgical patients. Indian J Anaesth. 2012;56(5):454-62.
57. Rath GP, Dash HH. Anaesthesia for neurosurgical procedures in paediatric patients. Indian J Anaesth 2012;56(5):502-10.
58. Karnik HS. Fluid management in infants and children during intracranial surgery. J Neuroanaesthesiol Crit Care. 2017;4(04):S24-9.
59. Starship. (2016). Fluid, diuretic and nutrition management in children having cardiac surgery. [Online] Available from https://starship.org.nz/guidelines/fluid-diuretic-and-nutrition-management-in-children-having-cardiac-surgery/ [Last accessed June, 2025].
60. Cheung YF. Fluid management. In: Cheung YF (Ed). Congenital and Paediatric Acquired Heart Disease in Practice. Springer, Singapore; 2023. pp 463-4.
61. Castañuela-Sánchez V, Hernández-Suárez A, García-Benítez L, Díaz-García L, Martínez-Jasso G, Macedo-Quenot AP. Fluid overload as a predictor of morbidity

and mortality in pediatric patients following congenital heart surgery. Bol Med Hosp Infant Mex. 2022;79(3):187-192.

62. Dhar M, Rawat J, Payal YS, Agrawal S, Sharma R, Gupta V. Impact of early postoperative oral hydration in paediatric patients undergoing elective surgery after general anaesthesia. A randomised controlled trial. Indian J Anaesth. 2025;69(4):365-71.
63. Feld LG, Neuspiel DR, Foster BA, Leu MG, Garber MD, Austin K, et al. Subcommittee on fluid and electrolyte therapy. Clinical Practice Guideline: Maintenance Intravenous Fluids in Children. Pediatrics. 2018;142(6):e20183083.

CHAPTER 5

# Recent Advances in Anaesthesia for Paediatric Laparoscopic Surgeries

*Suvarna Kaniyil, Malavika Kulkarni, Raksha Kundal, Manoj Kumar*

## ABSTRACT

Anaesthetic management of paediatric laparoscopic surgery is challenging, especially in neonates and infants. A thorough knowledge about the physiological effects of laparoscopy is essential to deliver safe anaesthetic care. Physiological effects of pneumoperitoneum and extremes of positioning are exaggerated in neonates. Limiting intra-abdominal pressure to 6–12 mm Hg and flow of gases to <1 l/min is required. Intravenous access should be secured above the diaphragm as pneumoperitoneum can impair blood flow in the inferior vena cava. Slow insufflation and limiting the duration of extreme positions during laparoscopic surgery are essential to prevent complications.

***Keywords:*** Anaesthesia, Paediatric, Pneumoperitoneum, Position, Laparoscopic surgery.

## INTRODUCTION

Laparoscopic surgery has become the standard surgical approach for many paediatric abdominal and pelvic procedures due to its advantages such as faster recovery, reduced postoperative morbidity and shortened hospital stay. A thorough understanding of the paediatric physiology and anaesthetic considerations including the effects of laparoscopy is essential for safe anaesthetic care and improved patient outcome.

## PHYSIOLOGICAL CONSIDERATIONS

Laparoscopic surgeries in paediatric patients are associated with physiological changes similar to those in adults but are significantly influenced by the child's age and cardiopulmonary status. These changes are caused by a combination of factors such as the increase in intra-abdominal pressure (IAP), the extreme patient posture during surgery, the insufflation gas used, and the surgical procedure itself. These physiological effects are more pronounced in neonates and infants.

### Effects of Pneumoperitoneum

Pneumoperitoneum is achieved by insufflating gas, most commonly carbon dioxide ($CO_2$), into the abdominal cavity, which pushes the abdominal wall outward, causes the diaphragm to rise, increases IAP, and decreases thoracic volume. The restricted diaphragmatic excursion, along with reduced thoracic and lung compliance, decreases the functional residual capacity (FRC) and vital capacity while increasing peak airway pressures. In smaller children, early closure of the smaller airways can occur as the closing volume is closer to the FRC, leading to basal atelectasis, resulting in ventilation-perfusion mismatch and hypoxia. Neonates and infants, who already have reduced respiratory reserves, decompensate more quickly compared to adults.

A sudden rise in the IAP due to rapid gas insufflation or trocar insertion can trigger a vasovagal reflex, causing bradycardia. This is common in paediatric patients due to higher vagal tone. Increased IAP compresses the inferior vena cava (IVC), aorta, and splanchnic and renal vasculature, shifting peripheral vascular volume to the central compartment, initially increasing venous return and cardiac output.[1] However, subsequent IVC compression and venous pooling in the lower limbs reduce cardiac output. Pneumoperitoneum increases both systemic and pulmonary vascular resistance, increases heart rate, and can cause arrhythmias. Higher IAP (>15 mm Hg) can significantly increase afterload, reduce preload and decrease cardiac output. These cardiovascular changes are particularly challenging in neonates and children with pre-existing cardiac diseases.

Raised IAP also increases the risk of regurgitation, necessitating aspiration prophylaxis. Compression of the renal vasculature lowers renal blood flow and function to some extent.

## Effects due to Insufflation Gas

$CO_2$ is commonly used for insufflation because it is non-toxic, non-flammable, readily soluble in blood, easily removed by the lungs and reasonably priced.[2] As $CO_2$ is a typical by-product of cellular metabolism, it is harmless at physiological levels. The absorption rate of $CO_2$ is determined by its partial pressure gradient between the peritoneal cavity and blood and the diffusion coefficient. Due to the relatively large surface area of the thin-walled peritoneum, neonates and infants experience greater absorption during pneumoperitoneum, leading to significantly elevated levels of $CO_2$, which can result in hypercarbia and subsequent respiratory acidosis. Increasing the respiratory rate is required to improve ventilation and maintain the partial pressure of $CO_2$ at or near normal levels.

Mild hypercarbia has little influence on haemodynamics, but moderate to severe hypercarbia has both direct and indirect effects on the cardiovascular system. Acidosis can affect myocardial function, reducing cardiac output, impairing the function of cardiac ion channels, disrupting the heart's electrical conduction system and raising the risk of arrhythmias. All these effects can be detrimental in paediatric patients as they have reduced cardiac reserves.

Pneumoperitoneum, hypercarbia and high systemic vascular resistance along with Trendelenburg position, result in increased cerebral blood flow, raising intraocular and intracranial pressure (ICP).[3] Pre-existing ventriculoperitoneal shunt and elevated ICP are relative contraindications to laparoscopic surgeries, necessitating close monitoring of these variables to prevent any further rise in ICP. The continuous insufflation of large volumes of cold, non-humidified $CO_2$ directly into the abdominal cavity increases the risk of hypothermia in paediatric patients. Active warming measures such as forced air warming, warmed intravenous fluids and use of warmed humidified $CO_2$ for insufflation will maintain normothermia intraoperatively.[4]

### Effects due to Patient Position

Placing the patient in the Trendelenburg or reverse Trendelenburg position is essential for optimal surgical field visibility in the abdomen and pelvis. Trendelenburg position exaggerates the effects of increased IAP with pneumoperitoneum causing the diaphragm and abdominal contents to move cephalad, which reduces pulmonary compliance, and raises peak airway pressure. Conversely, the reverse Trendelenburg position has beneficial ventilatory effects but can have detrimental haemodynamic consequences.

## ANAESTHETIC MANAGEMENT

### Pre-anaesthetic Evaluation and Premedication

The preoperative evaluation and standard nil per oral instructions are similar to that followed for any paediatric surgical case. The anaesthetic plan should also be customised to address the specific concerns of the disease. Sedative premedication is decided based on the patients' age and their anxiety levels. It is generally administered to children older than 8–9 months of age as they are prone to experience separation anxiety.[5] Oral or nasal premedication is preferred in children with midazolam (0.5–0.75 mg/kg oral, 0.2–0.3 mg/kg nasal) or dexmedetomidine (1–4 μg/kg nasal).[6] Triclofos, ketamine, clonidine or short-acting opioids like fentanyl may also be selected depending on institutional protocols. It is preferable to obtain venous access in the upper limb as increased IAP can cause compression of the IVC and in the possibility of inadvertent vascular injury, the administered medications may not reach the heart. Anticholinergic medication such as atropine or glycopyrrolate may be used therapeutically to treat bradycardia occurring in response to the creation of pneumoperitoneum or during visceral manipulation.

### Induction of General Anaesthesia

The most widely practised anaesthetic technique is general anaesthesia (GA) with endotracheal intubation and controlled ventilation. Sevoflurane is the ideal volatile agent for inhalational induction in children when venous access is not in place followed by neuromuscular blockade achieved with intravenous atracurium or vecuronium.

### *Airway Management*

Traditionally, cuffed endotracheal tubes and of late, the microcuff tubes are being used for airway management in paediatric laparoscopic surgeries as they offer a more predictable ventilation and reduce the risk of aspiration of gastric contents. Second generation supraglottic airway devices (SADs) such as i-gel® and laryngeal mask airways (LMAs) such as LMA® Proseal™ (better airway seal pressures and integral gastric drainage tube) have emerged as alternative options for shorter procedures in older children, though it is important to be aware that the increased IAP and Trendelenburg position during laparoscopy may result in decline in pulmonary compliance and ineffective ventilation.[7,8] The use of these devices in children is therefore limited to short duration surgeries requiring the use of low IAP and mild tilt.

### *Decompression of Stomach*

Placement of oro- or nasogastric tube is necessary to empty the stomach, prevent inadvertent trocar injury to stomach after pneumoperitoneum and facilitate the visualisation of intra-abdominal contents.

## Intraoperative Monitoring

Apart from standard monitoring, respiratory parameters such as the end-tidal $CO_2$, peak inspiratory pressure, exhaled tidal volumes, compliance and pressure volume curve should be closely monitored as pneumoperitoneum and positioning affect the respiratory mechanics. Invasive monitoring is not necessary routinely, however, post-induction invasive pressures (invasive blood pressure and central venous pressure) and urine output may be monitored based on the cardiovascular status and complexity of the surgical procedure. Due to the limited workspace for surgeons in small children, the access of the anaesthesiologist to the patient's airway and intravenous lines will be often restricted by the surgeon and laparoscopic instruments; hence intravenous extension tubing will be necessary to administer drugs from a distance.

## Maintenance

Anaesthesia is maintained using controlled ventilation with the use of muscle relaxant, intravenous opioids and an inhalational agent such as sevoflurane or isoflurane in oxygen-air combination or by total intravenous anaesthesia.[5,9] It is preferable to avoid the use of nitrous oxide for the maintenance of anaesthesia because it produces bowel distension during prolonged surgeries which impairs the surgical exposure. It also increases post-operative nausea vomiting (PONV) and increases the size of gas emboli if any.

## Peritoneal Insufflation Pressures and Surgery

The mechanical insufflators used in children are the same as those used for adults, but flow rates should be at a slower rate of <1 l/min. The intracavitary pressure should be kept as low as 6–8 mm Hg in neonates and infants and 10–12 mm Hg in children.[10,11] The advantages of low insufflation pressures include reduced cardiopulmonary compromise, better control of alveolar ventilation and a reduced risk of $CO_2$ embolism. The insufflation is begun gradually and increased up till optimal IAP and working conditions are obtained.

## Positioning

Extreme precaution is necessary during positioning the patient to avoid nerve compression and soft-tissue injuries. Appropriate padding of pressure points, avoiding a chin tilt of >15° and neutral positioning of major joints is necessary. Endobronchial migration of the endotracheal tube is a potential risk during laparoscopy due to short trachea in neonates and infants, upward displacement of the diaphragm caused by increased IAP and steep Trendelenburg position. Endobronchial intubation should be suspected whenever there is a sudden increase in the airway pressure, decrease in peripheral oxygen saturation ($SpO_2$) with or without associated hypercarbia.[5] The risk of cerebral oedema and upper airway oedema due to prolonged steep Trendelenburg position should also be kept in mind.

## Ventilation

Volume-controlled ventilation (VCV) has been preferentially used for GA and has the merit of a guaranteed preset tidal volume. However, it presents the risk of increased airway pressure when pulmonary compliances change. Unlike VCV, pressure-controlled ventilation (PCV) has lower risk of barotrauma because the peak airway pressure is preset; however, it cannot ensure optimum tidal volume as it is dependent on the pulmonary compliance which in turn is influenced by IAP. The application of positive end-expiratory pressure of about 4–5 cm of water is required to prevent basal atelectasis. Pressure-controlled ventilation volume-guaranteed (PCV-VG) is a newer mode of ventilation on anaesthesia workstations which delivers a preset tidal volume at the lowest required airway pressure and is being frequently used during GA. This mode makes use of a decelerating flow and constant pressure. For these reasons, PCV and PCV-VG modes are superior to VCV mode in providing adequate oxygenation at lower peak inspiratory pressures during laparoscopic surgeries.[12]

### Fluid Management

Intraoperative fluid losses are less compared to open procedures. Administration of maintenance fluid should be sufficient in minimally invasive surgeries. Hidden hypovolaemia and haemodynamic consequences of raised IAP may be overcome by the administration of 10–20 ml/kg of balanced salt solutions prior to peritoneal insufflation.[5]

### Maintenance of Normothermia

Intraperitoneal insufflation of large volumes of cold, non-humidified $CO_2$ with increased oxygen consumption predisposes children for intraoperative hypothermia. Therefore, core temperature monitoring with active and passive body warming measures is necessary. The application of warm and humidified $CO_2$ insufflation for the creation of pneumoperitoneum during abdominal laparoscopic procedures has been found to reduce the incidence of hypothermia.[4]

### Analgesia

In general, laparoscopic surgeries being minimally invasive, are associated with smaller incision and less tissue trauma requiring lesser analgesics. Apart from incisional pain, referred pain from diaphragmatic irritation and nerve traction from positioning needs to be addressed. A multimodal analgesic approach is essential for optimal care. The analgesic modalities that can be adopted include local anaesthetic infiltration, non-steroidal anti-inflammatory drugs, paracetamol, opioids and regional techniques such as rectus sheath block, transversus abdominis plane block and neuraxial techniques such as caudal, spinal or epidural block.

## POSTOPERATIVE CARE

Upon the completion of surgery, normocarbia must be ensured prior to extubation. The high incidence of PONV in laparoscopic surgeries should be addressed prophylactically with a combinations of drugs like ondansetron and dexamethasone. The residual gas in abdomen can cause shoulder tip pain; however, it is less in children.[9] Postoperative pain should be addressed well, as described earlier.

## REGIONAL ANAESTHESIA FOR LAPAROSCOPY

There is a recent surge in regional anaesthesia (RA) usage in many adult laparoscopic surgeries because of the advantages such as reduction in the postoperative morbidity following GA, shortened hospital stay and cost-effectiveness. Nevertheless, its routine use is still debated.[7] Reports of RA for paediatric laparoscopy are limited. These include a report on the use of spinal anaesthesia for laparoscopic pyloromyotomy in infants and another report on its application in a case of inguinal hernia repair.[13,14] Further, well-conducted studies are required to establish the safety of RA for routine use in paediatric laparoscopic surgeries.

## COMPLICATIONS

Complications are related to the physiological alterations caused by pneumoperitoneum, extremes of positions and the surgical intervention itself. Pneumoperitoneum and extreme positioning can cause haemodynamic/respiratory disturbances such as hypotension/hypertension, hypercarbia or hypoxia. Rapid gas insufflation during the creation of pneumoperitoneum can trigger a reflex vagal response, resulting in severe bradycardia or arrhythmia which usually respond to the cessation of stimulus and deflation of pneumoperitoneum. Subcutaneous emphysema, a common and usually self-resolving complication, can occurs from improper cannula placement, prolonged operative time, or increased IAP.

Rare complications include gas embolism, tension pneumothorax, capnothorax, capnomediastinum and capnopericardium. Capnothorax is a potentially life-threatening complication indicated by the rise in the end-tidal $CO_2$ and airway pressure, a decline in $SpO_2$ and reduced air entry on the affected side. Deflation of pneumoperitoneum and improving the ventilation with application of positive end-expiratory pressure usually suffices for mild cases, but moderate to severe capnothorax may require chest tube insertion.[15] $CO_2$ embolism, though rare, can be a potentially fatal complication, caused by the inadvertent injection of $CO_2$ into a large vein, artery or solid organ. Transoesophageal echocardiography and Doppler are sensitive tools for detecting gas embolism.[16]

Upper airway obstruction can occur due to pharyngeal emphysema or airway oedema from prolonged Trendelenburg position; hence, evaluating the upper airway before extubation is beneficial.[7] Injuries to vascular or solid organs during surgical interventions should be born in mind. Concealed bleeding from vascular injury can sometimes present postoperatively. Prophylactic antiemetics such as ondansetron and dexamethasone are useful for addressing the increased incidence of PONV in laparoscopic surgeries.

## RECENT ADVANCES

Paediatric laparoscopic surgery ranges from minimally invasive foetal surgery and micro-laparoscopic surgery in newborns to robotic laparoscopic surgery in adolescents. Recent advances include single-incision endoscopic surgery (SILS), gasless laparoscopy and robotic/computer-assisted laparoscopic surgery.[17]

One of the distressing features of paediatric laparoscopic surgery is the limited workspace available in children. Robotic/computer-assisted surgery addresses this challenge by providing enhanced precision and manoeuverability.[16] Technological advances in prenatal diagnostics has improved the early detection of foetal anomalies for timely corrective foetal surgery. Foetoscopic endoluminal hiatal occlusion for congenital diaphragmatic surgery, foetal cystoscopy to treat urinary tract obstructions are some of them. Artificial intelligence and augmented reality in paediatric surgery are emerging as future advancements.

## CONCLUSION

In this era of minimally invasive surgery, laparoscopic techniques have become the standard approach for many procedures even in paediatric patients. Understanding the physiological effects of pneumoperitoneum and extreme positioning is crucial in laparoscopic surgery. Effective collaboration between surgeon and anaesthesiologists regarding perioperative plans, including insufflation pressure and patient positioning, is essential for achieving optimal patient outcomes.

## REFERENCES

1. Atkinson TM, Giraud GD, Togioka BM, Jones DB, Cigarroa JE. Cardiovascular and ventilatory consequences of laparoscopic surgery. Circulation. 2017; 135(7):700-10.
2. Yu T, Cheng Y, Wang X, Tu B, Cheng N, Gong J, et al. Gases for establishing pneumoperitoneum during laparoscopic abdominal surgery. Cochrane Database Syst Rev. 2017;6(6):CD009569.
3. Huettemann E, Terborg C, Sakka SG, Petrat G, Schier F, Reinhart K. Preserved CO(2) reactivity and increase in middle cerebral arterial blood flow velocity during laparoscopic surgery in children. Anesth Analg. 2002;94(2):255-8, table of contents.
4. Dean M, Ramsay R, Heriot A, Mackay J, Hiscock R, Lynch AC. Warmed, humidified $CO_2$ insufflation benefits intraoperative core temperature during laparoscopic surgery: A meta-analysis. Asian J Endosc Surg. 2017;10(2):128-36.
5. Veyckemans F. Pediatric anesthesia: basic principles-state of the art-future. In: Bissonette B (Eds). Anesthesia for Laparoscopic Procedures, 1st edition. USA: Peoples Medical Publishing House; 2011. pp. 968-80.
6. Heikal S, Stuart G. Anxiolytic premedication for children. BJA Educ. 2020;20(7):220-5.
7. Bajwa SJ, Kulshrestha A. Anaesthesia for laparoscopic surgery: General vs regional anaesthesia. J Minim Access Surg. 2016;12(1):4-9.
8. Bandyopadhyay A, Puri S, Ashok V. Supraglottic airway device versus tracheal tube for pediatric laparoscopic surgery-A systematic review and meta-analysis. Paediatr Anaesth. 2023;33(11):905-12.
9. Gupta R, Singh S. Challenges in paediatric laparoscopic surgeries. Indian J Anaesth. 2009;53(5):560-6.

10. Joon P, Mandelia A, Dhiraaj S, Singh TK, Shamshery C, Mishra P. Physiological and anesthetic considerations of safe and optimal pneumoperitoneal pressures for laparoscopic surgeries in children. J Indian Assoc Pediatr Surg. 2024;29(1):13-8.
11. Truchon R. Anaesthetic considerations for laparoscopic surgery in neonates and infants: a practical review. Best Pract Res Clin Anaesthesiol. 2004;18(2):343-55.
12. Jo YY, Kwak HJ. What is the proper ventilation strategy during laparoscopic surgery? Korean J Anesthesiol. 2017;70(6):596-600.
13. Islam S, Larson SD, Kays DW, Irwin MD, Carvallho N. Feasibility of laparoscopic pyloromyotomy under spinal anesthesia. J Pediatr Surg. 2014;49(10):1485-7.
14. Chiao F, Boretsky K. Laparoscopic Surgery in Infants Under Spinal Anesthesia Block: A Case Report of 3 Cases. A A Pract. 2019;12(5):168-70.
15. Spinelli G, Vargas M, Aprea G, Cortese G, Servillo G. Pediatric anesthesia for minimally invasive surgery in pediatric urology. Transl Pediatr. 2016;5(4):214-21.
16. Park EY, Kwon JY, Kim KJ. Carbon dioxide embolism during laparoscopic surgery. Yonsei Med J. 2012;53(3):459-66.
17. Meinzer A, Alkatout I, Krebs TF, Baastrup J, Reischig K, Meiksans R, et al. Advances and Trends in Pediatric Minimally Invasive Surgery. J Clin Med. 2020;9(12):3999.

CHAPTER 6

# Emergency Surgeries in Paediatrics: Be Prepared for any Emergency

*Avnish Bharadwaj, Shamshad Beegum TS, Sarvjeet Kaur, Akshita Singla, Shikha Gupta*

## ABSTRACT

A broad spectrum of paediatric emergencies exists, encompassing conditions from birth defects to gastrointestinal issues (acute abdomen), foreign body ingestion and trauma. Enhanced recovery after anaesthesia represents a novel approach aimed at expediting the recovery of infants and children following anaesthesia. Emergency cases in paediatric anaesthesia demand specialised training, particularly in airway management, perioperative fluid therapy, monitoring, post-anaesthesia recovery, analgesia and critical care management. Neonatal cases involving congenital anomalies carry a high risk of morbidity and mortality following emergency surgery, making preparedness in these cases critically important. This article explores the critical aspects of managing emergency paediatric surgeries, with a focus on preoperative preparation, adaptability in challenging circumstances, special considerations in paediatric anaesthesia, effective teamwork and communication and continuous learning for improvement.

***Keywords:*** Anaesthesia, Emergency, Paediatric, Surgery.

## INTRODUCTION

As anaesthesiologists specialising in paediatric care, we encounter a wide array of emergency scenarios in the operating room. The nature of paediatric emergencies necessitates not only clinical expertise but also a comprehensive understanding of the unique challenges and considerations involved. Emergencies in paediatric patients require a high level of preparedness, adaptability, and teamwork from anaesthesiologists.[1] These surgeries encompass a variety of situations, many of which are life-threatening and often involve multiple organ system failures.[1] Unlike elective cases, where adequate preoperative evaluation and meticulous planning are possible, emergency surgeries require heightened attention and vigilance for rapid preoperative evaluation, nil per oral status, fluid and blood transfusions and the availability of appropriate monitoring equipment and facilities in line with recent resuscitation guidelines.[2] Recent advances in paediatric anaesthesia aim to improve patient safety and introduce newer methods of perioperative care.[2] Emergency surgeries include procedures such as appendectomy, intussusception, volvulus, intestinal obstruction, perforation, testicular or ovarian torsions, foreign body aspiration, post-tonsillectomy bleed, trauma and fractures including limb-saving surgeries, degloving injuries, congenital anomalies such as congenital diaphragmatic hernia, tracheo-oesophageal fistula, pyloric stenosis, biliary atresia, among others.[2] These surgeries require specialised expertise and preparedness from anaesthesiologists.[3] Neonates and infants are at a greater risk of anaesthesia-related cardiac arrest compared to older children.[1] Effective communication and co-operation between the entire healthcare team, including surgeons, anaesthetists, nursing and intensive care unit staff are of paramount importance to ensure the best possible care for these tiny humans.[4]

## PREPARATION: METICULOUS PLANNING FOR EMERGENCIES

The unpredictability of these emergencies underscores the critical importance of meticulous preparation.[5] Preparation is fundamental in achieving successful outcomes in emergency paediatric surgeries. From trauma cases to acute abdominal conditions to congenital anomalies, the ability to swiftly transition from assessment to intervention is essential. Trauma is a leading cause of mortality and morbidity in children aged 1–14 years. Trauma cases and limb-saving surgeries in paediatric patients demand detailed preoperative planning to optimise outcomes.[5] Ensuring the rapid availability of blood and blood products along with cell salvage techniques helps in improving the prognosis. Children are more susceptible to multiple organ injuries due to their smaller body size and larger body surface area. Anaesthesiologists must be proficient in trauma resuscitation protocols and be prepared to address life-threatening injuries.[5] Rapid assessment and stabilisation of airway, breathing and circulation while remaining vigilant for associated injuries is crucial.[1]

Essential steps include preoperative evaluation, anticipating potential complications, and ensuring the availability of specialised equipment, monitoring devices, fluid and blood products tailored for paediatric patients.[2] In the realm of emergency paediatric anaesthesia, knowledge of developmental physiology is crucial.[3] Understanding age-specific differences in anatomy, pharmacokinetics and responses to stressors is vital for the safe and effective delivery of anaesthesia.[6] Being updated in paediatric anaesthesia principles and current guidelines form the basis of successfully managing these patients.[7] Preparation begins well before the emergency case arrives in the operating room. Special considerations are given to age-specific pharmacokinetics and physiological differences that influence anaesthesia management.[7] The preoperative assessment involves a comprehensive evaluation of the patient's medical history, airway assessment, cardiovascular stability and any comorbid conditions.[8]

The paediatric anaesthesia cart is a crucial resource during emergencies. It should be well-stocked and organised with age-appropriate equipment for airway management (e.g. various sizes of laryngoscopes, endotracheal tubes, supraglottic airway devices and tracheostomy tubes), vascular access (e.g. appropriately sized intravenous catheters, intraosseous needles and central line kits) and monitoring devices (e.g. paediatric-sized blood pressure cuffs, pulse oximeters, arterial cannulas and capnography) tailored for paediatric patients.[3,8] Emergency drugs should be available on the anaesthesia cart. Various case studies and scenarios illustrate the importance of preparation in optimising outcomes for paediatric emergencies.[6] Thus, preparation forms the base of handling any paediatric emergency. It should be done as quickly and as diligently as possible in minimum time. The plan of anaesthesia, plan B and drug dosages can also be calculated beforehand.

## Physiological and Pharmacological Concerns in Paediatric Patients

Paediatric patients require specialised care due to their unique physiological characteristics and vulnerability. Factors such as airway management, fluid management and temperature regulation must be meticulously addressed.[4] Rapid assessment of the physiological status of the patient, particularly in the presence of congenital abnormalities, is of utmost importance.[6] Children are more prone to severe dehydration and hypothermia, which necessitates careful management.[7]

Airway management in children can be challenging due to anatomical differences, requiring expertise in paediatric intubation techniques.[8] The choice of anaesthetic agents and techniques must prioritise safety while minimising potential adverse effects.[3]

Understanding the pharmacokinetics of commonly used anaesthetic agents in children is essential for safe and effective anaesthesia delivery.[3,7] The higher metabolic rates and large volume of distribution can affect drug clearance and heat production.[4] Consequently, loading doses of drugs need to be larger, and the duration of action may be prolonged.[7] Lean body mass can predict the dose requirement for most children better than mg/kg calculations.[6] This is of particular importance in overweight and obese children; nevertheless, obesity in children is a new global epidemic. Further, the minimum alveolar concentration of volatile agents is higher in children compared to adults.[3]

Preterm infants are at risk of post-operative apnoea. This may be due to complex actions of residual anaesthetic suppression on an immature respiratory drive. Infants need to be carefully monitored in the post-operative period. If apnoea develops, the infant needs to be ventilated with positive pressure to maintain heart rate and saturation. Post-operative apnoea can be managed by the use of oral or intravenous caffeine or continuous positive airway pressure. The use of regional anaesthesia is advocated to reduce this risk.[6]

Due to their larger body surface area relative to body weight, paediatric patients are more vulnerable to hypothermia, necessitating vigilant temperature monitoring and maintenance.[4,6] Warming devices must be used during the perioperative period to prevent hypothermia.[8]

Moreover, paediatric patients are more susceptible to fluid shifts and haemodynamic instability.[8] Precise fluid management tailored to individual needs is crucial to prevent complications such as hypovolaemia or fluid overload.[8] Perioperative fluid therapy should be administered with isotonic solutions. Recent guidelines in perioperative fluid resuscitation have shifted the paradigm to the use of isotonic salt solutions with plasmaLyte and Ringer's lactate being the fluids of choice with lesser concentration of dextrose (1–2%).[9] The famous 4:2:1 rule of Holliday and Segar is still followed for the calculation of maintenance fluid.[9,10] In the post-operative period, the fluid requirement drops down to 2:1:0.5 instead of 4:2:1. Early oral feeding is encouraged. Alternatively, fluid can be administered according to the Rule of 10 in emergency scenarios. 10 ml/kg of isotonic fluid (Ringer's lactate) is administered, and further on, the rate of infusion is based on clinical parameters, e.g. heart rate, blood pressure, capillary refill time, perfusion index, pleth variability index, estimation of ongoing losses, etc. Starvation fluid is calculated by multiplying the hours of starvation with the calculated maintenance fluid per hour. Half of it is given in the first hour and the remaining is given as one-fourth in the next two consecutive hours. Any additional losses such as evaporative losses, blood loss and nasogastric tube aspirate are replaced. In special situations (laparotomy, severe pre-existing dehydration), the fluid administration rate can be much higher.

Pre-school children are at risk of post-operative agitation and delirium due to various factors, including pain, fear, and hunger.[11] Children receiving propofol anaesthesia are at a lower risk of delirium compared to those receiving volatile anaesthetic agents, especially sevoflurane.[5]

Anaesthesiologists play a vital role in ensuring optimal pain management and haemodynamic stability during these procedures.[7] In limb-saving surgeries, anaesthesiologists may need to implement regional anaesthesia techniques or multimodal analgesia strategies tailored to paediatric patients to minimise perioperative pain and optimise recovery. These surgeries require meticulous attention to perioperative pain control and potential intraoperative positioning challenges. Anaesthetic considerations include optimising regional anaesthesia techniques or balanced anaesthesia approaches to enhance post-operative outcomes.[12]

Furthermore, psychological considerations must not be overlooked. Providing reassurance and comfort to both the child and the family amidst the chaos of an emergency situation is a critical aspect of the anaesthesiologist's role.[12]

## Adaptability: Dynamic Decision-making in High-stress Environments

Emergencies rarely unfold as anticipated.[5] The ability to adapt rapidly to changing circumstances is fundamental.[2] This includes making swift decisions on anaesthetic techniques, fluid management and pharmacological interventions tailored to the paediatric patient's specific needs.[3] Paediatric patients can deteriorate quickly due to their limited physiological reserves, necessitating rapid decision-making.[1] Anaesthesiologists must design their anaesthetic plans based on real-time patient responses and the evolving surgical requirements.[3,12] This may involve choosing the appropriate induction agents, implementing regional anaesthesia techniques, modifying ventilation strategies or addressing unforeseen complications promptly.[1] In emergencies, flexibility extends beyond clinical skills.[3] A key aspect of adaptability is maintaining composure under pressure.[12] Effective stress management and decision-making skills are essential during high-stakes situations.[12] Additionally, effective communication and collaboration with the surgical team, nursing staff and other specialists are vital for seamless coordination and optimal patient outcomes.[4,12]

## Preoperative Assessment

The preoperative evaluation includes a rapid yet thorough history-taking and physical examination, which serve as the cornerstone of anaesthetic management planning.[1,7] The main goals of preoperative evaluation are to establish whether the child is fit or unfit for surgery, check for the presence of any diseases requiring preoperative treatment that may affect anaesthetic management, optimisation as far as possible in a limited time, decide on the mode of anaesthesia for the procedure to prevent them from complications of emergency surgery and establish a rapport with the child and their parents to alleviate anxiety.[6,7]

Early recognition and treatment of life-threatening conditions such as airway obstruction, inadequate breathing, intra-abdominal and intracranial haemorrhage significantly increase the survival rate following major trauma.[1] The assessment of injury severity is primarily conducted using the Paediatric Trauma Score, which includes assessments of airway, blood pressure, level of consciousness, nature of wounds and fractures.[1,7]

Over the last decade, significant changes have been made in the preoperative care of children.[8] Enhanced Recovery After Surgery (ERAS) protocols focus on preoperative, intraoperative and post-operative care.[6] Pre-admission counselling and education are encouraged by ERAS recommendations, and communication and trust-building form an important component of ERAS protocols in paediatrics. Effective communication extends to families in paediatric cases.[8]

## Consent and Ethical Aspects

Emergency surgeries in paediatrics carry a high risk and require informed consent, which must be properly communicated to the patient's parents or guardians and documented accordingly.[7] Communication with the families is paramount in paediatric cases. Building trust and rapport through transparent discussions about the procedure, potential risks and expected outcomes can alleviate anxiety and foster a supportive environment.[6] Anaesthesiologists should provide empathetic and transparent explanations about the procedure, potential risks and expected outcomes to alleviate anxiety and build trust.[12]

The ethical practice of medicine weighs the respect for autonomy, particularly in those who are competent to make medical decisions. However, children are not autonomous in making decisions about their treatment. The legal age of autonomy is 18 years, but the decision-making capacity in children is variable. A 2-year-old child cannot make decisions, whereas children aged 12–14 years may be capable of making decisions about their treatment.[13] In these children, the value of assent cannot be undermined. Assent is the agreement of someone not able to give legal consent to participate in the activity. Verbal assent is carefully obtained by calmly and diligently explaining the child about the nature of the emergency and presenting good options. A child who understands what is to be done is more co-operative during the procedures. Emancipated minor status and mature minor doctrine is followed in some countries but is not legal in India.

Key points for consideration include ensuring that the surgeon and anaesthesiologist accurately discuss the surgical management and potential alternatives, disclose common risks that are more likely to occur during the perioperative period and disclose serious risks due to their potentially severe consequences. Informed refusal is also significant, with some patients having the right to refuse certain treatments, such as blood transfusions, in special situations like those involving Jehovah's Witnesses.[13]

## Airway Evaluation

Assessment of the airway is crucial for maintaining airway safety.[3] Airway complications continue to be a significant contributing factor to perioperative cardiac arrest (21%) and brain death, as reported by the Paediatric Perioperative Cardiac Arrest (POCA) registry and the American Society of Anesthesiologists (ASA).[1] The Mallampati scoring system is not reliable in non-cooperative children, and the more reliable Colorado Paediatric Airway Score (COPUR) (Chin, Opening mouth, Previous intubation difficulty and obstructive sleep apnoea, Uvula, Range of movements) is recommended.[3] The NECTARINE (Neonate and Children Audit of Anaesthesia Practice in Europe) multi-centre trial found a high incidence of difficult airways in children, leading to severe hypoxaemia and emphasising the need for a preoperative airway management plan.[7]

Now, video laryngoscopes play a pivotal role in paediatric difficult airway management, improving first-attempt success rates and reducing complications.[9] Uncuffed endotracheal tubes are preferred in children under 8 years of age due to the risk of mucosal injuries causing subglottic stenosis.[4] The availability of microcuff tubes has made them the airway device of choice even in infants. Microcuff tubes have been designed specifically for paediatric anatomy which along with providing a sealed airway reduce the risk of tracheal trauma. Emergency tracheostomy may be required in children presenting with difficult airway, airway trauma or neonates with subglottic stenosis.

### Fasting Guidelines

Recent international consensus has shifted from conservative, prolonged fasting durations to more liberal policies that allow clear fluids up to 1 hour before the administration of anaesthesia.[8,9] In most emergent cases, the child may not be fasting, necessitating careful discussion and analysis of the risk-benefit ratio regarding the aspiration risk. Gastric ultrasound plays a significant role in establishing the safety of liberal feeding practices in children.[8] Nevertheless, a gastric ultrasound though not commonly done currently, can be done to know the status of gastric emptying.

## INTRAOPERATIVE MANAGEMENT

Intravenous access is often a significant challenge in paediatric emergency procedures, especially in small children and neonates. The peripheral veins in the dorsal venous plexus of the hand are usually preferred, with alternatives including the veins of the antecubital fossa and external jugular veins. In neonates and infants, scalp veins may be accessed, though leg veins are generally avoided to prevent immobilisation of the child. If time allows, local anaesthetic cream [Eutectic Mixture of Local Anaesthetics (EMLA)] can be applied 30–45 minutes before venous cannula insertion, though it may cause vasoconstriction, complicating cannulation. Venous cannulation via the umbilical vein is a life-saving procedure in neonates. Ultrasonography-guided intravenous access may be obtained in difficult cannulation cases. Alternatively, a light emitting diode handheld vein finder may be used in emergencies to locate the peripheral veins for cannulation. Intraosseous access is indicated if other attempts fail, especially during circulatory access in cardiac arrest scenarios.[10]

### Rapid Sequence Induction and Aspiration Risk

*Nil Per Oral (NPO) status:* Guidelines for preoperative fluid management and fasting have evolved, with recommendations minimising preoperative fasting and allowing clear fluids up to 1 hour before anaesthesia.[11] Rapid sequence induction (RSI) is typically preferred for emergency surgeries, combined with ventilation and endotracheal intubation. While cricoid pressure is traditionally used to reduce aspiration risk, it may be challenging in children due to anatomical differences, and alternative methods, such as controlled RSI without cricoid pressure, are increasingly favoured.[11]

## Induction of Anaesthesia

Inducing anaesthesia may be distressing for children, necessitating careful planning based on the type of emergency case.[7] Separation anxiety is a significant factor, and appropriate premedication is essential to alleviate stress before induction. Sedative premedication, such as midazolam or ketamine should be used cautiously in emergency cases.[11] However, ERAS protocols do not recommend pharmacological premedication for anxiolysis, particularly long-acting drugs, unless the child exhibits significant anxiety.[8]

For children without an intravenous line, inhalational induction using sevoflurane is safe, reliable and quick. But this carries a risk of significant aspiration.[8] Intravenous induction, if an intravenous cannula is available, is preferred, particularly in patients at risk of aspiration. The choice of anaesthesia depends on the case and individual circumstances, with propofol and ketamine commonly used as induction agents.[11]

## Intravenous Fluids and Blood Transfusion

Fluid resuscitation should begin as early as possible.[10] In practice, a maintenance solution of 5% dextrose and 0.45% saline was most commonly used to compensate for ongoing losses.[11] However, studies have shown higher risk of hyponatraemia with the use of hypotonic salt solutions. Also, the use of 5% dextrose has been associated with higher incidence of hyperglycaemia which is as detrimental as hypoglycaemia. Thus, recent fluid therapy guidelines suggest use of balanced salt solutions with addition of dextrose only if indicated. An ideal balanced salt solution does not exist, so presently plasmaLyte/Ringer's lactate is the maintenance fluid of choice with the addition of 1–2% dextrose if required.

Cross-matched blood should be available before surgery begins, and intraoperative blood transfusions may be necessary depending on the rapidity and volume of blood loss, preoperative haemoglobin levels and the patient's overall condition, particularly cardiac status.[13] Blood and blood products are the ideal replacement for ongoing blood losses. Adequate blood loss replacement is crucial to reducing morbidity and mortality.[13] If hypovolaemia is not responsive to fluid therapy, blood transfusion should be considered. However, care has to be taken to avoid transfusion-related adverse effects.

Blood loss ≥20 ml/kg should be replaced with equal volume of packed red blood cells.

The required transfusion volume of packed red blood cells in children can also be calculated as follows: body weight (kg) × desired increment in haemoglobin (g/dl) × 5.

Transfusion trigger is usually accepted to be around a haemoglobin level of 7–8 g/dl in children having intraoperative loss. A haemoglobin level of 7 g/dl is acceptable if there is no active on-going loss and stable clinical parameters. Current evidence for optimum haemoglobin threshold in neonates is controversial and evolving (12 g/dl).[13]

$$\text{Maximum allowable blood loss (MABL)} = EBV \times (H0 - H1)/H0$$

(EBV = estimated blood volume; H0 = starting haematocrit; H1 = lowest acceptable haematocrit)

Transfusion of 8 ml/kg whole blood raises the haemoglobin by 1 g/dl.

Transfusion of 4 ml/kg packed cells raise the haemoglobin by 1 g/dl.

Formula for calculation of volume of blood to be transfused in paediatric surgical patients:
Volume (ml) to be transfused = (Desired Haemoglobin – Actual Haemoglobin) × Weight (kg) × Blood Volume (ml/kg)/Hematocrit of transfused blood.

## Temperature Maintenance and Warming

Maintaining body temperature is crucial in paediatric patients. Methods include using sheets, blankets, and caps, particularly during hospital transfers. Monitoring of dual temperature including core body temperature using oesophageal/rectal probe and skin temperature should be done. The ambient temperature in the operating theatre should ideally be maintained between 20 and 23°C to prevent hypothermia. Minimising exposure of large areas of skin before surgery begins and humidifying ventilation gases can also help to reduce heat loss.[14] Use of carbon fibre or forced warm air blanket is useful in maintaining body temperature.

## Monitoring

In paediatric emergencies, non-invasive monitoring such as pulse oximetry, capillary refill time, temperature and urine output are essential for evaluating circulatory volume status. Invasive monitoring techniques such as invasive blood pressure monitoring using arterial cannulation and serial monitoring of arterial blood gases can be done. Recent advancements include Masimo signal extraction technology, which overcomes challenges of body movement and low perfusion during pulse oximetry. Non-invasive co-oximetry of pulse (SpHb) and near-infrared spectroscopy for cerebral oxygenation during cardiac repair are also beneficial in reducing mortality.[12]

### Special Case Scenarios

Certain paediatric emergencies require specific anaesthetic approaches. For instance, congenital diaphragmatic hernia demands immediate intubation and careful ventilatory strategies to prevent pulmonary barotrauma. In cases of omphalocele or gastroschisis, maintaining body temperature and fluid resuscitation is critical. Other conditions, such as tracheo-oesophageal fistula or oesophageal atresia, require precise airway management, often involving intubation with the tube positioned to maintain ventilation without exacerbating the condition.[9]

### Ear, Nose and Throat Emergencies

Ear, nose and throat (ENT) emergencies, such as laryngomalacia or subglottic stenosis, require careful airway management, often with the patient maintaining spontaneous respiration.[9] High-frequency jet ventilation may be utilised in certain cases, combined with careful anaesthetic management to ensure airway patency.[3] Post-tonsillectomy bleed patients present as full stomach and are at a higher risk for the aspiration of blood.

### Acute Abdomen

Careful and rapid initial assessment needs to be done. Adequate and aggressive fluid resuscitation is required to cover third-space losses. Fluid resuscitation has to be managed to avoid both under- and overhydration. Rapid sequence intubation has to be done.

### Regional Anaesthesia

Spinal anaesthesia is a safe and effective alternative in neonates and infants, particularly for lower abdominal surgeries. It is associated with haemodynamic stability and a reduced hormonal stress response during the perioperative period, making it a valuable technique in managing post-operative pain.[9] Spinal anaesthesia provides dense analgesia in children with inguinal hernia or lower abdominal surgeries. It may be used as the sole anaesthetic technique in inadequately fasted babies. However, there is a faster regression of spinal anaesthesia in children. Caudal block, epidural catheters, erector spinae plane blocks and paravertebral blocks can be used for both intraoperative and post-operative analgesia.

## POST-OPERATIVE MANAGEMENT AND ANALGESIA

Post-operative care varies depending on the hospital's location and resources. Ideally, the recovery area should be well-equipped with oxygen, suction, good lighting and proximity to nursing stations. Fluid therapy and blood transfusions should be continued as needed, with careful monitoring of the patient's condition.[14]

Multimodal analgesia should be the cornerstone of post-operative care. Keeping the child pain-free alleviates anxiety and helps in faster recovery. Various regional blocks can be given during the intraoperative period which can provide very good post-operative analgesia. Patient-controlled analgesia (PCA) pumps for on demand analgesia can be used. But they require round the clock monitoring. These PCA pumps can be nurse-controlled or parent-controlled. Bolus epidural injections and elastomeric pumps can also be used.

## CONTINUOUS LEARNING AND IMPROVEMENT

Paediatric emergency surgeries offer valuable learning opportunities for anaesthetists. Participation in paediatric anaesthesia workshops, simulations and continuing education programmes is essential to stay at the forefront of advancements in paediatric critical care. Regular debriefings after critical cases allow for knowledge sharing and identification of areas for improvement in protocols, equipment or team dynamics. Continuous learning and commitment to excellence are crucial in delivering the highest standard of care when it matters most.[15]

## CONCLUSION

Paediatric emergency surgeries require a comprehensive, multidisciplinary approach. As anaesthesiologists, our role extends beyond our technical expertise. It encompasses our readiness, providing tender loving care, adaptability and teamwork to manage high pressure and critical situations. We can significantly improve the outcomes of our tiny humans during critical moments by adhering to these principles and setting up defined protocols. A strong commitment to continuous learning and pursuit of excellence can ensure the highest standard of care when it is most needed. This can make a life-saving difference in paediatric emergencies.

## REFERENCES

1. Wald SH. Paediatric Anaesthetic Emergency Data Manual. Anesthesiology. 2017;127:911.
2. Pani N, Panda CK. Anaesthetic consideration for neonatal surgical emergencies. Indian J Anaesth. 2012;56(5):463-9.
3. Maheshwari M, Sanwatsarkar S, Katakwar M. Pharmacology related to paediatric anaesthesia. Indian J Anaesth. 2019;63(9):698-706.
4. National Guideline Alliance (UK). Communication by healthcare staff: Babies, children and young people's experience of healthcare: Evidence review B. London: National Institute for Health and Care Excellence (NICE); 2021. (NICE Guideline, No. 204.)
5. Remick K, Gausche-Hill M, Joseph MM, Brown K, Snow SK, Wright JL; American Academy of Pediatrics Committee on Pediatric Emergency Medicine

and Section on Surgery; American College of Emergency Physicians Pediatric Emergency Medicine Committee; Emergency Nurses Association Pediatric Committee. Pediatric Readiness in the Emergency Department. Pediatrics 2018;142(5):e20182459. Erratum in: Pediatrics. 2019;143(3):e20183894.

6. Rai E, Naik V, Singariya G, Bathla S, Sharma R, Pani N. Recent advances in paediatric anaesthesia. Indian J Anaesth. 2023;67(1):27-31.
7. Newton M. Anaesthesia for emergency paediatric general surgery. Update in Anaesthesia. [online] Available from https://resources.wfsahq.org/wp-content/uploads/uia30-Anaesthesia-for-emergency-paediatric-general-surgery.pdf [Last accessed June, 2025].
8. Mitchell M. Anaesthesia for common paediatric emergency surgeries. Surg Clin North Am. 2017;97:223-32.
9. Frykholm P, Schindler E, Sümpelmann R, Walker R, Weiss M. Preoperative fasting in children: review of existing guidelines and recent developments. Br J Anaesth. 2018;120(3):469-74.
10. Scott-Warren VL, Morley RB. Paediatric vascular access. BJA Education. 2015;15:199-206.
11. Mathew A, Rai E. Pediatric perioperative fluid management. Saudi J Anaesth. 2021;15(4):435-40.
12. Lee H, Kim JT. Pediatric perioperative fluid management. Korean J Anesthesiol. 2023;76(6):519-30.
13. Bharadwaj A, Khandelwal M, Bhargava SK. Perioperative neonatal and paediatric blood transfusion. Indian J Anaesth. 2014;58(5):652-7.
14. Machovec KA, Weldon BC. Thermoregulation in pediatric anesthesia. In: Kaye AD, Fox CJ, Diaz JH (Eds). Essentials of Pediatric Anesthesiology. United Kingdom: Cambridge University Press; 2014. pp. 400-405.
15. Everett TC, MacKinnon R, de Beer D, Taylor M, Bould MD. Ten years of simulation-based training in pediatric anesthesia: The inception, evolution, and dissemination of the Managing Emergencies in Pediatric Anesthesia (MEPA) course. Paediatr Anaesth. 2017;27:984-90.

CHAPTER 7

# Perioperative Cardiac Arrest in Paediatrics

*Anita Malik, Malavika Kulkarni, Preethy J Mathew, Ankit Desai*

## ABSTRACT

Paediatric perioperative cardiac arrest, a rare critical event, is the cessation of adequate mechanical cardiac activity, requiring cardiopulmonary resuscitation with or without defibrillation. Despite advances in anaesthesia, perioperative cardiac arrest in the paediatric population continues to occur. Younger age, significant comorbidities, congenital heart disease, emergency surgery, and prematurity have been consistently identified as predictors of perioperative cardiac arrest in children. Delineating potential risk factors and correctable causes of perioperative cardiac arrest may facilitate improvements in perioperative techniques and outcomes, leading to a decrease in morbidity and mortality. The Royal College of Anaesthetists Guidelines for Provision of Anaesthetic Services recommend training in advanced life support to all anaesthetists who provide care to children that covers their expected range of clinical practice and responsibilities. The practice of simulations of intraoperative cardiac arrest and common operating room emergencies promotes the teamwork skills and identifies latent situations that predispose to medical errors in multidisciplinary operating room teams. Newer modalities such as point-of-care ultrasound (POCUS) are being increasingly utilised to prevent and treat reversible causes of cardiac arrest in the perioperative period.

***Keywords:*** Cardiac arrest, Life support, Paediatric, Perioperative, Resuscitation.

## INTRODUCTION

Paediatric perioperative cardiac arrest, a rare critical event, is the cessation of adequate mechanical cardiac activity, requiring cardiopulmonary resuscitation (CPR) with or without defibrillation; however, the duration differs in different studies ranging from 60 minutes after anaesthesia until 24–48 hours after the completion of anaesthesia.[1-4] The reported incidence of paediatric perioperative cardiac arrest in developed countries ranges from 2.9 to 7.9 per 10,000 anaesthetics,[2,5,6] while in developing countries differs between 2.7 and 22.9 per 10,000 anaesthetics.[4,7]

Keeping in view the patient's comorbidities, allocation of resources and an appropriate communication between clinicians, the paediatric American Society of Anesthesiologists Physical Status (ASA-PS) classification could be used to enhance the consistency of the scoring for better perioperative care. With advances in technology and healthcare, obtaining a paediatric ASA-PS classification that most accurately and reliably reflects the categories of paediatric patients cared for, can provide more accurate data capture.[8]

The Royal College of Anaesthetists Guidelines for the Provision of Anaesthetic Services (GPAS) recommend training in advanced life support to all anaesthetists who provide care to children that covers their expected range of clinical practice and responsibilities. Multidisciplinary and scenario-based annual training should help to maintain these competencies.[9]

## RISK FACTORS OF PERIOPERATIVE CARDIAC ARREST

Delineating potential risk factors and correctable causes of perioperative cardiac arrest may facilitate improvements in perioperative techniques and outcomes, leading to a decrease in morbidity and mortality.[10] Children with cardiac disease are at high risk of cardiac arrest due to unique characteristics and different physiologies. Congenital anomalies, low physiological reserve and emergency high-risk surgery in neonates are correlated with a higher risk of cardiac arrest.[11,12]

Risk factors for cardiac arrest and associated mortality include prematurity, lower weight, younger age, (under 12 months having higher odds of cardiac arrest), single-ventricle physiology, pulmonary arterial hypertension, arrhythmias, genetic syndrome, cognitive impairment, longer duration of surgery, comorbidities, surgical complexity, higher vasoactive-inotropic score, mechanical ventilation preceding cardiac arrest and factors related to institutional characteristics and resources.[11] Children who have anaesthesia induction in the intensive care unit are at high risk for perioperative cardiac arrest due to higher ASA-PS and other factors such as patient (individual pathophysiology), procedural and institutional characteristics.[2]

## CAUSES OF PERIOPERATIVE CARDIAC ARREST

According to an update from the Paediatric Perioperative Cardiac Arrest (POCA) registry, cardiovascular causes include hypovolaemia associated with and without blood loss, air embolism, electrolyte imbalance; respiratory causes such as airway obstruction, laryngospasm, difficult intubation, oesophageal or endobronchial intubation, inadvertent or premature extubation, inadequate ventilation or oxygenation, bronchospasm, pneumothorax and aspiration; medication-related causes such as halothane/sevoflurane-induced cardiovascular depression, other single or combination medication, allergic reaction and intravascular injection of local anaesthetic; equipment-related causes including those involving central catheter, kinked or plugged endotracheal tube, peripheral intravenous catheter and breathing circuit.[13]

Anaesthesia-related factors in cardiac arrest from hypovolaemia due to blood loss include underestimation of blood loss, pre-existing hypovolaemia or anaemia, inadequate peripheral venous access, central venous catheter not present or not transduced, arterial catheter not present or malfunctioning, delay in obtaining blood from the blood bank, insufficient help available to treat blood loss, development of coagulopathy, and unappreciated or undertreated hypocalcaemia.[13]

In children with congenital heart disease, the incidence is highest, and cardiac tamponade and isolated severe hypotension are reported to be the causes of cardiac arrest in cardiac surgery or cardiological procedures, while severe hypoxaemia, bradycardia and major haemorrhage are reported in non-cardiac surgery.[6]

The evolution of anaesthesia practices appears to have influenced the distribution of causes, with a notable reduction in medication-related arrests and an increase in cardiovascular and respiratory causes.[14]

## PREVENTION OF PERIOPERATIVE CARDIAC ARREST

Availability of the paediatric specific ASA-PS grading system now avoids the underestimation of physical status in children, a common problem affecting the critical event.[8] The Paediatric Cardiac Critical Care Consortium collaborative's introduction of cardiac arrest prevention bundle (quality improvement programme) have been shown to reduce the rates of cardiac arrest in children with congenital heart disease.[15] For greater standardisation of clinical practice, a quality improvement project implementation has been shown to reduce the anaesthesia attributable cardiac arrest incidence.[16] The practice of simulations of intraoperative cardiac arrest and common operating room emergencies has been found to promote the teamwork skills and identify latent situations that predispose to medical errors in multidisciplinary operating room teams undergoing crisis management training.[17]

Most paediatric cardiac arrest cases result from an inability to stop the progression of respiratory failure, shock, or both into cardiac arrest situations. According to the 7th National Audit Project of the Royal College of Anaesthetists, the incidence of perioperative cardiac arrest was found to be highest in neonates (27, 26%), infants (36, 35%) and in children with congenital heart disease (44, 42%). The reasons for non-cardiac causes of perioperative cardiac arrest included severe hypoxaemia (20, 22%), bradycardia (10, 11%), and major haemorrhage (9, 8%).[6] The survival rate of children who develop cardiac arrests in hospitals is only approximately 43%.[18] Therefore, rapid identification and intervention are crucial to prevent cardiac arrest and achieve favourable outcomes.

## MANAGEMENT OF PERIOPERATIVE CARDIAC ARREST

### Intraoperative Cardiac Arrest

*Recognition and immediate response to perioperative paediatric cardiac arrest:* Cardiac arrest is defined as the 'cessation of cardiac mechanical activity determined by unresponsiveness, inability to palpate a central pulse and apnoea'. This definition was first put forth in the paediatric Utstein guidelines in 1995, which formed definitions and templates to define critical events during cardiac arrest.[19]

This is ascertained intraoperatively by identifying arrest rhythm on the monitor. Arrest rhythms include asystole, pulseless electrical activity (PEA), ventricular fibrillation (VF), and pulseless ventricular tachycardia (VT), including torsades de pointes. Asystole and PEA are the most commonly identified rhythms in children aged <12 years.

Rapid response to the initiation of high-quality CPR comprising chest compressions and rescue breaths can significantly improve outcomes after paediatric perioperative cardiac arrest.

Perioperative paediatric cardiac arrest resuscitation follows the American Heart Association Pediatric Advanced Life Support (AHA PALS) algorithm. High-quality CPR is the cornerstone of basic and advanced life support for cardiac arrest management.

## *Sequence of Basic Life Support in Infant and Child*

The sequence of basic life support in an infant and child is as follows:

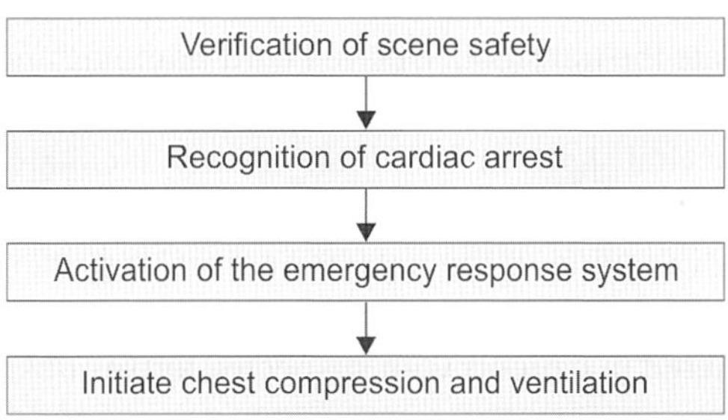


- Chest compression-ventilation ratio should be 30:2 with a single rescuer or 15:2 with two rescuers without an advanced airway in place.
- Continuous chest compression should be delivered at a rate of 100–120/min with one breath every 2–3 seconds with an advanced airway in place. Each rescue breath is delivered over 1 second with a visible chest rise.
- The depth of compression needs to be one-third the antero-posterior diameter of the chest (approximately 5 cm in children in the age range of 1 year to puberty), and about 4 cm during infancy.
- The compression technique preferred in infants is the two-finger technique for a single rescuer or the two-thumb encircling hands technique with two rescuers. In the case of children older than 1 year, it is the two hands or one hand over the lower half of the sternum.
- Sufficient time needs to be given to permit complete chest recoil and limit interruptions between chest compressions.

- The next action would be to use the automated external defibrillator/ manual defibrillator at the earliest.

*Assessing the effectiveness of high-quality CPR:* Essentials of high-quality CPR are good team dynamics along with the appropriate rate and depth of compression, permitting sufficient time for adequate chest recoil with minimal interruption and avoiding excessive ventilation. Continuous monitoring of end-tidal carbon-dioxide ($EtCO_2$) with an advanced airway in place and arterial waveform with an arterial catheter in-situ not only guides us to assess the quality of chest compressions, but also in the identification of return of spontaneous circulation (ROSC). During CPR, the goal is to obtain an $EtCO_2$ of >10–15 mmHg and ROSC is indicated with an abrupt increase in $EtCO_2$ beyond 40 mmHg.

### *Important Recent Concepts of Neonatal Resuscitation*

Neonatal resuscitation guidelines apply specifically to newborn babies transitioning from foetal to neonatal life. However, these guidelines may be applicable to the entire neonatal period (birth to 28 days). The neonatal resuscitation algorithm has not changed since 2015 and provides structural support for neonatal resuscitation.[20]

Every healthy newborn baby should have a trained and equipped person assigned to facilitate the transition. Delayed cord clamping and active warming should be implemented. All neonatal resuscitation equipment to provide warmth, monitor vital signs, maintain the airway, facilitate ventilation and provide circulatory support should be readily available whenever necessary, and continuous evaluation of the baby for normal respiratory function and stimulation may be necessary to facilitate respiratory effort. Suctioning should be considered in patients with suspected airway obstruction.

*Evaluation of heart rate:* Heart rate (HR) is assessed initially by auscultation and/or cord palpation. Pulse oximetry and electrocardiography are important additives in neonates and can serve as a guide for oxygen therapy to meet resuscitation goals.

*Guidelines for oxygen therapy:* Positive pressure ventilation (PPV) remains the primary means of providing support for apnoeic newborns, bradycardia or inadequate respiratory effort.

Positive pressure ventilation should be initiated with air (21% oxygen) for term and late preterm babies and with up to 30% oxygen in preterm babies.

*Initiation of chest compressions:* Despite 30 seconds of adequate PPV, if the HR persists at <60 beats/min, chest compressions should be started. The compression-to-ventilation ratio is 3:1 (with 90 compressions per minute and 30 PPV per minute) using the two-thumb encircling hands technique for chest compression.

*Mode of vascular access:* The umbilical venous route is the chosen route of vascular access in the newborn. However, the intraosseous route should be considered when intravenous access is not possible.

*Administration of medications:* Epinephrine should ideally be administered intravenously if HR drops to <60 beats/min despite 60 seconds of chest compressions and adequate PPV. If the HR remains <60 beats/min, intravenous or intraosseous epinephrine (10–30 μg/kg/dose) may be administered every 3 minutes. Epinephrine may be administered via the tracheal tube (50–100 μg/kg/dose) if intravenous/intraosseous access cannot be obtained.

*Fluid resuscitation:* In conditions where blood loss is anticipated based on history and examination and there is no response to epinephrine, volume expansion is indicated with isotonic crystalloids (normal saline) or blood if neonates are not responsive to resuscitation and volume depletion is a possibility.[21]

### *Advanced Life Support Measures*

Early recognition and prevention of impending cardiac arrest are important cornerstones of advanced life support. The principles of advanced life support are also applicable in the event of cardiac arrest, after establishing basic life support. The key steps include (1) identifying the cause of haemodynamic collapse and its management, (2) identifying and managing the cardiac rhythm, and (3) maintaining oxygenation and carbon dioxide elimination during resuscitation.

Intraoperative haemodynamic collapse can occur for a multitude of reasons, as elaborated earlier in this chapter. Close monitoring of vitals usually warns of impending collapse. Preoperative hypovolaemia and ongoing intraoperative blood loss are other factors that should be considered. At least two wide-bore vascular accesses are critical for volume resuscitation, if not already secured. Intra-arterial blood pressure monitoring should be instituted whenever possible. It is imperative to have adequate cross-matched blood and blood products in the operating room. Serial haematocrit, electrolyte and blood gas analyses are useful for monitoring physiological derangement intraoperatively.

Disturbances in cardiac rhythm may be haemodynamically stable or unstable, depending on systemic blood pressure and peripheral perfusion. One of the haemodynamically stable cardiac dysrhythmias that requires prompt intervention is supraventricular tachycardia (SVT). The Valsalva manoeuvre and ice application to the face can be used to treat haemodynamically stable SVT in infants and children.[21] Pharmacologic therapy includes a rapid bolus of intravenous adenosine (0.05–0.10 mg/kg) to expect a sinus rhythm within 20 seconds.[22] Amiodarone may be used as a second-line agent to treat haemodynamically stable SVT refractory to vagal manoeuvres and adenosine. Synchronised cardioversion starting with a dose of 0.5–1 J/kg is recommended if the patient with SVT becomes haemodynamically unstable.[22] If unsuccessful, the cardioversion dose can be increased to 2 J/kg.

Wide-QRS tachycardia in children who are otherwise haemodynamically stable is treated similar to SVT.[22] If the diagnosis of VT is confirmed, intravenous amiodarone may be administered at a dose of 5 mg/kg (maximum dose of 300 mg/dose) for 20–30 minutes. If VT persists, amiodarone may be repeated or procainamide may be considered. However, amiodarone and procainamide should not be administered together, because their combination may increase the risk of hypotension. Synchronised cardioversion remains the treatment of choice for unstable VT. Amiodarone may be considered for the treatment of haemodynamically unstable VT.

Cardiac tachyarrhythmia without a pulse could be a VF/pulseless VT. The treatment of choice is prompt defibrillation at an initial dose of 2 J/kg (biphasic or monophasic waveform) using a manual defibrillator. If VF or pulseless VT does not respond to defibrillation, intravenous amiodarone is recommended. Intravenous epinephrine is recommended for all pulseless rhythms, including asystole and PEA, along with chest compressions.

*Airway and oxygenation:* If an advanced airway is not in place, placement of an endotracheal tube is preferable. Laryngeal mask airway may be an acceptable alternative airway adjunct during paediatric cardiac arrest. Although there is insufficient evidence to support any specific fractional inspired oxygen concentration, the AHA recommends 100% oxygen until ROSC. Once the circulation is restored, oxygen saturation should be monitored to titrate inspired oxygen.

*Vascular access and drug routes during cardiac arrest:* Children in cardiac arrest should receive 10 μg/kg epinephrine as the first and subsequent intravascular dose. Routine administration of high-dose (100 μg/kg) intravascular epinephrine is not recommended and may be harmful.[22] Establishing additional vascular access during resuscitation in children can be difficult. If additional access is required, the intraosseous route can be considered, although it is limited by a lack of reported experience in children. Intravascular injection of drugs, including intraosseous, is preferable for administration via the tracheal route. The recommended tracheal dose of atropine (0.03 mg/kg), epinephrine (0.1 mg/kg) or lidocaine (2–3 mg/kg) is higher than the vascular dose. Central venous access may be considered after ROSC.

*Post-resuscitation care:* Vasoactive drugs should be considered to improve haemodynamic status in the post-cardiac arrest phase. The choice, timing and dose of specific vasoactive drugs must be individualised and guided by available monitoring data. Hyperventilation after cardiac arrest may be harmful and should therefore be avoided. The target for post-resuscitation ventilation is normocapnia. Short periods of hyperventilation may be indicated only as a temporising measure for children with signs of impending cerebral herniation.

Temperature control is an important management aspect. Induction of hypothermia (32–34°C) for 12–24 hours may be considered in children who remain comatose after resuscitation from cardiac arrest.[22] The blood glucose concentration should be checked during or immediately after cardiac arrest to maintain normoglycaemia.

## Post-operative Cardiac Arrest

Despite advances in anaesthesia, perioperative cardiac arrest continues to occur in the paediatric population. Most cardiac arrests were recorded in neonates and infants (36% and 26%, respectively), and more than half of these were associated with congenital heart disease.[6] The 104 children who reported to the National Audit Project 7 (NAP7) registry, when compared with the 3,429 paediatric cases in the NAP7 activity survey, were more often male (68, 65% vs. 2023, 59%), younger, sicker and more comorbid (ASA-PS 1–2:13, 13% vs. 2,908, 85%). They also had higher rates of urgent or immediate surgery (52, 50% vs. 573, 17%), non-elective surgery (74, 71% vs. 1,023, 30%), major or complex surgery (66, 63% vs. 298, 9%) and general anaesthesia (99, 97% vs. 2,982, 90%). Cardiac surgery was the most prevalent speciality (30, 29%), followed by ear, nose and throat surgery (14, 13%); interventional cardiology (12, 12%); and lower gastrointestinal surgery (11, 11%).[6] Most cardiac arrests present with a non-shockable rhythm, and sustained ROSC is achieved after <20 minutes of resuscitation.[6] According to the Wake-up Safe initiative, of all reported adverse events (2,544 events), the most common adverse events were cardiac arrest (646, 31.6%), respiratory complications (598, 29.2%) and medication events (345, 16.9%). Of all anaesthesia-related events (612 events), medication events were the most common (239, 31.9%), followed by respiratory complications (181, 24.1%), and cardiac arrests (139, 18.5%). Overall, 85% of anaesthesia-related serious adverse events were deemed somewhat or almost certainly preventable.[23]

The causes of cardiac arrest in the postoperative period include major haemorrhage, severe hypoxaemia and bradyarrhythmia. Misplaced or obstructed tracheal tubes, accidental tracheal extubation and failure to reintubate leading to a ‘cannot intubate, cannot oxygenate’ scenario are important causes of cardiac arrest. Another important cause of non-return to spontaneous circulation is the use of atropine or glycopyrrolate for bradyarrhythmias instead of adrenaline.[6]

Debriefing should be routinely performed after any paediatric perioperative cardiac arrest. Fewer than half of all paediatric reports to NAP7 were debriefed, and this was less common when the child was successfully resuscitated. Failure to review cases is likely to mean that individuals and organisations will miss key lessons and opportunities to improve patient safety.

Newer modalities, such as point-of-care ultrasound (POCUS), are being increasingly utilised to prevent and treat reversible causes of cardiac arrest in the perioperative period.[24] Conditions such as volume status, bleeding, cardiac tamponade and tension pneumothorax can be diagnosed earlier and should be incorporated into routine practice. Clinicians can directly visualise cardiac contractility and central arterial pulsatility with POCUS. The apical 4-chamber (A4), subxiphoid (SX) and femoral artery views may be used when defibrillator pads or active compressions preclude parasternal cardiac views.[25] However, these manoeuvres are time-sensitive and should follow the 10-second rule. The Royal College of Anaesthetists has published comprehensive guidelines for the provision of anaesthetic services with specific recommendations for paediatric services.[9] However, there are challenges associated with POCUS, including potential interruptions in chest compressions during image acquisition and the need for operator proficiency.[26]

## CONCLUSION

Younger age, significant comorbidities, congenital heart disease, emergency surgery and prematurity have been consistently identified as predictors of perioperative cardiac arrest in paediatrics. Indian data are largely lacking, and a registry to record cases of cardiac arrest is needed to improve outcomes related to this age group. Most paediatric cardiac arrest cases result from an inability to stop the progression of respiratory failure, shock or both into cardiac arrest situations. Therefore, rapid identification through close monitoring of vitals as well as clinical situation vigilance, usually warns of impending collapse. Timely appropriate interventions are crucial to prevent perioperative cardiac arrest and achieve favourable outcomes.

## REFERENCES

1. Habre W, Disma N, Virag K, Becke K, Hansen TG, Jöhr M, et al. Incidence of severe critical events in paediatric anaesthesia (APRICOT): a prospective multicentre observational study in 261 hospitals in Europe. Lancet Respir Med. 2017;5:412-25.
2. Jansen G, Borgstedt R, Irmscher L, Popp J, Schmidt B, Lang E, et al. Incidence, mortality, and characteristics of 18 pediatric perioperative cardiac arrests: an observational trial from 22,650 pediatric anesthesias in a German tertiary care hospital. Anesth Analg. 2021;133:747-54.

3. Christensen RE, Lee AC, Gowen MS, Rettiganti MR, Deshpande JK, Morray JP. Pediatric perioperative cardiac arrest, death in the off hours: a report from Wake Up Safe, the pediatric quality improvement initiative. Anesth Analg. 2018;127:472-7.
4. Khoso N, Ghaffar WB, Abassi S, Khan FA. Pediatric anesthesia severe adverse events leading to anesthetic morbidity and mortality in a tertiary care center in a low- and middle-income country: a 25-year audit. Anesth Analg. 2021;132:217-22.
5. Flick RP, Sprung J, Harrison TE, Gleich SJ, Schroeder DR, Hanson AC, et al. Perioperative cardiac arrests in children between 1988 and 2005 at a tertiary referral center: a study of 92,881 patients. Anesthesiology. 2007;106:226-37; quiz 413-4.
6. Oglesby FC, Scholefield BR, Cook TM, Smith JH, Pappachan VJ, Kane AD, et al. Peri-operative cardiac arrest in children as reported to the 7th National Audit Project of the Royal College of Anaesthetists. Anaesthesia. 2024;79(6):583-92.
7. Gobbo Braz L, Braz JR, Modolo NS, do Nascimento P, Brushi BA, Raquel de Carvalho L, et al. Perioperative cardiac arrest and its mortality in children. A 9-year survey in a Brazilian tertiary teaching hospital. Paediatr Anaesth. 2006;16:860-6.
8. Ferrari L, Leahy I, Staffa SJ, Berry JG. The pediatric-specific American Society of Anesthesiologists physical status score: a multicenter study. Anesth Analg. 2021;132:807-17.
9. Royal College of Anaesthetists. (2023). Guidelines for the Provision of Anaesthetic Services. [online] Available from https://www.rcoa.ac.uk/safety-standards-quality/guidance-resources/guidelines-provision-anaesthetic-services [Last accessed June 2024].
10. Foz C, Staffa SJ, Brown ML, DiNardo JA, Nasr VG. Predictors and outcomes of perioperative cardiac arrest in children undergoing noncardiac surgery. BJA Open. 2023;8:100244.
11. Sperotto F, Gearhart A, Hoskote A, Alexander PMA, Barreto JA, Habet V, et al. Cardiac arrest and cardiopulmonary resuscitation in pediatric patients with cardiac disease: a narrative review. Eur J Pediatr. 2023;182:4289-308.
12. Sperotto F, Daverio M, Amigoni A, Gregori D, Dorste A, Allan C, et al. Trends in in-hospital cardiac arrest and mortality among children with cardiac disease in the intensive care unit: a systematic review and meta-analysis. JAMA Netw Open. 2023;6(2):e2256178.
13. Bhananker SM, Ramamoorthy C, Geiduschek JM, Posner KL, Domino KB, Haberkern CM, et al. Anesthesia-related cardiac arrest in children: Update from the pediatric perioperative cardiac arrest registry. Anesth Analg. 2007; 105:344-50.
14. Lampugnani, Lerman J, Grasso C, Moscatelli A. Cardiac arrest in children. Curr Anesthesiol Rep. 2017;7(2):1-8.
15. Alten J, Cooper DS, Klugman D, Raymond TT, Wooton S, Garza J, et al; PC4 CAP Collaborators. Preventing cardiac arrest in the pediatric cardiac intensive care unit through multicenter collaboration. JAMA Pediatr. 2022;176(10):1027-36.
16. Hohn A, Trieschmann U, Franklin J, Machatschek JN, Kaufmann J, Herff H, et al. Incidence of peri-operative paediatric cardiac arrest and the influence of a specialised paediatric anaesthesia team: Retrospective cohort study. Eur J Anaesthesiol. 2019;36:55-63.

17. Gros E, Shi R, Hasty B, Anderson T, Schmiederer I, Roman-Micek T, et al. In situ interprofessional operating room simulations: empowering learners in crisis resource management principles. Surgery. 2021;170(2):432-9.
18. American Heart Association and American Academy of Pediatrics. Pediatric Advanced Life Support Provider Manual: Part 5—Recognizing and Managing cardiac arrest. 2021;71-88.
19. Zaritsky A, Nadkarni V, Hazinski MF, Foltin G, Quan L, Wright J, et al. Recommended guidelines for uniform reporting of pediatric advanced life support: The Pediatric Utstein Style: A statement for healthcare professionals from a task force of the American Academy of Pediatrics, the American Heart Association, and the European Resuscitation Council. Resuscitation. 1995;30:95-115.
20. Aziz K, Lee CHC, Escobedo MB, Hoover AV, Kamath-Rayne BD, Kapadia VS, et al. Part 5: Neonatal Resuscitation 2020 American Heart Association Guidelines for Cardiopulmonary Resuscitation and Emergency Cardiovascular Care. Pediatrics. 2021;147(Suppl 1):e2020038505E.
21. Kariuki E, Sutton C, Leone TA. Neonatal resuscitation: current evidence and guidelines. BJA Educ. 2021;21(12):479-85.
22. Topjian AA, Raymond TT, Atkins D, Chan M, Duff JP, Loyner BL, et al. Pediatric Basic and Advanced Life Support. 2020 American Heart Association Guidelines for Cardiopulmonary Resuscitation and Emergency Cardiovascular Care. Circulation. 2020;142:S469-S523.
23. Haché M, Sun LS, Gadi G, Busse J, Lee AC, Lorinc A, et al. Outcomes from wake up safe, the pediatric anesthesia quality improvement initiative. Paediatr Anaesth. 2020;30:1348-54.
24. Boretsky K. Perioperative point-of-care ultrasound in children. Children (Basel). 2020;7(11):213.
25. Leviter JI, Chen L, O'Marr J, Riera A. The feasibility of using point-of-care ultrasound during cardiac arrest in children: Rapid apical contractility evaluation. Pediatr Emerg Care. 2023;39(5):347-50.
26. Copetti R. Clinical integrated ultrasound in peri cardiac arrest and cardiac arrest. J Clinic Experiment Cardiol. 2012;S10-003.

CHAPTER 8

# Regional Anaesthesia in Paediatrics: Maximising Safety and Efficacy Through Advanced Techniques

*Mukesh Kumar Prasad, Ridhima Sharma, Payal Jain, S Sanjay Prabhu*

## ABSTRACT

Paediatric regional anaesthesia has evolved significantly, offering safer and more effective pain management for children undergoing surgery. This chapter focuses on recent advances in peripheral nerve blocks, particularly the use of ultrasound guidance, which enhances precision and mitigates risks. Ultrasound, combined with nerve stimulation, improves the accuracy of block placement, reducing complications such as nerve injury and intravascular injection. The chapter also highlights the role of advanced equipment, multimodal analgesia, and adjuvants to optimise outcomes while minimising local anaesthetic doses. By integrating the latest evidence-based practices, this chapter aims to provide the tools to ensure safe and effective techniques for effective peri-/intraoperative pain management in paediatric subsets.

***Keywords:*** Anaesthesia, Local anaesthetic, Paediatric, Peripheral nerve blocks, Regional, Safety, Spinal anaesthesia.

## INTRODUCTION

Paediatric regional anaesthesia has evolved significantly over the past few decades, offering safer and more effective options for pain management in children undergoing surgical procedures. With advancements in technique, technology, and understanding of paediatric physiology, the landscape of regional anaesthesia in paediatric patients has expanded, enabling clinicians to reduce the risks and optimise outcomes.[1] Paediatric regional anaesthesia provides profound and prolonged analgesia perioperatively, reduces the side effects of opioids and non-steroidal anti-inflammatory drugs (NSAIDs) and positively impacts the stress response and cellular, metabolic, immunological, hormonal and haemostatic aspects.[2]

This chapter aims to explore the latest techniques in paediatric regional anaesthesia, focusing on strategies to enhance safety, efficacy and patient satisfaction. By delving into innovative approaches and evidence-based practices, the chapter seeks to equip healthcare professionals with the knowledge and skills necessary to provide superior perioperative pain management for paediatric patients.

## SAFETY IN PERIPHERAL NERVE BLOCKS

*'The more distal, the safer it becomes'*—Peripheral nerve blocks have an excellent risk-to-benefit ratio, making them a well-established technique among anaesthesiologists.[3] A nearly six-fold increase in the complication rate has been demonstrated for central versus peripheral techniques. Anatomical variations in growing children make landmark-guided approaches less reliable, especially when the margin of safety is narrow. The Paediatric Regional Anaesthesia Network (PRAN) is a collaborative group of several paediatric hospitals that acts as a registry for regional procedures in children. In 2018, the data collected between 2007 and 2015 was reported and it included 104,393 blocks placed on 91,701 paediatric patients.[3] The most common single-injection block was caudal, and the most common single-shot peripheral nerve block was a femoral block. The widespread popularity of adjuvants and ambulatory catheters has increased the duration of blocks and made them more cost-effective.

The French-Language Society of Paediatric Anaesthesiologists has conducted studies that have demonstrated no increased incidence of adverse effects when general anaesthesia techniques were supplemented by regional anaesthesia. Interestingly, the overall incidence of regional anaesthesia-related complications was <0.9 of 1,000 anaesthetic procedures performed.[4,5]

According to a survey conducted by PRAN, the overall incidence of neurological complications was 2.4 per 10,000 blocks. These were mainly sensory issues that were resolved in <3 months. None of the patients had permanent motor deficits. The incidence of severe local anaesthetic systemic toxicity (LAST) (cardiac arrest/seizures) was 7 per 10,000 blocks. Most of them were in infants, <6 months of age and after a bolus dose of local anaesthetic.[5]

## INDICATIONS OF PERIPHERAL NERVE BLOCKS

With the appropriate knowledge, skill and expertise, the indications for blocks in adults also apply to paediatric patients. Some of the indications for peripheral nerve blocks include:

- As a sole technique for anaesthesia (though children will require some sedation along with this)
- Along with general anaesthesia, to provide intraoperative and post-operative analgesia
- Chronic pain conditions
- Analgesia in traumatic pain (e.g. femoral nerve or fascia iliaca block for femoral fractures).
- To improve perfusion in an ischaemic limb

## ADVANCED EQUIPMENT AND TECHNIQUES FOR PAEDIATRIC NERVE BLOCKS

The use of appropriate equipment for successful paediatric blocks cannot be overstated:

- An appropriately sized short-bevel echogenic needle (4 cm/5 cm/10 cm) with a blunt tip improves the sensation of passage through the tissues (a sharp-tip needle can be helpful for fascial plane blocks).
- A short extension tube should be attached to the needle to avoid unnecessary movement while delivering the drug.
- The use of a nerve stimulator is encouraged for deep-seated nerve blocks (lumbar plexus blocks), and to help decide the endpoint of injection, i.e. needle-nerve contact (0.2 mA–0.4 mA).
- A nerve stimulator with adequate current output capable of eliciting percutaneous stimulation (e.g. 5 mA/1 ms) for surface mapping can be used.
- The use of injection pressure monitoring equipment can help to decrease intra-neural injection.[6]
- The landmark-guided approach has been surpassed by ultrasound, which offers key advantages despite requiring operator skill and training. Dual guidance (peripheral nerve stimulation along with ultrasound) should be encouraged.[7]
- Linear probes with a small footprint (25 mm in length) are necessary for performing blocks in infants and children weighing <15 kg.
- A needle tracking system can be used to improve visualisation of the needle axis, reducing the chances of unintended punctures.
- For children with very superficial structures, a 5 mm sterile ultrasound gel pad may help to focus the ultrasound beam better.

## PRE-BLOCK ASSESSMENT

- The patient and family should be assessed and prepared for the proposed surgery and anaesthetic technique.
- A thorough history, examination (local/systemic) and investigations as appropriate are required. Any preoperative neurological deficits need to be documented clearly.
- A more distal block is preferred, given that it is safer.
- Assessment of the requirement and application of a single-shot or continuous block technique using a catheter should be done.
- Taking informed consent from the guardians and assent from the child after explaining the pros and the cons is necessary. It is also important to have a backup plan for analgesia in case the block fails. Strategy for multimodal analgesia, including the use of pre-emptive analgesia, should be encouraged.

## PERIOPERATIVE MANAGEMENT FOR MAXIMISING SAFETY AND EFFICACY OF NERVE BLOCK

Some basic precautions are to be followed to ensure that the regional anaesthetic technique is performed safely and effectively.

- An experienced anaesthesiologist and skilled assistant are keys to a successful technique.
- As part of the World Health Organisation Surgical Safety Checklist, consent and the side of surgery are checked. A time-out before proceeding with the block is mandatory.
- *Nerve block:* Awake or sedated? The vast majority of children are unlikely to co-operate with an awake needling technique. Thus, the use of deep sedation or general anaesthesia (spontaneous respiration) is highly recommended except in premature infants posted for minor surgeries where the risk of post operative apnoea overpowers the benefit of general anaesthesia. The risk of complications associated with an awake block is higher than blocks performed under general anaesthesia.
- The child, ultrasonography machine, equipment and the anaesthesiologist should be positioned ergonomically.[8]
- Application of a eutectic mixture of local anaesthetic cream over the needle insertion site is recommended 45 minutes prior to insertion.
- Distracting the child using phones, videos, or music can be tried, or anxiolytic agents such as midazolam, propofol or remifentanil can be used.[9]
- Peripheral nerve blocks should be given under full aseptic conditions using chlorohexidine/povidone-iodine solution. This solution, after having sufficient contact, should be wiped dry before needle insertion so as to prevent chemical meningitis and contact dermatitis. The area cleaned should be sufficient to perform a mapping/scout scan and for a better view of the anatomy.
- A multimodal approach to pain management is encouraged, especially if the block covers only a few aspects of pain, e.g. the transversus abdominis plane block is useful for somatic pain, not visceral pain.
- Hydro-dissection technique with saline to identify the final target location can be used to prevent reaching the toxic dose in the paediatric age group.
- In-plane approach with continuous tip visualisation is encouraged to mitigate nerve injury.
- Strict adherence to dosing guidelines and the use of ultrasonography is recommended.
- Ideal body weight is used for the calculation of the maximal allowable dose of local anaesthetic **(Table 1)**.
- Toxicities of different local anaesthetic drugs are additive. A different local anaesthetic should not be used if a maximal dose of one local anaesthetic

**TABLE 1:** Maximal allowable dose of local anaesthetic.

| *Local anaesthetic* | *Maximum allowable dose* |
|---|---|
| Bupivacaine/levobupivacaine without epinephrine | 2.5 mg/kg |
| Lidocaine with epinephrine | 7 mg/kg |
| Lidocaine | 5 mg/kg |

has already been used. Alternatively, if two local anaesthetics are to be mixed in equal volume, using only 50% of the maximum recommended dose of each local anaesthetic is important.

- Infants under 6 months of age require at least 30% reduction in the maximal dose due to increased free fractions and decreased elimination. On the other hand, a larger volume of distribution counteracts the increased potential for toxicity caused by the larger free non-protein bound fraction.
- The paediatric population has incomplete myelination at birth, and myelination can take 12 years to complete, thus allowing lower concentrations of local anaesthetic to be used.
- It should be remembered that the descending inhibitory pathways are immature, allowing unmodulated nociceptive inputs to the ascending spinal pathways, leading to greater pain experienced by this subset of the population.
- Immature liver function and high cardiac output make infants highly vulnerable to local anaesthetic toxicity.[10,11]
- In children, the general anaesthetic can mask neurological manifestation's and cardiac manifestations are noticed first or in conjunction with neurological signs. Treatment remains the same as for adults. Ideally, the least effective local anaesthetic concentration should be used so as not to mask the symptoms of compartment syndrome.[12]
- Various adjuvants are used in neuraxial and peripheral nerve blocks, prolonging the duration and decreasing the local anaesthetic drug dosages **(Table 2)**.[13]

The post-operative analgesia management should be clearly documented and verbally handed over to the ward staff and parents or caregivers. Rescue drugs for analgesia, an antiemetic, and the proposed time and date to stop the peripheral nerve catheter infusion should be well documented. When the peripheral nerve catheter infusion is stopped, the patient should be loaded with simple analgesics to ease the transition.

## COMMONLY PERFORMED PERIPHERAL NERVE BLOCKS

As stated, all the blocks that are given in an adult can be given in the paediatric age-group with due caution. The list of most performed blocks is given in **Table 3**.

**TABLE 2:** Commonly used additives and recommended doses in paediatric regional anaesthesia.

| *Additive (route of administration)* | *Mechanism of action* | *Recommended doses* | *Maximum doses* | *Side effects* |
|---|---|---|---|---|
| *Morphine (epidural)* | Local action on the spinal cord | 30 μg/kg | 50 μg/kg | Nausea, vomiting, respiratory depression |
| *Morphine (intrathecal)* | Local action on the spinal cord | 10 μg/kg | 20 μg/kg | |
| *Fentanyl (epidural)* | Local action on the spinal cord | 1–1.5 μg/kg | 2.5 μg/kg | |
| *Fentanyl (intrathecal)* | Local action on the spinal cord | 0.2 μg/kg | 25 μg/kg | |
| *Clonidine (epidural or along peripheral nerves)* | α-2 agonist | 1–1.5 μg/kg | 2 μg/kg | Sedation, bradycardia, hypotension |
| *Ketamine (epidural or occasionally along peripheral nerves)* | NMDA antagonist | 0.5 mg/kg | 1 mg/kg | Sedation, odd behaviour, agitation or restlessness |

(NMDA: N-methyl-D-aspartate)

**TABLE 3:** Commonly performed blocks in children.

| *Name of the block* | *Indications* | *Dose* | *Remarks* |
|---|---|---|---|
| *Head and neck blocks* | | | |
| Supraorbital/ supratrochlear nerve block | Frontal craniotomies, excision of abscess | 1–2 ml 0.25% bupivacaine with 1:200,000 epinephrine | Analgesia and anaesthesia |
| Maxillary nerve block | Cleft lip surgery, nasal septal repair, and endoscopic sinus surgery | 1–2 ml 0.25% bupivacaine with 1:200,000 epinephrine | Analgesia and anaesthesia |
| Mandibular nerve block/mental nerve block (most commonly blocked) | | 1–2 ml 0.25–0.5% bupivacaine with 1:200,000 epinephrine | Analgesia and anaesthesia |
| Greater occipital nerve block | Posterior fossa craniotomies, chronic occipital neuralgia | 1.5–2 ml 0.25–0.5% bupivacaine with 1:200,000 epinephrine | Analgesia and anaesthesia |

*Contd...*

*Contd...*

| *Name of the block* | *Indications* | *Dose* | *Remarks* |
|---|---|---|---|
| Superficial cervical plexus block | Tympanomastoid surgery, otoplasty, thyroid surgery, procedures on anterior portion of the neck, cochlear implant | 1–3 ml of 0.25–0.5% bupivacaine with epinephrine 1:200,000 | Analgesia and anaesthesia |
| Arnold nerve block (auricular branch of vagus) | Myringotomy | 0.5–1 ml of 0.25% bupivacaine with epinephrine 1:200,000 | Analgesia |
| *Upper limb blocks* | | | |
| *Interscalene block* | Shoulder and proximal arm surgery | 0.3–0.5 ml/kg | *Limited use* |
| Supraclavicular block | Surgery below the shoulder and deltoid, such as in the hand, forearm, elbow or arm | 0.3–0.5 ml/kg* | • Always use Doppler to identify potentially dangerous vessels in the proposed needle trajectory. Peripheral catheter can easily be fixed<br>• Analgesia and anaesthesia |
| Infraclavicular block | Surgery below the shoulder and deltoid, such as in the hand, forearm, elbow or arm | Same as above | • Applied if C/I to supraclavicular approach. Peripheral catheter can easily be fixed<br>• Analgesia and anaesthesia |
| Axillary nerve block | Elbow, forearm surgery | Same as above | • Transarterial approach not recommended. 40–50% chance of missing the musculocutaneous nerve with this approach<br>• Analgesia and anaesthesia |
| Wrist block (radial, median and ulnar) | Surgical procedures on the hand or fingers | 0.1–0.3 ml/kg* | Absence of motor block, tourniquet pain not mitigated |

*Contd...*

*Contd...*

| *Name of the block* | *Indications* | *Dose* | *Remarks* |
|---|---|---|---|
| *Lower limb blocks* | | | |
| Lumbar plexus | Surgeries of the hip, proximal femur and anterior thigh | 0.5 ml/kg* | • Chances of intrathecal/ epidural spread, hypotension, and iliopsoas or renal haematoma<br>• Use dual guidance (USG + PNS) |
| Femoral | Femur fracture<br>Slipped capital femoral epiphysis | 0.2–0.4 ml/kg* | Analgesia and anaesthesia |
| Fascia illaca | Femur fracture<br>Slipped capital femoral epiphysis | 0.5 ml/kg* | Mainly used for analgesia |
| Adductor canal | Knee arthroplasty/ arthroscopy<br>Saphenous vein stripping or harvesting<br>Medial foot or ankle surgery | 0.5 ml/kg* | Analgesia |
| Sciatic nerve block | Tendon transfers/ lengthening | 0.3–0.5 ml/kg* | Analgesia and anaesthesia |
| Ankle | Syndactyly surgery | 0.1–0.2 ml/kg* | Analgesia and anaesthesia |
| *Truncal blocks* | | | |
| Transversus abdominis plane (TAP) block (unilateral/ bilateral) | Abdominal surgeries | 0.2–0.3 ml/kg* | Analgesia |
| Rectus sheath block | Midline incisions, umbilical hernia repair | 0.2 ml/kg* | Analgesia |
| *Other peripheral nerve blocks* | | | |
| Penile block | Circumcision | 0.1 ml/kg | Analgesia |

*0.25%/0.5% bupivacaine/levobupivacaine or 0.2%/0.5% ropivacaine
(C/I: contraindication; PNS: peripheral nerve stimulator; USG: ultrasonography)

## NEWER NERVE BLOCKS

### Pectoral Nerve Blocks

#### *Introduction*

Pectoral nerve blocks (PECS) are ultrasound-guided superficial thoracic wall blocks first described by Blanco in 2012.[14] PECS cover the following nerves—lateral pectoral, medial pectoral, long thoracic nerve, thoracodorsal nerve, intercostal nerves and intercostobrachial nerve.

#### *Indications*

PECS I and II are widely used for analgesia after various surgeries involving the anterior thorax like breast surgeries, axillary dissection, anterior thoracotomies, pacemaker implantation, anterior shoulder surgery, tumour resection, rib fracture and minimally invasive cardiothoracic surgery.[15]

#### *Technique*

The patient is kept supine with the arm abducted 90° or kept by his/her side. Under all aseptic precautions, a linear high-frequency ultrasound probe is placed under the clavicle in the midclavicular line with an inferolateral angulation. The axillary vessels, 2nd rib, pectoralis major and minor muscles are identified. While moving inferolaterally towards the axilla, the 3rd and 4th ribs and serratus anterior muscle are identified below the pectoralis minor.

For the PEC I, the needle is inserted in an in-plane technique from medial to lateral direction in an oblique manner until the tip enters the plane between the pectoralis major and minor muscles between the 3rd and 4th ribs and the drug is deposited. For PEC II, the needle is then advanced into the plane between the pectoralis minor and serratus muscles between the 3rd and 4th ribs depositing drug there **(Figs. 1 and 2)**. Bupivacaine 0.25–0.5 mg/kg or ropivacaine 0.2–0.3 mg/kg, based on weight and age of the child can be used as the local anaesthetic.

#### *Important Considerations*

Although rare, pneumothorax can occur due to improper needle placement. Proper ultrasound guidance to visualise the needle tip and the use of normal saline spread to identify the needle tip can avoid pneumothorax.

### Modified Thoracoabdominal Paravertebral Block

Modified thoracoabdominal paravertebral (M-TAPA) block is an interfascial plane block used to provide analgesia for anterior and lateral thoracoabdominal wall surgeries.[16] In M-TAPA, the local anaesthetic is administered just below the costal cartilage, deep to the origin of the

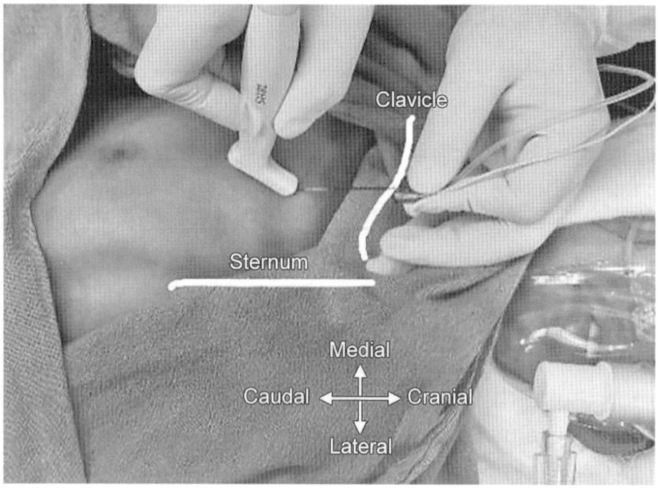


**Fig. 1:** Patient image and needle position for PEC block. (PEC: pectoral nerve) *(For color version, see Plate 3)*

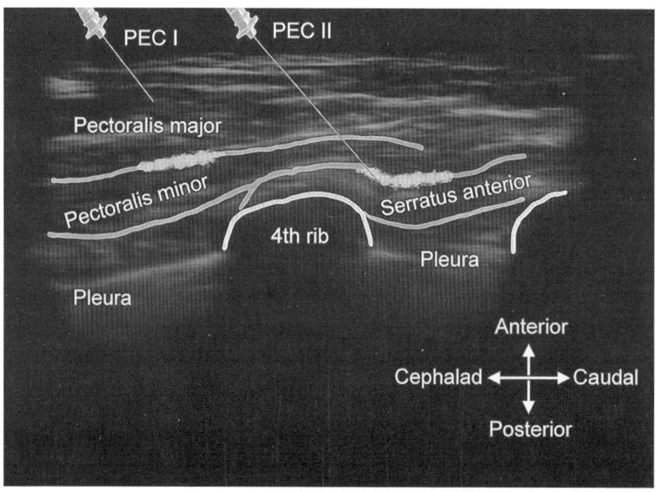


**Fig. 2:** Ultrasound image of PEC block. *(For color version, see Plate 3)*

transversus abdominis muscle. The anterior and lateral cutaneous branches of the T5–T12/L1 thoracoabdominal nerves are blocked.

## *Indications*

Modified thoracoabdominal paravertebral block can used for post-operative analgesia in several abdominal procedures, such as ventral hernia repair, laparoscopic appendectomy and laparoscopic cholecystectomy.

## *Technique*

The patient is positioned supine or in a lateral decubitus position, depending on the site of surgery and the anaesthetist's preference. A high-frequency linear

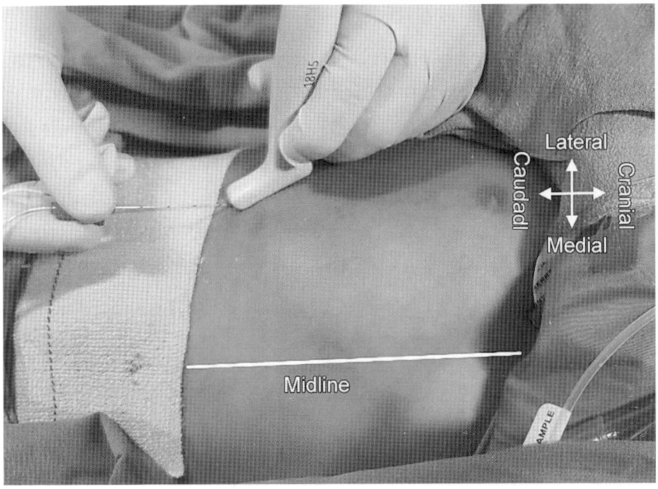


**Fig. 3:** Patient image and needle position for M-TAPA block. (M-TAPA: modified thoracoabdominal paravertebral) *(For color version, see Plate 4)*

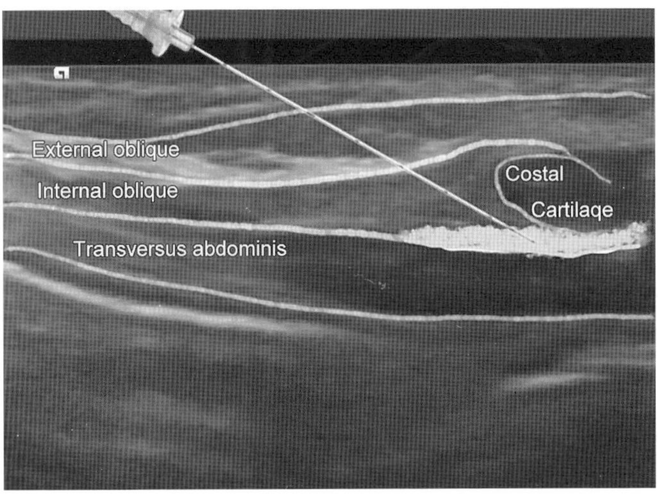


**Fig. 4:** Ultrasound image of M-TAPA block. *(For color version, see Plate 4)*

ultrasound probe is placed in the sagittal plane at the 10th costal margin, and the external oblique, internal oblique and transversus abdominis muscles are identified from superficial to deep orientation. In the midclavicular line at the level of the 10th rib (arcus costarum), a needle is inserted in-plane and the drug is deposited between the upper fascia of the transversus abdominis muscle and the lower fascia of the costochondral tissue **(Figs. 3 and 4)**. 0.25% bupivacaine 0.25–0.5 ml/kg (with a maximum dose of 2–3 mg/kg) or 0.2–0.5 mg/kg ropivacaine with a maximum total dose of 3 mg/kg can be used. Adjuvants can be added to prolong the analgesic effect.

## Quadratus Lumborum Block

The quadratus lumborum block (QLB), first described by Blanco in 2007, is a fascial plane block used for somatic and visceral analgesia during abdominal surgeries. This technique targets the posterior abdominal wall's quadratus lumborum (QL) muscle.[17] It has been increasingly used in paediatric patients for its potential to provide effective analgesia in the abdominal and pelvic regions, as well as during and after surgery. The local anaesthetic drug is deposited in and adjacent to the QL muscle to anaesthetise the thoracolumbar nerves (T6-L3).

### *Indications*

QLB is indicated for various paediatric surgeries that require post-operative abdominal or pelvic pain management. Some common indications include:

- Abdominal surgeries such as herniorrhaphy, appendectomy, abdominal laparotomy and ileostomy
- Urologic surgeries such as pyeloplasty, nephrectomy and orchiopexy
- Pelvic surgeries, including hip surgeries and certain pelvic tumour resections
- Pain management after abdominal trauma

### *Technique*

The child is positioned lateral, prone or supine with lateral tilt. An appropriate probe, usually a low-frequency probe, is positioned transversely above the iliac crest. The rectus abdominis and three layers of the abdominal wall muscles are identified and traced posteriorly, and the deep fascia of the transversus abdominis and the thoracolumbar fascia are connected. The QL and latissimus dorsi muscles can be traced medially or posteriorly to the transversus abdominis. On medial advancement of the probe over the transverse process, the erector spinae muscle is visible posteriorly, and the psoas major muscle is seen anteriorly to the QL muscle. There are various approaches for QLB.

- *QL1 (lateral QL block/posterior transversus abdominis plane block):* The needle is inserted in-plane with anterior/lateral to posterior/medial direction, and the drug is deposited lateral to the QL muscle between the aponeuroses of internal oblique and transversus abdominis muscles.
- *QL2 (posterior QL block):* The needle is inserted in-plane with lateral/anterior to medial/posterior direction, and the drug is deposited posterior to the QL muscle inside the middle layer of the thoracolumbar fascia, between the QL and either the latissimus dorsi or erector spinae muscles.
- *QL3 (anterior/transmuscular/subcostal):* The needle is inserted in-plane in a posterior/medial to anterior/lateral direction through the QL muscle

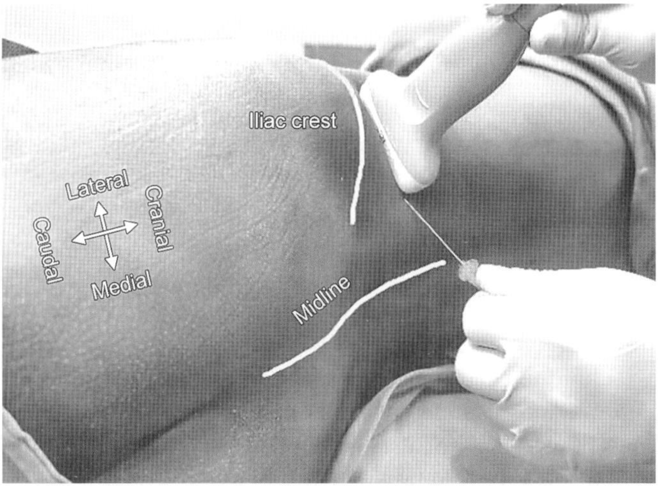


**Fig. 5:** Patient image and needle position for QL block. (QL: quadratus lumborum) *(For color version, see Plate 5)*

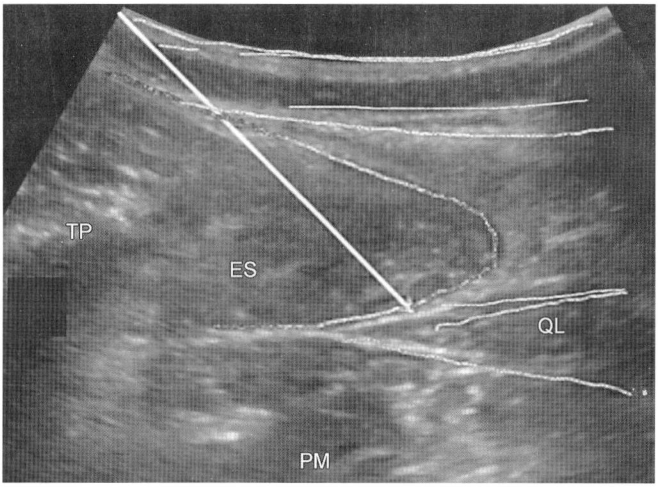


**Fig. 6:** Ultrasound image of QL block. (ES: erector spinae; PM: psoas major; QL: quadratus lumborum; TP: transverse process) *(For color version, see Plate 5)*

and the drug is deposited medial to the QL muscle, between the QL and psoas major muscles **(Figs. 5 and 6)**.

## *Drug Dosing*

Local anaesthetics used for QLB in paediatrics include bupivacaine, ropivacaine with or without adjuvants.

- Bupivacaine (0.25–0.5%) in a dose of 0.2–0.5 ml/kg, not exceeding a total of 2 mg/kg
- Ropivacaine (0.2–0.5%) in a dose of 0.2–0.5 ml/kg, not exceeding 3 mg/kg

### Important Considerations

- Lumbar plexus injury can occur during needle placement which can be avoided with careful needle tip placement.
- Bleeding and needle trauma of surrounding retroperitoneal structures (e.g. pleura, kidney, liver and spleen) are possible.
- Hypotension may occur due to spread of drugs into the paravertebral space causing sympathetic block.

### Erector Spinae Plane Block

The erector spinae plane block (ESPB), first described by Forero in 2016, is a novel technique used in both adult and paediatric patients.[18] Its use in children has not only been described for perioperative pain management for various types of surgeries but also in managing non-surgical pain. It involves injecting a local anaesthetic in the fascial plane deep to the erector spinae muscle.

### Indications

Pain management in thoracic and cardiac surgery, rib fractures, abdominal surgery such as inguinal hernia repair, nephrectomy, pyeloplasty, hip surgery, laparoscopic surgery, spine surgery, genitourinary surgery and chronic pain conditions.

### Technique

The patient is placed in the lateral, sitting or prone position. The block is performed at the thoracic (T5-T8) or lumbar (L2-L5) levels. An appropriate ultrasound probe is kept initially in the midline of the spine with a transverse orientation to visualise the spinous processes. The transverse process is located while moving the probe in the lateral direction. The various structures identified from superficial to deep are the trapezius, rhomboid, and erector spinae muscles and the transverse process of the respective vertebra. An out-of-plane approach can be used maintaining the probe in a transverse orientation, with the needle placed in a cranio-caudal or caudo-cranial direction. Otherwise, an in-plane approach can be used after a 90° rotation of the probe. After contacting the needle with the transverse process, the drug is deposited in a plane deep into the erector spinae muscle **(Figs. 7 and 8)**.[19]

Local anaesthetics such as bupivacaine (0.25% or 0.5%) in a dose of 0.5–1.0 ml/kg (maximum total dose of 2.5 mg/kg for a single shot), ropivacaine (0.2% or 0.5%) in a dose of 0.5–1.0 ml/kg (maximum total dose 3 mg/kg for single shot) and lidocaine (1% or 2%) in a dose of 0.5–1.0 ml/kg (maximum total dose 5 mg/kg for a single shot) can be used. The duration of action can be prolonged by adding adjuvants such as epinephrine, dexamethasone or clonidine.

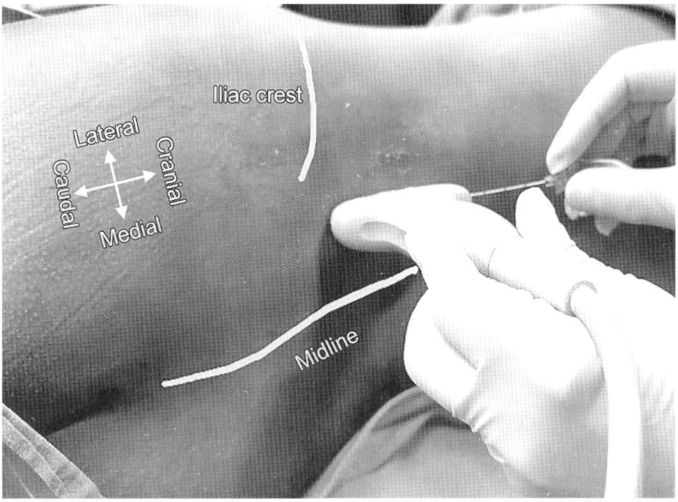


**Fig. 7:** Patient image and needle position for ESP block. (ESP: erector spinae plane) *(For color version, see Plate 6)*

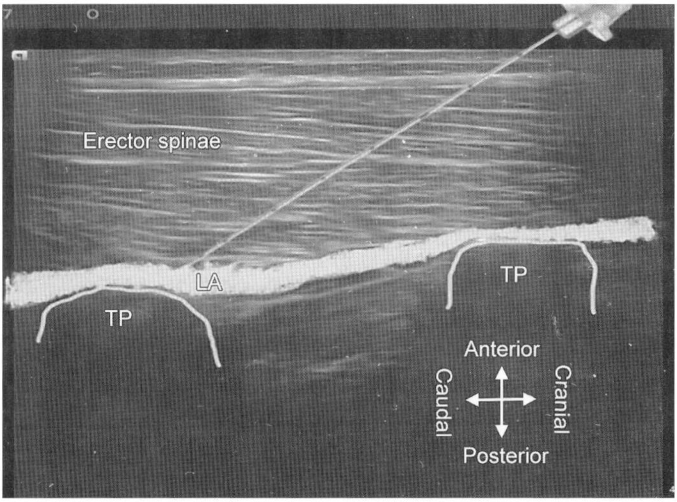


**Fig. 8:** Ultrasound image of ESP block. (ESP: erector spinae plane; LA: local anaesthetic; TP: transverse process) *(For color version, see Plate 6)*

## Sacral Erector Spinae Plane Block/Sacral Multifidus Plane Block

The sacral ESPB is an emerging regional anaesthesia technique for pain management in paediatric patients. It involves injecting local anaesthetic into the fascial plane below the erector spinae muscles at the sacral level. This block provides analgesia for lower abdominal, pelvic and lower limb surgeries.

## Indications

Post-operative analgesia in paediatric patients for perineal or perianal surgery such as hypospadias and chordee repair, circumcision, anoplasty, anal fistulectomy, pilonidal sinus excision, gender reassignment surgery, sacral teratoma excision and excision of the coccyx.

## Technique

It is administered by placing the ultrasound probe longitudinally at the body's midline, above the sacrum and targeting the 4th median crest. The median approach provides bilateral spread of the drug providing bilateral analgesia with a single injection.[20]

The child is placed in a prone or lateral decubitus position. A high-frequency linear ultrasound probe is placed longitudinally to visualise the sacral vertebrae in the midline and the overlying erector spinae muscle. A block needle is introduced in-plane from the cranial to the caudal direction towards the S3 level ultrasound probe, aiming to reach the plane between the erector spinae muscle and the sacrum **(Figs. 9 and 10)**.

*Sacral multifidus plane block* is a modification of the sacral ESPB where two separate injections are given between the sacrum and the erector spinae muscle, but in a parasagittal plane (given in the midline in sacral ESPB). A linear ultrasound probe is kept in the horizontal direction over the sacrum identifying the median crest in the midline while identifying two intermediate crests on either side of the midline. The centre of the probe is slid laterally to either of the intermediate sacral crests. The probe is then rotated 90° to a parasagittal plane. A block needle is introduced in-plane from the cranial to

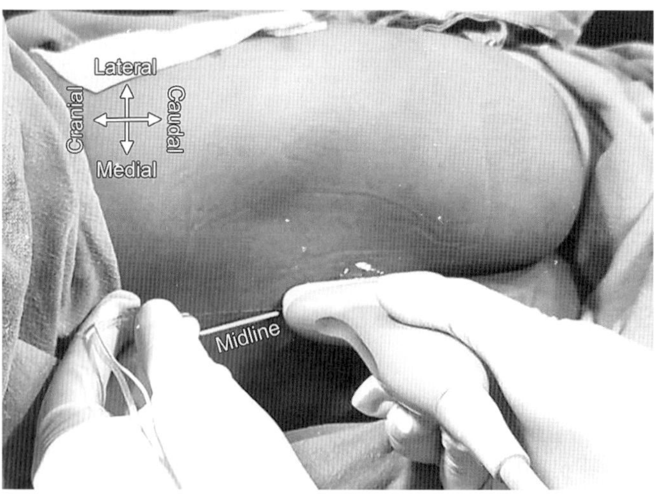


**Fig. 9:** Patient image and needle position for sacral erector spinae plane block.
*(For color version, see Plate 7)*

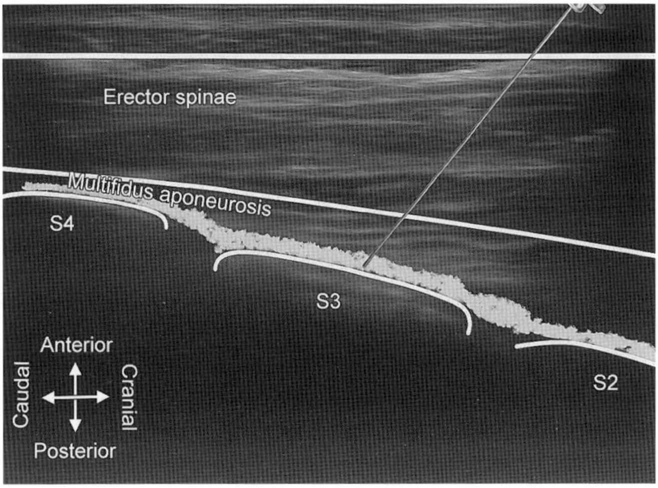


**Fig. 10:** Ultrasound image of sacral erector spinae plane block.
*(For color version, see Plate 7)*

the caudal direction, and the drug is deposited in the fascial plane between the erector spinae muscle and the sacral vertebra.

0.2–0.5 mg/kg of 0.25% bupivacaine with a maximum dose of around 2 mg/kg or 0.2–0.5 mg/kg of 0.2%/0.5% ropivacaine with a maximum total dose of 3 mg/kg can be used as the local anaesthetic. The duration of action can be prolonged with the addition of adjuvants like epinephrine.

## External Oblique Intercostal Fascial Plane Block

The external oblique intercostal fascial plane (EOIFP) block is a technique that targets the fascial plane between the external oblique muscle and the intercostal muscles which provide blockade of the lateral and anterior cutaneous branches of the intercostal nerves from T6/7 to T10/11.[21] This block is particularly useful in paediatric anaesthesia, as it provides excellent analgesia for upper abdominal and thoracoabdominal surgeries.

### *Indications*

- Anterolateral and upper abdominal surgeries
- Thoracoabdominal procedures, including rib fractures, chest tube placements and thoracotomies
- Post-operative pain management in upper abdominal and chest wall surgeries
- For analgesia after blunt abdominal or thoracic trauma

### *Technique*

The patient is placed supine with the ipsilateral arm in abduction. The linear probe is placed between the midclavicular and anterior axillary lines over

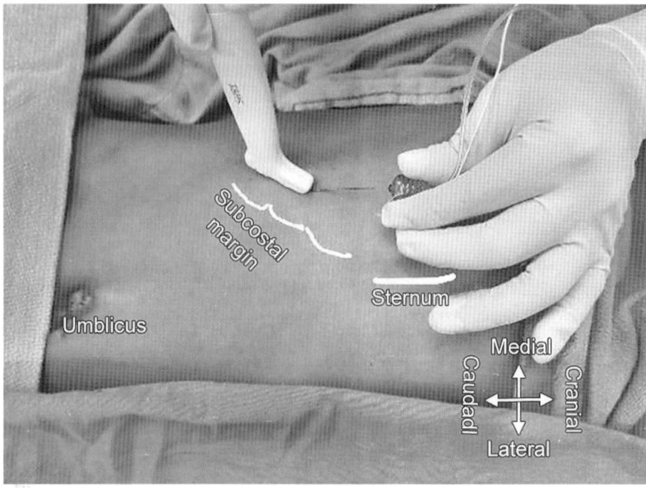


**Fig. 11:** Patient image and needle position for EOIFP block. (EOIFP: external oblique intercostal fascial plane) *(For color version, see Plate 8)*

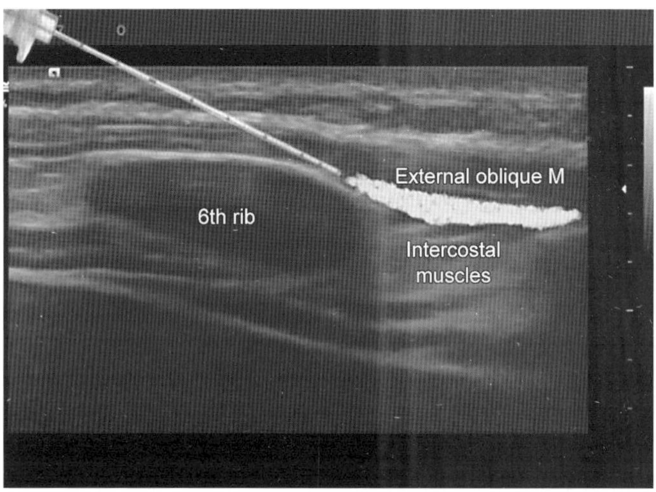


**Fig. 12:** Ultrasound image of EOIFP block. *(For color version, see Plate 8)*

the 6th rib in the paramedian sagittal plane. The cephalad end of the probe is slightly rotated towards the midline to view the ribs in the short axis. The anatomical structures identified from superficial to deep are the subcutaneous tissue, external oblique muscle, intercostal muscles, ribs, pleura and lungs. Under all aseptic precautions, a 5 cm echogenic needle is inserted using in-plane approach from the cranial end until the tip lies in the plane between the external oblique muscle and intercostal muscles between the 6th and 7th ribs and the drug is deposited in the plane in incremental doses, ensuring proper spread along the fascial plane **(Figs. 11 and 12)**. The volume injected is typically around 0.2–0.5 ml/kg, but this varies depending on the child's size and the surgery's nature. Local anaesthetics such as bupivacaine (0.25–0.5%) and ropivacaine (0.2–0.5%) can be used along with adjuvants such as clonidine (1–2 µg/kg) or dexamethasone (0.1 mg/kg) to prolong the block or enhance its analgesic effect.

## COMPLICATIONS OF NERVE BLOCKS

- *Intravascular injection and haematoma* can be avoided by ensuring accurate needle placement under ultrasonographic guidance.
- *LAST* can be avoided by proper dosing and avoiding intravascular injection. Drug dosing must be calculated based on the child's weight and age to minimise the risk of toxicity.
- *Infection* can be avoided using strict aseptic technique.
- *Insufficient block* can be supplemented with opioids or other regional anaesthesia techniques.
- *Nerve injury,* though rare, can occur due to incorrect needle placement or excessive pressure during injection.

Levobupivacaine and ropivacaine can be used as relatively safe alternatives to prevent complications of bupivacaine.

Continuous monitoring of vital signs during and after the procedure is essential to detect early signs of complications.

## PERIPHERAL NERVE CATHETERS—HOW TO ENHANCE THE SUCCESS RATE?

- A space can be created around the nerve to insert a catheter.
- Stimulating nerve catheters can be used for confirmation of position.
- Scanning should be done in all the planes feasible to locate and confirm the tip of catheter.
- The length of the catheter beyond the needle tip should not be >2–3 cm.
- It is important to check the catheter for any kinks prior to insertion, as this creates significant resistance. This can alter the infusion rates when elastomeric pumps are used.
- Leakage of the catheter especially at the insertion point should be avoided.
- Tunnelling or tissue glue should be used in order to prevent catheter dislodgement.
- The typical rate of infusion for 0.125% levobupivacaine or ropivacaine is set at 0.1–0.3 ml/kg/hour. For fascial plane blocks that require volume to work, a local anaesthetic bolus regime may be preferable to running an infusion.

## PAEDIATRIC CENTRAL NEURAXIAL BLOCK

Central neuraxial anaesthesia remains a valuable tool in the armamentarium of paediatric anaesthesia. Spinal and epidural blocks can be used as the primary anaesthetic or provide significant post-operative pain relief in addition to general anaesthesia. Caudal epidural anaesthesia is commonly used for lower abdominal, urological and orthopaedic procedures in outpatient surgeries. In addition, thoracic and lumbar epidural infusions (via catheter) can offer analgesia for chest and upper abdominal procedures. Spinal anaesthesia has been estimated to be at par with general anaesthesia in terms of neuro-developmental outcomes in infants, and there exists the benefit of intrathecal technique, particularly in cases of respiratory impairment.

## Anatomical and Physiological Considerations

There are several anatomical considerations for neuraxial anaesthesia in infants and children.

- There is less caudal angulation of the thoracic spinous process in infants.
- The conus medullaris will extend to L4 (premature infants) and L3 in a term neonate; nonetheless, by 1 year of age, it will be nearer its adult location of L1.
- To minimise the risk of spinal cord injury, dural puncture should be performed below the termination of the spinal cord—specifically, below the L2–L3 level in neonates and infants.
- The dural sac extends lower in premature infants and neonates (to around S4), and by the age of 2 years, it will develop to its adult location at S2.
- The absence of thoracic kyphosis in infants results in greater cephalad spread of injected drugs, outspreading the dermatomal coverage of a central neuraxial block
- The cerebrospinal fluid (CSF) volume of an infant (4 ml/kg) is twice that of an adult (2 ml/kg).
- Additionally, infants have a greater proportion of CSF in the spinal canal compared to adults. This distribution, along with higher cardiac output, contributes to increased local anaesthetic dose requirements and shorter spinal anaesthesia duration in infants and children.
- The vascularity of the pia mater, along with greater cardiac output, causes faster local anaesthetic reabsorption and, therefore, less block duration.
- The immaturity of the sympathetic autonomic nervous system in infants indicates that the sympathectomy of the central neuraxial block will not result in hypotension, vasoplegia, or cardiovascular instability as observed in adults.

## Spinal Anaesthesia

- Spinal anaesthesia can be used as the sole anaesthetic technique for providing anaesthesia, with this being a preferred option in preterm-born neonates.

**TABLE 4:** Local anaesthetic dosage for spinal block in infants/children.

| *Local anaesthetic (concentration)* | *Weight <5 kg* | *Weight 5–15 kg* | *Weight >15 kg* | *Duration (min)* |
|---|---|---|---|---|
| Bupivacaine (0.5%) | 0.1–0.12 ml/kg or 0.5–0.6 mg/kg | 0.08 ml/kg or 0.4 mg/kg | 0.06 ml/kg or 0.3 mg/kg | 80 min |
| Ropivacaine (0.2%) | 0.1–0.2 ml/kg or 0.5–1 mg/kg | 0.1 ml/kg or 0.5 mg/kg | 0.1 ml/kg or 0.3–0.4 ml/kg | 96 min |

- Used for inguinal, urological and lower limb surgery
- Spinal blocks with plain bupivacaine in neonates and infants will provide a 45–60 minutes duration of surgical anaesthesia.
- The duration of the block can be extended by the addition of an adjunct/combination with an epidural (caudal) injection of a local anaesthetic.
- Contraindications include localised infection, degenerative axonal diseases and suspected raised non-communicating intracranial pressure.
- Ultrasound can be useful while giving the block for depth and level estimation or to rule out abnormal low-lying cord.
- Local anaesthetic dosage for spinal block in infants/children is mentioned in **Table 4**.
- The recommended dosage regimens for fentanyl (0.2 μg/kg), clonidine (1 μg/kg) and adrenaline (2–4 μg/kg) have been shown to prolong spinal analgesia effectively when administered with bupivacaine.

## Equipment for Spinal Anaesthesia

Paediatric spinal needles (25 mm, 25 G) are preferred to adult needles due to the following reasons: lower dead space, smaller bevel profiles and better precision and accuracy when manipulated. Needle introducers used from hypodermic needles may carry the risk of epidermoid cyst within the spinal canal due to implantation of skin cells during needling. Lumbar puncture is performed at the L4/L5 or L5/S1 interspace, as identified by Tuffier's line or a pre-procedure ultrasound scan.

## Technique of Spinal Anaesthesia

- Fully flex the lumbar spine of the child, while keeping the head in neutral or slightly extended position where the airway is not secured.
- Sucrose on a pacifier may provide some sedation.
- Local anaesthesia (topical) may be placed at the intended puncture site before taking the child into the operating room to decrease pain at the time of needle insertion.
- Lateral decubitus positioning is typical; however, the sitting position is also described.

## Complications of Spinal Anaesthesia

- Total spinal anaesthesia
- Failed block
- Subcutaneous infection
- Epidural haematoma
- Post-dural puncture headache especially in dehydrated babies and in hot weather
- Backache
- Meningitis

## Epidural Anaesthesia

- Depth of the epidural space can be estimated in two ways. The 'rule of thumb' is that the distance from skin to lumbar epidural space in children weighing over 10 kg is 1 mm/kg. However, it is more accurately estimated by a pre-procedure ultrasonography.
- The epidural space contains less fibrous tissue and fluidic fat in children. Hence, threading catheters from the caudal space to higher levels is easier.
- Several methods are available for optimising catheter tip posting. These include electrocardiographic guidance, epidurography, nerve stimulation and ultrasonography. Data from the PRAN show that one or more of these are used in 47% of neonatal neuraxial catheters.
- To assess for intravascular injection, a test dose of 0.1 ml/kg (up to 3 ml) of local anaesthetic solution, such as 0.25% bupivacaine with 5 μg/ml of epinephrine is given. The response is considered positive if there is an increase in heart rate by >10 beats/min (may be blunted In infants and neonates, due to immature autonomic responses), an increase in systolic blood pressure by >15 mm Hg or a 25% change in T-wave amplitude. A false-positive test is anticipated if the child is in a very light plane of anaesthesia, or when there is any noxious stimulus like incision or airway manipulation.
- Loading with bupivacaine/ropivacaine at a dose of 1.5–2 mg/kg followed by an infusion (0.2 mg/kg/hour) is considered suitable for post-operative analgesia in abdominal surgeries.

## Caudal Block

- Caudal blocks are commonly used in paediatric regional anaesthesia with low failure and complication rates. The American Society of Regional Anesthesia and Pain Medicine (ASRA)/European Society of Regional Anaesthesia and Pain Therapy (ESRA) recommend ropivacaine (0.2%) or levobupivacaine/bupivacaine (0.25%), with volumes not exceeding 1 ml/kg body weight (maximum dose: ropivacaine 3 mg/kg, bupivacaine 2 mg/kg).

- The epidural space extends from the foramen magnum to the sacral hiatus and can be accessed through the sacrococcygeal ligament that covers the sacral hiatus.
- A needle or a catheter is passed through the sacrococcygeal ligament into the epidural space for injection of local anaesthetic drugs.
- Sacral anatomy in children and infants is unique, with an absent sacral pad of fat in this age group, and sacral ossification is not complete until 8 years of age.
- The classic Armitage regimen of caudal dosing: Bupivacaine 0.25% at 0.5 ml/kg for sacrolumbar block, 1 ml/kg for abdominal block, and 1.2 ml/kg for mid-thoracic block.

### Safety Considerations of Neuraxial Block

- A neuraxial blockade is generally indicated to expand post-operative analgesia and decrease the need of intravenous opioid requirement.
- Central neuraxial blockade in amalgamation with general anaesthesia has the potential to decrease anaesthetic requirements and opioid consumption, thereby, enhancing recovery and offering better post-operative pain control.
- There exists a higher risk of toxicity in children from local anaesthetics due to low plasma concentrations of α1-acid glycoprotein (AGP) and immaturity of the cytochrome (CYP) P450 system.
- A low AGP concentration in paediatric subset leads to a higher free fraction of (non-protein-bound) circulating local anaesthetics.
- CYP maturity occurs during the period of adolescence. Bupivacaine is metabolised through the *CYP3A4* subtype, reaching maximum clearance at the age of 1 year.
- Ropivacaine is metabolised by *CYP1A2* and may not attain maximum clearance before 6–8 years age.

## MYTHS, LIMITATIONS AND CONTROVERSIES IN PAEDIATRIC REGIONAL ANAESTHESIA

- It is a common misconception that infants do not feel pain. However, it is proved beyond doubt that children from 20 weeks in utero have fully developed pain pathways to feel pain, in fact, with a lower threshold, compared to older children and adults.
- Regional anaesthesia plays a crucial component in providing multimodal analgesia. Nevertheless, it is important to be aware that it is only one element of the various strategies for good pain relief, and over-reliance on regional anaesthesia should be avoided.
- As opposed to adult practice, it is imperative to emphasise that regional blocks should be conducted under general anaesthesia or deep sedation

in order to decrease the risk of post-operative neurologic symptoms in children of all ages.

- Though regional anaesthesia in paediatrics is relatively safe, and ultrasonography has revolutionised the way of performance of the blocks, ultrasonography-guided blocks do not always prevent complications. This depends on the competence of the anaesthetist and inherent limitations of ultrasonography (may lack the resolution to differentiate epineurium from perineurium, may encourage regular needle position adjustments to get to the target site and multiple injections aiming to cover the nerve circumferentially).[22]
- Caudal block is easy and reliable, but it has limitations such as short duration, anatomical variations, higher risk of complications, urinary retention, mobility issues and a failure rate.
- Non-verbal and cognitively impaired children may present unique challenges such as the inability to articulate symptoms of compartment syndrome, leg weakness after a caudal and difficulties in assessing pain scores and response to analgesia.
- Due to the diverse population, dosing errors are common in paediatric regional anaesthesia, and due to physiological reasons, they have a higher risk of toxicity from local anaesthetics.
- There is no clear consensus on the test dose, and the heart rate response to an adrenaline-containing test dose is non-specific, given that children have a higher baseline heart rate.
- It is important to administer local anaesthetic doses incrementally. An increase in T-wave amplitude is more reliable, and hence, vigilant attention to the electrocardiography trace during the injection is recommended.

## CONCLUSION

Regional anaesthesia in paediatrics has evolved significantly, offering numerous advantages such as improved pain control, reduced opioid consumption and faster recovery. It also becomes a key element of the enhanced recovery after surgery pathway. Advances in techniques, including ultrasound guidance and catheter-based approaches, have enhanced the safety and efficacy of regional blocks in children. However, meticulous patient selection, appropriate dosing and adherence to strict safety protocols remain paramount in preventing complications. Ongoing research, education and training, are essential to further refine these techniques and ensure optimal outcomes for paediatric patients. Anaesthetists can continue to improve the standard of care and provide safer and more effective regional anaesthesia for children by integrating evidence-based practices with technological advancements and adhering to best practices.

## REFERENCES


1. Derbyshire SW. "Fetal Pain: Do We Know Enough to Do the Right Thing?" Reprod Health Matters. 2008;16: 117-26.
2. Goksan S, Hartley C, Emery F. fMRI reveals neural activity overlap between adult and infant pain. eLife. 2015;4:06356.
3. Walker BJ, Long JB, Sathyamoorthy M. Complications in paediatric regional anesthesia: an analysis of more than 100,000 blocks from the paediatric regional Anesthesia network. Anesthesiology. 2018;129:721-32.
4. Neal JM. Ultrasound-guided regional anesthesia and patient safety: update of an evidence-based analysis. Reg Anesth Pain Med. 2016;41:195-204.
5. Lin JA, Blanco R, Shibata Y. Advances of techniques in deep regional blocks. Biomed Res Int. 2017:7268308.
6. Lin JA, Lu HT. A convenient alternative for monitoring opening pressure during multiple needle redirection. Br J Anaesth. 2014;112:771-2.
7. Mahrous RSS, Ahmed AAA, Ahmed AMM. Comparison between ultrasound-guided caudal analgesia versus peripheral nerve blocks for lower limb surgeries in pediatrics: A randomized controlled prospective study. Local Reg Anesth. 2022;15:77-86.
8. Hafeman M, Greenspan S, Rakhamimova E. Caudal block vs transversus abdominis plane block for pediatric surgery: a systematic review and meta-analysis. Front Pediatr. 2023;11:1173700.
9. Failla MD, Gerdes MB, Williams ZJ. Increased pain sensitivity and pain-related anxiety in individuals with autism. Pain Rep. 2020;5:e861.
10. Dontukurthy S, Tobias JD. Update on Local Anesthetic Toxicity, Prevention and Treatment During Regional Anesthesia in Infants and Children. J Pediatr Pharmacol Ther. 2021;26:445-54.
11. Bosenberg A. Benefits of regional anesthesia in children. Paediatr Anaesth. 2012;22:108.
12. Frawley G, Bell G, Disma N. Predictors of failure of awake regional anesthesia for neonatal hernia repair: data from the general anesthesia compared to spinal anesthesia study comparing apnea and neurodevelopmental outcomes. Anaesthesiology. 2015;123:55-65.
13. Suresh S, Ecoffey C, Bosenberg A, Lonnqvist PA, de Oliveira GS Jr, de Leon Casasola O, et al. The European Society of Regional Anaesthesia and Pain Therapy/American Society of Regional Anesthesia and Pain Medicine recommendations on local anaesthetics and adjuvants dosage in paediatric regional anesthesia. Reg Anesth Pain Med. 2018;43:211-6.
14. Blanco R. The 'pecs block': a novel technique for providing analgesia after breast surgery. Anaesthesia. 2011;66:847-48.
15. Elhaddad AM, Hefnawy SM, El-Aziz MA, Ebraheem MM, Mohamed AK. Pectoral nerve blocks for transvenous subpectoral pacemaker insertion in children: a randomized controlled study. Korean J Anesthesiol. 2023;76:424-32.
16. Erten E, Bahadir G, Kara U, Simsek F, Atasever HE, Kina SF, et al. Modified thoracoabdominal nerve block through perichondrial approach for laparoscopic appendectomy in children: a randomized trial. Signa Vitae. 2024:20;89-96.
17. Park I, Park JH, Shin HJ, Na HS, Koo BW, Ryu JH, et al. Postoperative analgesic effects of the quadratus lumborum block in pediatric patients: a systematic review and meta-analysis. Korean J Pain. 2024;37:59-72.

18. Forero M, Adhikary SD, Lopez H, Tsui C, Chin KJ. The erector spinae plane block: a novel analgesic technique in thoracic neuropathic pain. Reg Anesth Pain Med. 2016;41:621-7.
19. Lucente M, Ragonesi G, Sanguigni M, Sbaraglia F, Vergari A, Lamacchia R, et al. Erector spinae plane block in children: a narrative review. Korean J Anesthesiol. 2022;75:473-86.
20. Aksu C, Gürkan Y. Sacral erector spinae plane block with longitudinal midline approach: could it be the new era for pediatric postoperative analgesia? J Clin Anesth. 2019;59:38-9.
21. Elsharkawy H, Kolli S, Soliman LM. The external oblique intercostal block: anatomic evaluation and case series. Pain Med. 2021;22:2436-42.
22. Ivani G, Suresh S, Ecoffey C, Bosenberg A, Lonnqvist PA, Krane E, et al. The European Society of Regional Anaesthesia and Pain Therapy and the American Society of Regional Anesthesia and Pain Medicine Joint Committee Practice Advisory on controversial topics in pediatric regional anesthesia. Reg Anesth Pain Med. 2015;40:526-32.

CHAPTER 9

# Total Intravenous Anaesthesia in Paediatrics: Stay Informed on the Latest Techniques!

*Ekta Rai, HM Krishna, Dilip Chavan, Ina Smriti, Shikha Sharma*

## ABSTRACT

Total intravenous anaesthesia (TIVA) is emerging as a promising technique in paediatric anaesthesia, offering several advantages over traditional inhalational methods. Anaesthesiologists may precisely manage the degree of anaesthesia with TIVA with reduced risks of complications such as post-operative nausea and vomiting and a quicker and more seamless recovery. TIVA is recommended for children who have hypotonia, have a clinical risk of anaesthesia-induced rhabdomyolysis, or have a family history of malignant hyperthermia. Propofol, opioids, ketamine and dexmedetomidine are among the medications that can be used for TIVA in children. Knowing the impact of different age-groups on drug dosing helps in the maintenance of TIVA. A clear, methodical approach is required for safe medication administration procedures via TIVA/target-controlled infusion and these procedures should preferably be standardised. Real-time feedback is helpful in titrating TIVA infusions. The TIVA approach can be environment-friendly as it allows to avoid the impact of the harmful effects of anaesthetic gases, especially when used in paediatric patients.

***Keywords:*** Drugs, Infusion, Paediatric, Pharmacodynamics, Pharmacokinetics, Propofol, Total intravenous anaesthesia.

## INTRODUCTION

Imagine a small youngster, nervous about an imminent surgery, grasping a parent's hand. Traditionally, this child's trip into anaesthesia might have included a mask and the disturbing odour of anaesthetic gases—a frightening experience for even the bravest small ones. Consider a second situation in which that same child is carefully guided into a state of relaxation via a simple intravenous tube, eliminating the necessity for the scary mask. This is the promise of total intravenous anaesthesia (TIVA) in paediatrics, provided the intravenous catheter placement is not a traumatic experience. By delivering anaesthetic agents directly intravenously, TIVA eliminates the sensory overload often accompanying inhalational methods. TIVA is leaping forward in the world of paediatric anaesthesia, though in the current scenario, <10% of paediatric anaesthesiologists are using TIVA in their regular practice.[1] It is emerging as a promising technique in paediatric anaesthesia, offering several advantages over traditional inhalation methods.

The concept of TIVA in general anaesthesia began in adult patients following advancements in intravenous anaesthetic drugs in the 1970s to 1980s. However, its application in paediatrics was limited due to lack of suitable drugs and concerns about safety and efficacy. The introduction of propofol, a short-acting hypnotic agent in 1989, revolutionised TIVA. Propofol's rapid onset and quick recovery profile made it suitable for use both in adults and children. This period marked the beginning of the more widespread use of TIVA in paediatric anaesthesia. With improvements in monitoring technology, such as pulse oximetry, capnography and electroencephalogram (EEG)-based depth of anaesthesia monitors, anaesthesiologists could better manage the administration of TIVA in children. Additionally, the development of more precise infusion pumps allowed for a safer and more controlled delivery of intravenous anaesthetics.

Research in paediatric anaesthesia expanded, leading to more studies validating the safety and efficacy of TIVA in children. Anaesthetic techniques were refined, and protocols were developed specifically for paediatric patients, making TIVA a more common practice in this population.

In the modern era, the use of TIVA in paediatric patients has become routine in high-resource settings. New drugs and combinations, as well as adjuncts, have been introduced to improve outcomes and minimise side effects. The focus has also been on tailoring anaesthesia to individual patient needs, enhancing recovery and reducing the risk of post-operative complications.

The benefits of TIVA extend far beyond comfort. This approach provides anaesthesiologists with precise control over the depth of anaesthesia, significantly reducing the risk of post-operative nausea and vomiting (PONV) and facilitating a quicker, smoother recovery. This allows children to resume their activities early. For parents and caregivers, the assurance of a safer, more predictable anaesthetic course is invaluable.

TIVA is used in paediatric anaesthesia for a variety of reasons, providing specific advantages in certain clinical scenarios; however, there are certain situations where its use may be contraindicated.

## INDICATIONS FOR TOTAL INTRAVENOUS ANAESTHESIA

TIVA is indicated for physiological and clinical reasons. It is commonly applied to prevent various complications related to general anaesthesia.

*Physiological indications:* Children with asthma or other respiratory diseases benefit from TIVA because it avoids airway irritation by the use of inhalational agents and thus reduces the incidence of respiratory complications.[2,3] Children posted for neurosurgical surgeries benefit from TIVA due to its ability to reduce intracranial pressure more effectively than inhalational agents, providing a better operating environment for the surgeon. Stable haemodynamics, quick and clear-headed recovery with reduced PONV are the basic requirements for ambulatory anaesthesia. TIVA is the established way to provide anaesthesia for open airway surgeries in or around the airway (e.g. rhino-otolaryngological procedures) by obtunding airway reflexes and thus minimising the complications after extubation.

*Indications for reducing clinical complications:* TIVA is indicated for children with a family history of malignant hyperthermia, clinical risk of anaesthesia-induced rhabdomyolysis and in floppy children. These conditions are potentially life-threatening due to exposure to the triggering agents. TIVA is associated with a reduced incidence of PONV and is often preferred for children who are at high risk for PONV. TIVA provides a safe alternative to children with known allergies or adverse reactions to inhalational anaesthetics.

## CHALLENGES IN TOTAL INTRAVENOUS ANAESTHESIA

The absence of the necessary infusion pumps and monitoring equipment is one of the main reasons for the reserved usage of TIVA. In children with a fear of face masks, a serious fear of establishing intravenous access and poor or difficult venous access, the establishment and maintainence of an intravenous line can be challenging, making TIVA less feasible as an induction technique but still a maintenance option once the access is established. TIVA is not indicated if the child has known allergies or hypersensitivity to the medications commonly used in TIVA, such as propofol, and alternatives should be considered. Children with specific metabolic disorders, such as mitochondrial diseases, may have adverse reactions to certain intravenous anaesthetics like propofol. These conditions require careful consideration and potentially alternative anaesthetic strategies.

Cautious use is demanded in patients with severe cardiovascular instability. Most of the above alerts demand cautious use except for patient refusal, allergy to the medications, absence of the specific equipment and lack of monitoring required to check the depth of anaesthesia.

## PHARMACOLOGY OF COMMONLY USED DRUGS IN TOTAL INTRAVENOUS ANAESTHESIA

The drugs that can be used for TIVA in paediatrics are propofol, opioids (remifentanil, alfentanil and sufentanil), ketamine, dexmedetomidine and midazolam. An ideal drug for TIVA has the following characteristics: rapid onset of action, rapid recovery, potent, lipid-soluble, stable in solution, no tissue sloughing if extravasated, no/minimal adverse effects, cost-effectiveness and compatibility with agents it is likely to be mixed with.[4] Only propofol and remifentanil are widely used in paediatric target-controlled infusion (TCI). The salient features of the drugs used in paediatric TIVA are given in **Table 1**.

**TABLE 1:** Drugs used in total intravenous anaesthesia.[4,5]

| *Drug* | *Characteristic features* | *Dose* |
|---|---|---|
| *Propofol* | Quick onset and offset. Target plasma concentration is 3–4 μg/ml. The context-sensitive half-life in children is longer than in adults; 10.4 vs. 6.7 minutes after 1 hour infusion, 19.6 vs. 9.5 minutes after 4 hours infusion. | Bolus 1–2.5 mg/kg Infusion 13-11-9 mg/kg/h (10 min-10 min-subsequently) or 15-13-11-10-9 mg/kg/h (for 15 minutes, 15 minutes, 30–60 minutes, 1–2 hours and 2–4 hours |
| *Remifentanil* | Ultra-fast-acting opioid, rapid effect-site equilibration, fast onset/offset, short context-sensitive half-life of 2–3 minutes. Reduces propofol requirement by 40%. Children <8 years are less sensitive to its effects and may require higher doses. | • Bolus 0.5–1 μg/kg<br>• Infusion 0.1–0.5 μg/kg/min |
| *Alfentanil* | Fast onset. Context-sensitive half-life 10–45 minutes after 2 hours infusion Target concentration 90–120 ng/ml | • Bolus 10–50 μg/kg<br>• Infusion 1–5 μg/kg/min |
| *Sufentanil* | Highly potent, rapid onset and longer duration, and minimal histamine release | • Bolus 1–5 μg/kg<br>• Infusion 0.01–0.05 μg/kg/min<br>• 1/10th this dose for sedation |
| *Fentanyl* | Not suitable due to its relatively long CSHT | • Bolus 1–5 μg/kg<br>• Infusion 0.1–0.2 μg/kg/min |
| *Ketamine* | Advantages are less respiratory depression, bronchodilation, good analgesia, maintains sympathetic tone, can be used as sole anaesthetic. Larger clearance and, thus, short CSHT for <2 hours of infusion makes it a good option for short duration surgery | • Bolus 1 mg/kg<br>• Infusion 0.1–2.5 mg/kg/h |
| *Dexmedetomidine* | Less respiratory depression, opioid-sparing effect. Long context-sensitive half-life (250 minutes after 8 hours infusion) | • *Loading dose:* 0.5–1 μg/kg over 10–20 minutes<br>• Infusion 0.2–0.5 μg/kg/h |
| *Lidocaine* | Reduces TIVA dose by 10–20% | • Bolus 1–1.5 mg/kg<br>• Infusion 1.5 mg/kg/h |
| *Magnesium sulphate* | Reduces TIVA dose | • Bolus 30–50 mg/kg<br>• Infusion 10 mg/kg/h |
| *Midazolam* | May delay recovery especially in neonates, infants and critically sick patients. | • Bolus 0.1 mg/kg<br>• Infusion 0.1–0.3 mg/kg/h |

*Important note:* Neuromuscular blocking drugs *do not* reduce requirements of propofol, and their use can risk awareness if precautions are not taken.
(CSHT: context-sensitive half-time; h: hour; TIVA: total intravenous anaesthesia)

## Pharmacodynamics and Pharmacokinetics

The three-compartment model is described to understand TIVA. After administration of a drug intravenously, the drug distributes throughout the circulation, also binding to the proteins and lipids depending on its protein binding characteristics and lipid solubility **(Fig. 1)**. The volume of distribution in this compartment is V1 (central compartment or initial volume of distribution) and the concentration achieved is C1. Next, there is the distribution of this drug to the vessel-rich group like liver, abdominal viscera and muscles which is also called peripheral or rapid compartment. This volume of distribution is denoted as V2 and the concentration achieved is C2. Subsequently, the distribution of the drug happens to the scarcely perfused issues like the adipose tissue. This is represented as V3, and the concentration is achieved as C3. This is a large compartment. The rate constants for elimination or redistribution are denoted as K10 (excretion), K12 (redistribution from compartment 1 to 2) and K13 (redistribution from compartment 1 to 3). Similarly, K21 and K31 represent the movement of the drug back to the central compartment. The movement of the drug across the compartments is determined by the concentration of the drug, perfusion of the tissues and other factors. Clearance is the volume of blood from which the drug is eliminated per unit of time. Prolongation of the elimination of the drug (clinically offset of action) occurs when the volume of distribution is high or clearance is reduced or both.[6,7]

The concept of context-sensitive half-time is very relevant for TIVA. When the drug infusion is stopped, the drug moves back from the peripheral compartments back into the central compartment. From the central compartment, the drug is then eliminated. The half-life or time of the decrease in drug concentration in the plasma is dependent on the duration of the infusion (duration of the infusion is the context on which the half-life depends). By definition, context-sensitive half-time is the time required for blood or plasma concentrations of a drug to decrease by 50% after discontinuation of drug administration. Remifentanil is an exception

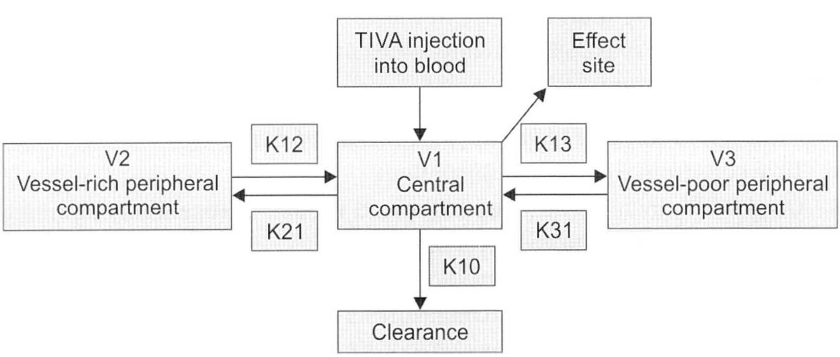


**Fig. 1:** Three-compartment model. (TIVA: total intravenous anaesthesia)

**TABLE 2:** Context-sensitive half-time of opioids in children.

| | *Context-sensitive half-time of named drug (minutes)* | | | |
|---|---|---|---|---|
| *Drugs infusion duration (minutes)* | *Remifentanil* | *Sufentanil* | *Alfentanil* | *Fentanyl* |
| 10 | 3–6 | 10 | 10 | 12 |
| 100 | 3–6 | 20 | 45 | 30 |
| 200 | 3–6 | 25 | 55 | 100 |
| 300 | 3–6 | 35 | 58 | 200 |
| 600 | 3–6 | 60 | 60 | — |

as its half-time becomes context-insensitive almost immediately after the initiation of the infusion because its elimination is rapid and complete. Drugs with low context-sensitive half-time are better suited for TIVA. The context-sensitive half-times of opioids in children are given in **Table 2**.

*Clinical relevance of context-sensitive half-lives:* The timing of stopping the infusion depends on the context-sensitive half-time. For most of the opioids other than remifentanil, with even short context-sensitive half-time, the infusions are stopped 30 minutes before the expected completion of the procedure.

The target-controlled infusion models or the manual infusion regimens replicate the principles of the bolus-elimination-transfer (BET) principle to adjust the infusion rate to maintain a steady estimated plasma concentration. Bolus dose aims to achieve the desired concentration in the central compartment and, hence at the effect-site quickly. This helps in achieving a steady state at the earliest (put to sleep fast; achieve analgesia fast).

The maintenance infusion is required to account for the equilibration/movement of the drug from the central compartment to the peripheral compartments as described in the three-compartment model. This infusion provides a continuous supply of the drug to the effect site and prevents a decrease in the concentration of the drug at the effect-site. Once the compartments get saturated with the drug, there is a need to reduce the rate of infusion to prevent an increase in the concentrations to excessive levels. Remifentanil achieves 75% of steady-state concentration after 5 minutes and 100% after 15–20 minutes.[8]

*Practical tips to consider regarding the infusion of drugs:*

- Take cues from the vitals of the patient.
- Do not blindly follow the mathematical model. Clinical judgement and manual interventions are necessary.
- Level of pre-operative anxiety, type and intensity of surgical stimulus, use of adjuvant drugs or regional anaesthesia must be considered.
- Drugs with long context-sensitive half-time are not suitable for TIVA.

The TCI models work on mathematical predictions aimed to achieve either a required plasma site concentration (Cp) or effect-site concentration (Ce). Usually, the difference between the estimated concentration by these models and the actual measured concentration is <25%. The user chooses the model and feeds in the patient's characteristics such as body weight, age and the concentration. Based on these inputs, the TCI pump determines the initial bolus dose and the subsequent infusion rates. The current paediatric models of TCI aim to achieve the required Cp. However, achieving the desired concentration at the effect-site is desirable. Since the Ce is not taken into account in paediatric models there would be a time lag between achieving the Cp and Ce.

Standard Cp values at steady state for propofol are as follows: propofol used alone—4–6 μg/ml, propofol with adjuncts (like regional anaesthesia or remifentanil)—3–4 μg/ml.

A combination of propofol and remifentanil in the same syringe (like 2.5, 5 and 10 μg remifentanil per ml of propofol) is often used by clinicians for TCI but is not widely recommended especially for patients under 10 kg. Though the drugs are combined, the TCI pump follows the pharmacokinetic (PK) model for propofol. So, remifentanil delivery would not be target-controlled.[9] Manual infusions are an alternative to TCI. The bolus dose and the infusion rates are set and adjusted by the user. There is no integrated PK model in the pump that adjusts the infusion rates automatically to achieve the desired Cp or Ce. **Table 1** gives details of some manual infusion schemes used in practice.[10]

*Clinical implications:* Various factors such as pre-operative anxiety, the desired depth of anaesthesia for the specific surgical stimulus, the use of adjuvants or regional blocks and individual variability between children and organ dysfunction and maturation affect the requirements while using the TIVA models, such as McFarlan TIVA model[10] (for 3–11 year old children) and Steur model[11] (<3 year-old children).

### *Dosages for Individual Drugs*

*Tips to consider:* Serum levels of the drugs used in TCI are not measured during TIVA. They are the estimated targets for the particular PK model being used in the pump. Processed EEG can be used as a guide for TIVA in children. It is strongly recommended when neuromuscular blocking drugs are being used with TIVA. However, EEG monitoring has limitations in the neonatal age group.

## Differences in the Pharmacodynamics and Pharmacokinetics of the Drugs in Paediatric Population

Based on the physiological differences as well as the differences in the PKs of various drugs, the paediatric age can be classified into three periods.[9]

In the neonatal age group, the hepatic enzymes are immature, leading to slowing down of the drug metabolism. This means that they need lower infusion rates in TIVA as compared to adults or older children. The PK variability is also higher in this age group. The changes in volume of distribution and clearance in this age group are non-linear accounting for the PK variability.

The second group is children (approximately the first 2–3 years of life). They have a larger central compartment and volume of distribution. This is greatest in infancy and decreases with age. Therefore, the requirement of a bolus dose of induction agent like propofol would be higher in this age group (to fill up the V1 and attain the required C1). The initial infusion rate also should be higher because the rate of clearance is higher, peaking at approximately 1 year of age. The context-sensitive half-life in children is longer than in adults (10.4 vs. 6.7 minutes after 1 hour of infusion of propofol and 19.6 vs. 9.5 minutes after 4 hours).[10]

The third group comprises children from about 3 years to puberty. In this group, the central compartment and the volumes of distribution are nearly twice that of adults and the clearance of the drugs is 50% higher. Elimination of drugs from the central compartment depends on hepatic glucuronidation and renal excretion.

Obese children need a special mention due to altered PKs. The dose calculations need to be based on lean body weight for induction of anaesthesia (for the initial bolus dose) and total body weight for maintenance infusion.[12-14]

Children need a larger bolus dose for induction and a higher initial maintenance rate. The maintenance rate needs to be reduced subsequently due to accumulation in the peripheral compartments. The context-sensitive half-life is more in children and hence, the infusion rates are tapered towards the end of long cases in order to avoid prolonged recovery times.

## Pharmacologic Interactions

The pharmacologic interactions include both pharmacodynamic and PK interactions.

*Pharmacodynamic interactions:* The effect-site concentration of amnesic agents required to produce unconsciousness is lower in the presence of opioids than when it is used in isolation. This reduction of amnesic agent improves the haemodynamic stability. In the study by Struys et al., remifentanil concentration of 4 ng/ml was found to reduce the Cp50 for loss of response to verbal command from 2.9 to 2.2 ng/mL.[4]

*Pharmacokinetic interactions:* Opioids increase the central volume (V1) and clearance of propofol. Propofol and midazolam inhibit the alfentanil metabolism by competing for the same cytochrome P450 enzyme isoform CYP3A4. High doses of propofol reduce the cardiac output and thus reduce the hepatic blood flow, which in turn leads to the reduction in the metabolism of propofol.[15]

*Practical tips to consider:* Pharmacodynamic interactions rather than PK interactions require a reduction in the target concentration of the drugs. It is important to be aware of the PK interactions, but in clinical doses, it does not ask for modification of the target concentrations.

## TARGET-CONTROLLED INFUSION

TIVA was initially administered to patients using a manual infusion regime. The first regimen used in adults was the '10-8-6 rule' from Bristol, United Kingdom, which is also known as the BET regime. This regime consists of a loading dose of propofol at 1 mg/kg, followed immediately by an infusion of 10 mg/kg/hour for 10 minutes, then 8 mg/kg/hour for the next 10 minutes, and finally, 6 mg/kg/hour thereafter.[16] Frequent adjustments in the drug infusion rate are necessary to maintain a constant plasma propofol concentration. Additionally, any desired increase in the target plasma propofol concentration requires the administration of a manual bolus and an increase in the infusion rate and a decrease in the target plasma propofol concentration necessitates temporarily stopping the infusion and reducing the rate.

Administering a manual infusion regimen presents several challenges. In surgery, when the need for different depths of anaesthesia and analgesia is required in response to different surgical stimulations, a rapid adjustment needs to be made in the infusion rates of the drugs. To address these issues, the TCI system was introduced.[17] TCI is a method of delivering anaesthetic drugs for TIVA to patients in a controlled manner. It refers to a system in which a drug is administered intravenously using a computer-controlled pump incorporated with a selected PK model to achieve a user-specified drug concentration within a particular body compartment or organ of interest. By incorporating PK models, the TCI systems can rapidly titrate the response as necessary and maintain steady concentrations during TIVA.

### Principles of Target-controlled Infusion and its Components

TCI is a drug-device combination. To understand its usage, we need to appreciate that it consists of a few components, namely an infusion device, drugs and relevant PK models.

- *Infusion device:* The TCI system consists of a user interface, a computer, a microprocessor and an infusion device. Using the age-appropriate PK models of opioids and anaesthetic drugs in the microprocessor, the computer models determine the drug dosage needed to reach and maintain a specific plasma concentration or effect-site concentration for anaesthesia in a patient.

- *Drugs:* Anaesthetic drugs that have been studied for use in the TCI system include propofol, remifentanil, sufentanil and alfentanil. The drugs have been discussed in detail under the subheading 'Drugs.'
- *Pharmacokinetic models:* A key concept in PK modelling for TCI is the three-compartment model, which accurately describes the behaviour of most anaesthetic drugs, and this has been discussed under PKs.

## Delivery of Drug via Target-controlled Infusion

To start the delivery of the drug from the machine to the patient, the clinician needs to set the target drug concentration and input the patient's details such as age, weight, and gender. The computer software then calculates the infusion rate required to achieve this target. The TCI system can automatically adjust the level of anaesthetic delivered into the bloodstream to achieve the target concentration rapidly. The rate of equilibration between the plasma and the effect-site depends on several factors. These include the factors that affect the drug's delivery to the effect-site (such as cardiac output and cerebral blood flow) and the drug's pharmacologic properties that determine how quickly it crosses the blood-brain barrier (lipid solubility and degree of ionisation).

Different age groups of patients exhibit distinct PK models for TIVA. These PK models are constructed based on plasma drug concentrations measured at various timepoints. Healthy children require relatively higher doses of intravenous agents per unit of body weight, and their maintenance infusion rates need to be higher than those adjusted for adult weight. This difference is due to variations in regional blood flow, body composition and body proportions between children and adults.

Accurate PK modelling plays a crucial role in the effective management of drug dosing regimens for patients receiving TIVA. The technology of TCI has evolved significantly and now TCI integrates multiple PK models and accommodates various drugs, enhancing anaesthetic management and marking a significant step towards precise and safe anaesthetic care, especially for children. Several commercial PK models for children are available, mainly the Kataria and Paedfusor models for propofol (uses age and weight as covariates). Paedfusor model can be used for those between 05–61 kg and 1–16 years of age, whereas Kataria can be used for those above 15 kg and between 3 and 16 years of age.[18] There are several differences between these two PK models **(Table 3)**.

Recently, the Eleveld PK model for propofol was introduced. It uses weight, age, post-menstrual age (PMA), height, gender, body mass index and presence/absence of concomitant anaesthetic drugs as covariates.[19] The Eleveld PK model demonstrates the compatibility of a single PK model across all age groups and hence can be labelled as 'one PK model for all.'

**TABLE 3:** Comparison of Kataria and Paedfusor PK model.

| *Demographic and PK parameters* | *Kataria model* | *Paedfusor model* |
|---|---|---|
| *Age* | 3–16 years | 1–16 years |
| *Weight* | 15–61 kg | 5–61 kg |
| *ke0* | 1.7/min | 0.8/min |
| *Vd* | 7.6 l | 9.2 l |
| *Clearance* | 0.74 l/min | 0.58 l/min |

(ke0: the blood effect-site equilibration rate constant; PK: pharmacokinetic; Vd: volume of distribution)

It can be used in patients as young as 27 weeks PMA up to elderly patients 88 years old with a weight range of 0.68–160 kg. The main benefit of a 'one PK model for all' model is not to perform better than other models, but instead to offer a solution for decreasing errors in model selection for clinicians who use a TCI pump. This advancement represents a significant step towards more precise and universally applicable anaesthetic management in diverse patient populations.

The Minto model is applied for remifentanil. It includes weight and height as the covariates and is applicable for children >12 years old and weighing >30 kg. In children younger than 12 years old and weighing <30 kg, the recommendation is to use mass rate infusion. This makes the use of Minto model less practical in the paediatric population.

## Mixifusors

Mixifusor is a technique of infusion of two or more drugs by mixing them in one syringe and infusing them through one infusion pump. It has come as an easy solution for limited resources and children as it significantly reduces extensions and dead spaces. There has been a trend of mixing propofol and remifentanil in paediatric anaesthesia. This practice is not favoured by the current guidelines due to the risk of layering of the drug, risk of drug errors, pharmacological incompatibility, bacterial contamination and legal implications.[20]

## TIVA and TCI: Ensuring Safe Delivery

Safe practices for the delivery of drugs by TIVA/TCI need a clear systematic approach and ideally should be standardised. The programming of the pump should be as per the drugs available. The infusion pumps must be calibrated regularly as per the guidelines of the manufacturers. The alarm limits should be set appropriately and is generally done by the company with the physician's input. The loading of a drug should be based on the weight and volume needed to be infused. Two-person checks will reduce medication-related errors. Understanding the details of the equipment minimises the error. While many infusions can perform weight-based dose calculations, the actual infusion rates should be checked before initiating the infusion. Appropriate dilution of drugs ensures accurate delivery as a very low-rate infusion like 0.5 ml/hour may not be reliable and consistent. Using drugs in lower dilution and ensuring a safe rate of infusion is safer than using very concentrated drugs requiring low infusion rates. Strict asepsis needs to be followed and change of the administration sets is recommended in prolonged infusions of propofol. Anti-reflux valves should be used to prevent the backflow of drugs in the intravenous line. The intravenous access and drug extensions should be visible and closer to the anaesthesiologists/physicians and must be inspected at regular intervals intraoperatively. Extensions with minimal possible dead space are preferred. In smaller children, intravenous access sites need to be carefully protected as the babies may be covered under the drapes to prevent hypothermia. Any obstruction (temporary or permanent) proximal to the intravenous access through which the infusion is running should be avoided. Non-invasive blood pressure cuff should not be applied on the same limb. Frequent misconnections leading to inefficient drug delivery have been reported in literature, leading to awareness during the procedures. To avoid this, all infusion lines should be visible and continuously monitored and checked every 15 minutes.[4] Once the need for infusion is over, one must flush the extension and intravenous access to avoid accidental administration of the residual drug in the ward or post-anaesthesia care unit.[21]

Overall safety related to TIVA and TCI can be enforced by structured TIVA training as a part of core anaesthesia training.

## MONITORING IN TOTAL INTRAVENOUS ANAESTHESIA

The real-time feedback towards the TIVA is very beneficial in titrating the infusion ensuring that neither excess nor less drug is administered as both can lead to complications such as haemodynamic instability and delayed awakening in higher than needed concentrations, whereas awareness is a possibility for less than required drugs.

This feedback can be in the form of vital signs, EEG waveforms and software-based numbers to assess the depth of anaesthesia. Currently, the feedback on the plasma or effect-site concentrations of the drug is completely based on the pharmacodynamic and PK model. There have been attempts to determine the correlation between expired levels of amnesic drug like propofol and EEG-based monitoring as well as propofol plasma concentrations calculated using paediatric PK models in paediatric anaesthesia.

- *Clinical parameters:* Clinical parameters like movements of the limbs and frowning can indicate the lack of adequate depth of anaesthesia. The movement can only be possible if the patient has not received muscle paralysis. Other clinical signs like sweating also can act as a guide for lack of adequate depth of anaesthesia. Clinical signs will not be able to guide in case of deeper than required plane of anaesthesia.

- *Haemodynamic parameters:* Changes in vital parameters are a good sensitive guide to the depth of anaesthesia but are not specific.
- *EEG-based feedback on the depth of anaesthesia:*[22] Processed electroencephalography (p-EEG) provides an independent system of depth of anaesthesia consistently and reliably in children >1 year of age. Bi-spectral index and entropy have been developed to improve the safety of anaesthesia under TIVA.
- *Expired drug levels:* This may be the future of the measurement of the depth of anaesthesia. There have been recent updates on the measurement techniques and some studies have attempted to establish the correlation between the expired propofol levels (exP), EEG-based depth of anaesthesia and plasma levels of propofol in patients on TIVA in adults. This measurement is based on multi-capillary column (MCC) combined with ion mobility spectrometry (IMS) system. The operating gas for the MCC-IMS is systematically processed from ambient air. The MCC-IMS estimates the exP with an accuracy of ±10% at 20 ppb.[23] Narcotrend index (NI) range of D0-E2 ensures correct depth of anaesthesia and the drugs are titrated to NI. However, the results of NI should be interpreted cautiously with the understanding of the limitations such as factors affecting the exP values. Nevertheless, this is an upcoming promising monitor for TIVA.

## TOTAL INTRAVENOUS ANAESTHESIA: LIMITATIONS

Understanding the limitations of TIVA will allow us to ensure its efficient and safe use. There are drug-related limitations, for example, propofol related side effects such as pain on injection, bacterial contamination on long-standing and propofol-related infusion syndrome (PRIS). The patient-related limitations include differences in the PKs and pharmacodynamics in children due to different profiles like obese children, children with liver or renal failure, difficulty level of cannulation, etc. The delivery-related limitations include long extensions with large dead space issues in the drug delivery systems. The depth of anaesthesia monitoring is financially demanding as it needs a separate set of dedicated equipment and thus awareness is a serious problem if TIVA is not practised as per guidelines. The favourable effect of TIVA on the environment is offset by the wastes generated, such as plastics.

### Propofol-related Infusion Syndrome

PRIS is a life-threatening condition which is usually seen in critically ill children receiving propofol either in high doses (0.5 mg/kg/hour) or for long duration (>48 hours) and it results in '*unexplained metabolic acidosis, rhabdomyolysis, or electrocardiographic (ECG) changes, with or without acute kidney injury (AKI), hyperkalaemia, lipidaemia, cardiac failure, fever, elevated liver enzymes or lactate*' leading to bradycardia and potential cardiac arrest. The most common clinical presentation is metabolic acidosis with ECG changes, with secondary features of lipidaemia, hyperkalaemia, AKI, fever, cardiac dysfunction, hepatomegaly with deranged transaminases and elevated lactate. The probable mechanism of action is direct mitochondrial respiratory chain inhibition, impaired fatty acid metabolism or interaction with the cytochrome system resulting in mitochondrial uncoupling. ECG findings for PRIS may show a Brugada-like pattern or ventricular or supraventricular tachycardia, or bradycardia in extreme conditions. The first step towards treatment is to stop the propofol infusion and initiate supportive management addressing the clinical features and monitor for the early warning signs. Ensuring adequate carbohydrate intake (68 mg/kg/min) and carnitine supplementation is important. Pacing in bradyarrhythmia, organ support such as haemodialysis for renal failure and extracorporeal membrane oxygenation for maintaining oxygenation is advised.

### Total Intravenous Anaesthesia: Environment Impact

TIVA eliminates the dangers of occupational exposure and harmful environmental effects related to volatile anaesthetic gases. It can be employed as an alternative to inhalational anaesthetics, although it is not without potential harmful environmental consequences.[24] Nonetheless, one must consider the overall environmental impact of TIVA, and agents such as propofol must be disposed off appropriately. TIVA in the paediatric population has a beneficial environmental impact because it has a lower carbon footprint than inhalational anaesthesia. The use of the TIVA technique, particularly in the paediatric patient group, can assist in protecting the environment from the detrimental effects of anaesthetic gases, ensuring a safe environment for future generations.[25]

## TOTAL INTRAVENOUS ANAESTHESIA: FUTURE TRENDS

- Addition of newer drugs such as remifentanil and ciprofol.[26]
- Newer monitors in the assessment of the depth of anaesthesia are being explored. The NI is under development.
- New models of TCI applicable to a wide range of age and weight are being developed. Investigation continues into the 'closed loop' systems where physiological data and p-EEG provide feedback directly to infusion pumps.[27]

## CONCLUSION

TIVA in children offers a safe and effective alternative to inhalational anaesthesia, providing advantages such as smooth emergence, less airway irritation and lower risk of PONV, while requiring the careful application of PKs and pharmacodynamics to ensure optimal outcomes.

## REFERENCES

1. Hill M, Peat W, Courtman S. A national survey of propofol infusion use by paediatric anaesthetists in Great Britain and Ireland. Paediatr Anaesth. 2008;18:488-93.
2. Lauder GR. Total intravenous anesthesia will supercede inhalational anesthesia in pediatric anesthetic practice. Paediatr Anaesth. 2015;25:52-64.
3. Von Ungern-Sternberg BS, Boda K, Chambers NA, Rebmann C, Johnson C, Sly PD, et al. Risk assessment for respiratory complications in paediatric anaesthesia: a prospective cohort study. Lancet. 2010;376:773-83.
4. Bajwa SJ, Vinayagam S, Shinde S, Dalal S, Vennel J, Nanda S. Recent advancements in total intravenous anaesthesia and anaesthetic pharmacology. Indian J Anaesth. 2023;67:56-62.
5. Struys MM, Vereecke H, Moerman A, Jensen EW, Verhaeghen D, Neve ND, et al. Ability of the bi-spectral index, autoregressive modelling with exogenous input-derived auditory evoked potentials, and predicted propofol concentrations to measure patient responsiveness during anesthesia with propofol and remifentanil. Anesthesiology. 2003;99(4):802-12.
6. Gaynor JBM, Ansermino JM. Paediatric total intravenous anaesthesia. BJA Educ. 2016;16(11):369-73.
7. Mogane P. Paediatric total intravenous anaesthesia and target-controlled infusion. South Afr J Anaesth Analg. 2022;28(5 Suppl 1):S55-60.
8. Nimmo AF, Absalom AR, Bagshaw O, Biswas A, Cook TM, Costello A, et al. Guidelines for the safe practice of total intravenous anaesthesia (TIVA). Anaesthesia. 2019;74:211-24.
9. Constant I, Rigouzzo A. Which model for propofol TCI in children? Paediatr Anaesth. 2010;20:233-9.
10. McFarlan CS, Anderson BJ, Short TG. The use of propofol infusions in paediatric anaesthesia: a practical guide. Paediatr Anaesth. 1999;9:209-16.
11. Steur RJ, Perez RS, DeLange JJ. Dosage scheme for propofol in children under 3 years of age. Paediatr Anaesth. 2004;14(6):462-7.
12. Mortensen A, Lenz K, Abildstrøm H, Lauritsen TLB. Anesthetizing the obese child. Paediatr Anaesth. 2011;21(6):623-9.
13. Diepstraten J, Chidambaran V, Sadhasivam S, Esslinger HR, Cox SL, Inge TH, et al. Propofol clearance in morbidly obese children and adolescents: influence of age and body size. Clin Pharmacokinet. 2012;51(8):543-51.
14. Cortinez LI, Anderson BJ, Penna A, Olivares L, Munoz HR, Holford NH, et al. Influence of obesity on propofol pharmacokinetics: derivation of a pharmacokinetic model. Br J Anaesth. 2010;105(4):448-56.
15. Roberts FL, Dixon J, Lewis GT, Tackley RM, Prys-Roberts C. Induction and maintenance of propofol anaesthesia. A manual infusion scheme. Anaesthesia. 1988;43 Suppl:14-7.
16. Struys MM, De Smet T, Glen JI, Vereecke HE, Absalom AR, Schnider TW. The history of target-controlled infusion. Anesth Analg. 2016;122:56-69.
17. Gepts E. Pharmacokinetic concepts for TCI anaesthesia. Anaesthesia. 1998;53(s1):4-12.

18. Hassan WMN, Mansor A, Zaini RHM. Anesthesia using target-controlled infusion of propofol during elective pediatric surgery: Kataria versus Paedfusor pharmacokinetic model. Anaesth Pain Intensive Care. 2018;22:207-11.
19. Eleveld DJ, Colin P, Absalom AR, Struys MMRF. Pharmacokinetic-pharmacodynamic model for propofol for broad application in anaesthesia and sedation. Br J Anaesth. 2018;120:942-95.
20. Absalom AR, Rigby-Jones AE, Rushton AR, Robert Sneyd J. De-mystifying the "Mixifusor". Paediatr Anaesth. 2020;30:1292-8.
21. Bowman S, Raghavan K, Walker IA. Residual anaesthesia drugs in intravenous lines—a silent threat? Anaesthesia. 2013;68(6):557-61.
22. Davidson AJ, Kwok T. Performance of BIS in children using the paediatric BIS Quattro sensor. Anaesth Intensive Care. 2008;36(6):807-13.
23. Heiderich S, Ghasemi T, Dennhardt N, Sümpelmann R, Rigterink V, Nickel K, et al. Correlation of exhaled propofol with Narcotrend index and calculated propofol plasma levels in children undergoing surgery under total intravenous anesthesia - an observational study. BMC Anesthesiol. 2021;21:161.
24. Varughese S, Ahmed R. Environmental and occupational considerations of anesthesia: A narrative review and update. Anesth Analg. 2021;133:826-35.
25. Koc S, Pecher S. New challenges for anesthesia due to the climate change. Anaesthesist. 2020;69:453-62.
26. Nair A, Seelam S. Ciprofol—A game-changing intravenous anaesthetic or another experimental drug. Saudi J Anaesth. 2022;16:258-9.
27. West N, Dumont GA, van Heusden K, Petersen CL, Khosravi S, Soltesz K, et al. Robust closed-loop control of induction and maintenance of propofol anesthesia in children. Paediatr Anaesth. 2013;23:712-9.

CHAPTER 10

# Role of Vasopressors and Inotropes in Critically Ill Infants: Know the Latest Developments to Provide the Best Care!

*Swati Daftary, Ranjith Karthekeyan, Ridhima Sharma, Varun Byrappa*


## ABSTRACT

Critically ill infants requiring vasopressors or inotropes, or both are in a state of shock, which can be best defined as a state of circulatory failure characterised by inadequate tissue perfusion to major organs. If not treated in good time, this can rapidly lead to multi-organ failure and death. Delays in vasopressor/inotrope administration in these critically ill infants are associated with an increased risk of mortality, especially in the first hour of treatment of septic shock.

Vasopressors are a powerful class of drugs that induce vasoconstriction and thereby an elevation in the mean arterial pressure (MAP). Vasopressors differ from inotropes, which increase cardiac contractility; however, many drugs have both vasopressor and inotropic effects. Most commonly used vasopressors and inotropes in infants are dopamine, dobutamine, epinephrine, norepinephrine, milrinone and levosimendan. A gestational age-based cutoff for 'normal' blood pressure goal, i.e. [MAP > gestational age], is used in many tertiary centres, especially in the first 3 days after birth. Dopamine is generally the first-line vasoactive drug. Epinephrine or norepinephrine infusions for refractory shock in neonates have been studied to a very limited extent. Refractory septic shock in paediatrics is demarcated as high blood lactate of >8 mmol/L with high vasoinotrope doses (Vasoactive inotrope score >200 µg/kg/min). Possibly revocable causes should be identified and treated in these children before considering extracorporeal support. Steroid supplementation is deemed important for maintaining sensitivity to catecholamines.

Clinicians mostly rely on vital signs and physical examinations to make decisions about therapy. Shortly after birth, an umbilical vein catheter can be used for resuscitation. The administration of vasopressors through peripheral lines until central access is achieved has been deemed safe. In the future, monitoring techniques such as functional echocardiography and near-infrared spectroscopy may provide physiologic data to optimise shock management.

In this chapter, we try to assess the role of vasopressors and inotropes in critically ill infants and learn about the latest developments to improve their outcomes.


***Keywords:*** Critical, Ill, Infants, Inotropes, Shock, Vasopressors.

## INTRODUCTION

Critically ill infants requiring vasopressors or inotropes, or both are in a state of shock, which can be best defined as a state of circulatory failure characterised by inadequate tissue perfusion to major organs. If not treated in good time, this can rapidly lead to multi-organ failure and death. Historically, the use of vasopressors and inotropes in neonates and infants was limited for fear of potential side effects as there was a lack of precise dosing, unavailability of critical monitoring and a lack of robust clinical studies.

Before the 1950s, children with shock would be treated with fluid bolus therapy, which led to increased mortality. The 1960s saw dopamine as the first inotrope cum vasopressor to be used in paediatric patients for the management of hypotension and shock. It remained as the first line of treatment for decades. Digoxin, an age-old inotrope, was commonly used for cardiac failure in paediatric patients. It has limited indications today because of a narrow therapeutic window, long half-life and multiple side effects. Recently, the advent of newer vasopressors and inotropes, monitoring technology, ongoing research and clinical innovations has led to improved outcomes in critically ill infants.

## PATHOPHYSIOLOGY OF SHOCK[1,2]

The clinical features of shock are basically due to the imbalance between oxygen consumption ($VO_2$) and oxygen delivery ($DO_2$). Once $VO_2$ increases or $DO_2$ decreases, O2ER (oxygen extraction ratio, ratio of $VO_2$ to $DO_2$) rises to maintain aerobic metabolism. Further increase in $VO_2$ or decrease in $DO_2$ at the critical value leads to tissue hypoxia and anaerobic metabolism, resulting in lactic acidosis, cell dysfunction and death. $DO_2$ depends on the cardiac output (CO) and the arterial content of oxygen. CO is decided by heart rate and stroke volume. Stroke volume is further dependent on preload, afterload, contractility and diastolic relaxation. Hence, it is better to start the appropriate vasopressor and/or inotropes early in cases of shock that do not respond to fluid boluses and optimised oxygen-carrying capacity.

## CLASSIFICATION OF SHOCK[2,3]

Shock can be classified based on the causative factors and presentation.

- Cardiogenic shock may be due to impaired contractility, dysrhythmia, valvular dysfunction and left ventricular outflow tract obstruction.
- Obstructive shock may be due to obstruction within or outside the circulatory system.
- Hypovolaemic shock due to excessive blood loss and fluid loss, as in gastrointestinal losses, diuresis, heat stroke, burns, diabetic ketoacidosis and third space loss.
- Distributive/vasodilatory shock as seen in neurogenic shock, adrenal failure, liver failure, anaphylaxis, septic shock, post-cardiopulmonary bypass vasoplegia, drugs and toxic exposures.

Shock can be further described by its stages, e.g. compensated, decompensated and irreversible.

*Septic shock* is further divided depending on the presentation as:
- *Cold shock:* Cold, clammy extremities, weak peripheral pulses and prolonged capillary refill (>3 seconds), narrow pulse pressure, high systemic vascular resistance (SVR).
- *Warm shock:* Hyperthermia, bounding peripheral pulses, brisk capillary refill, wide pulse pressure, hypotension and low SVR.

Depending on the response to treatment, septic shock is also classified as:
- *Fluid-sensitive*
- *Fluid-refractory:* Fails to improve with adequate volume resuscitation (>60 mL/kg).
- *Catecholamine-resistant:* Fails to improve with fluids and catecholamines.
- *Refractory septic shock*: Fails to improve with fluids, catecholamines and vasodilators.

Delays in vasopressor/inotrope administration in these critically ill infants are associated with an increased risk of mortality, especially in the first hour of treatment of septic shock. The rational use of these drugs based on their pharmacokinetic and pharmacodynamic properties is essential to achieve their optimal effects. Indications for vasopressors and inotropes in patients with shock vary depending on the aetiology and type of shock.

## CLASSIFICATION AND PHARMACOLOGY OF INOTROPES AND VASOPRESSORS

Inotropic agents are medications that enhance the heart's stroke work under specific pre-load and after-load conditions. They achieve this by influencing calcium interactions with different contractile proteins in the myocardium, ultimately affecting heart contraction **(Table 1)**.[4,5]

### Classification of Inotropes

Inotropes can be classified into three major groups depending on their mode of action.
1. *Class I drugs:* Increase intracellular calcium.
2. *Class II drugs:* Increase the sensitivity of actomyosin to calcium ions.
3. *Class III drugs:* Act through metabolic or endocrine pathways.

Some drugs will have multiple modes of action and belong to more than one class.[6]

In paediatric patients, commonly used inotropic agents include:
- Cardiac glycosides
- Beta-adrenergic agonists
- Selective phosphodiesterase III inhibitors

Digoxin, a well-known cardiac glycoside, is the classic example, with a lengthy track record of safe and successful application in infants and children.

**TABLE 1:** Inotropes and vasopressors.[4,5]

| *Medication* | *Dosage* | *Mechanism of action* | *Clinical uses* |
|---|---|---|---|
| *Dopamine* (Endogenous catecholamine precursor) | 0.5–2 µg/kg/min | Dopaminergic receptors agonism—proposed renotubular effects, intestinal and coronary vasodilation | ↑ BP |
| | ≥5–10 µg/kg/min | β-1 Adrenergic receptors agonism—mainly chronotropy | ↑ Urine output |
| | ≥10 µg/kg/min | α-1 Adrenergic receptors agonism—vasoconstriction | Has a modest effect on cardiac output |
| *Dobutamine* (synthetic catecholamine) | ≥3–15 µg/kg/min | β-1 Adrenergic receptor agonist—chronotropy and inotropy | ↑ Cardiac output without causing vasoconstriction, e.g. cardiogenic shock |
| | | β-2 Adrenergic receptor agonist—peripheral vasodilatation | Has an unpredictable effect on BP |
| *Epinephrine* (endogenous catecholamine) | ≥0.02–0.1 µg/kg/min | β-1 and some β-2 Adrenergic receptors agonism—chronotropy and inotropy, with a modest decrease in PVR | An inotrope with vasopressive action, e.g. septic shock and asphyxia |
| | ≥0.1 µg/kg/min | α-1 Adrenergic receptors agonism—vasoconstriction | At 0.02–0.05 µg/kg/min, may increase cardiac output more than SVR |
| *Norepinephrine* (endogenous sympathomimetic amine) | 0.02–0.4 µg/kg/min | α-1 (>β-1 > β-2) adrenergic receptors agonism—potent vasoconstriction (and mild inotropy) | A vasopressor which serves as an adjunct to other catecholamines at low doses<br>• Conditions with significant vasoplegia in refractory sepsis, postsurgical inflammation and asphyxia<br>• May have a mild pulmonary vasodilation effect |

*Contd...*

*Contd...*

| *Medication* | *Dosage* | *Mechanism of action* | *Clinical uses* |
|---|---|---|---|
| *Vasopressin* (exogenous vasopressin) | 0.0002–0.005 U/kg/min | V1a (>V2) receptors agonism—vasoconstriction | ↑ BP in catecholamine-resistant hypotension/shock |
| *Milrinone* (bipyridine derivative) | 0.25–0.75 µg/kg/min | Phosphodiesterase type III inhibition with increased cAMP levels—inotropy, lusitropy and pulmonary (and possible systemic) vasodilation | • An inotrope/lusitrope with mild pulmonary vasodilation (inodilator), e.g. pulmonary hypertension with ventricular dysfunction, post-PDA ligation<br>• Loading dose is not needed, whilst the onset of action may take 1–2 hours |
| *Levosimendan* (hydrazone, a pyridazinone and a nitrile) | 6–24 µg/kg/min bolus f/b infusion<br>0.1–0.4 µg/kg/min | Phosphodiesterase inhibitor and calcium sensitiser I | ↑ Stroke volume<br>↓ PVR, ↓ SVR<br>Causes vasodilatation and myocardial relaxation |

(BP: blood pressure; cAMP: cyclic adenosine monophosphate; PDA: patent ductus arteriosus; PVR: pulmonary vascular resistance; SVR: systemic vascular resistance; V1a, V2: vasopressin receptors; f/b: followed by; VR: vascular resistance)

In the paediatric population, dopamine, a mixed alpha- and beta-agonist, has been extensively utilised. However, there is a growing trend towards using both epinephrine and norepinephrine due to their enhanced potency and pressor activity, which are increasingly needed in clinical practice. The recent introduction of phosphodiesterase inhibitors such as amrinone and milrinone has expanded our therapeutic options. Apart from their modest inotropic effects, these agents, particularly milrinone and levosimendan, offer substantial pulmonary vasodilation as a beneficial component of their therapeutic profile.[4]

## INITIAL RESUSCITATION

As with all emergencies in critically ill infants, shock management begins with airway, breathing and circulation. Shortly after birth, an umbilical vein catheter can be used for resuscitation, but beyond this time, other peripheral or central venous access is essential for volume resuscitation, antibiotic administration and pressor therapy. Timely therapy, including rapid restoration of adequate tissue perfusion, has been shown to improve outcomes in adults and children with shock and should be the goal in critically ill infants as well.[7]

## Blood Pressure Targets

In contrast to term neonates, the definition of hypotension and shock in preterm neonates is less clear, particularly in the immediate newborn period. Blood pressure may be a poor indicator of systemic blood flow in preterm neonates, yet objective measures of adequacy of tissue perfusion and oxygen delivery are lacking. Another confounding variable in the management of neonatal shock is that inotrope use (dopamine and dobutamine) in hypotensive preterm neonates has not been shown to improve short or long-term outcomes significantly. These considerations notwithstanding, and in the absence of evidence of harm, some neonatologists advocate treating hypotension in preterm neonates to achieve a mean arterial pressure (MAP) of greater than or equal to 30 mm Hg. This goal MAP is based partly on a small study showing improved cerebral blood flow autoregulation above this threshold.[4] However, a gestational age-based cutoff for 'normal' blood pressure (goal MAP > gestational age) is used at many tertiary centres, especially in the first 3 days after birth.[8] Clearly, more studies are required to determine whether targeting a specific blood pressure improves outcomes in preterm infants.

## Vasoactive Agents

Dopamine is generally the first-line vasoactive drug, with a starting dose of 5–10 μg/kg/min and dose escalation as needed. For neonates with shock, which is unresolved with volume resuscitation and dopamine, several possibilities exist for additional therapy, including glucocorticoids, other catecholamines and inotropes/vasodilators. Epinephrine or norepinephrine infusions for refractory shock in neonates have been studied to a very limited extent. Neonates with vasodilatory shock may have a positive response to the alpha-adrenergic vasoconstrictive effect of these agents. A recent report on term neonates showed that the addition of noradrenaline to existing therapy (after fluid loading and dopamine or dobutamine infusion) resulted in increased blood pressure and decreased tissue lactate. Low-dose epinephrine was found to be as effective as low/moderate-dose dopamine for increasing blood pressure, cerebral blood volume and cerebral oxygen delivery in very low birth weight (VLBW) infants.[9] Patients with depressed myocardial function may benefit from an infusion of dobutamine for both inotropy and vasodilation. In a study of 42 preterm neonates with low systemic blood flow [as determined by low superior vena cava (SVC) flow] in the first 24 h after birth, dobutamine treatment improved and maintained systemic blood flow better than dopamine.[10]

As a caution, dobutamine, particularly in high doses, can increase myocardial oxygen demand due to β1 adrenergic stimulation. Dobutamine also has chronotropic actions, and severe tachycardia may lead to decreased CO, which may be corrected by decreasing the dose.[11] Milrinone, a phosphodiesterase inhibitor and inodilator, has not been studied in neonatal shock but has been used in paediatric patients with shock. In a study of patients aged 9 months to 15 years with volume-resuscitated catecholamine-resistant nonhyperdynamic septic shock, milrinone increased the cardiac index, stroke volume and $DO_2$. It decreased SVR without increasing the heart rate or blood pressure. Another alternative agent for treating septic shock is the vasoconstrictor, arginine-vasopressin (AVP) or its longer half-life analogue, terlipressin. In a report of six extremely low birth weight (ELBW) infants, AVP improved MAP and urine output in patients with septic shock but not in non-septic shock patients.[12]

Vasopressin produces vasoconstriction via V1 receptors and predominantly affects the splanchnic and skin circulation [coronary, central nervous system circulation is less potently vasoconstricted]. The pulmonary vasodilator effect is via pulmonary vascular endothelial V1 receptor-mediated nitric oxide release. Water reabsorption is via V2 receptors, which mediate aquaporin insertion in the renal collecting duct. Vasopressin is indicated as a first-line vasoconstrictor in the following patient populations:

- Term or preterm infants with hypotension [particularly low diastolic pressure or MAP, or both and known or suspected concurrent pulmonary hypertension.
- Hypotension in the presence of septal hypertrophy/hypertrophic obstructive cardiomyopathy [e.g. due to maternal diabetes].
- Hypotension due to vasodilator shock in the presence of sepsis/necrotising enterocolitis or massive haemorrhage until the intravascular volume status is restored using blood products.

Vasopressin should be used cautiously and only with echocardiographic guidance in patients with primary left ventricular dysfunction [increases afterload without positive inotropy] or infants in whom systemic circulation is dependent on right-to-left ductal shunt [e.g. aortic obstruction, vein of Galen malformation].[13]

## Therapeutic Endpoints

In the absence of widely available or well-tested methods for quantifying haemodynamic compromise in shock in infants, clinicians generally rely on vital signs and physical examination for decisions about therapy. Although the MAP may not reflect systemic blood flow, monitoring blood pressure and other measures, such as capillary refill time and urine output, provides indirect information on the adequacy of organ blood flow. Suggestions for cardiovascular therapeutic endpoints in term infants include a capillary refill time of <2 seconds, normal pulses without differential between peripheral and central pulses, warm extremities, urine output >1 ml/kg/h, low serum lactate and mixed venous saturation of >70%. Therapeutic endpoints in premature neonates have not been established, but the goals for term infants seem reasonable.[14] ELBW infants present the greatest challenge for determining therapeutic endpoints in shock. Assessment of MAP, urine output and capillary refill may not be particularly useful determinants of systemic blood flow in ELBW infants, particularly in the first 72 hours of life. In addition, the contribution of foetal haemoglobin may complicate the accurate determination of central venous oxygen saturation ($ScvO_2$) in neonates. $ScvO_2$ obtained using haemoglobin A calibration is 4–7% higher compared to $ScvO_2$, which accounts for foetal haemoglobin, implying that perhaps the goal $ScvO_2$ should be different in neonates than in older patients for optimum tissue $DO_2$. In the future, monitoring techniques such as functional echocardiography (FE) and near-infrared spectroscopy (NIRS) may provide physiologic data to optimise shock management. FE provides a bedside means to assess CO, peripheral vascular resistance, and organ blood flow in response to volume, colloid, and vasoactive medications. FE can also be used to assess SVC flow, which has been suggested as a surrogate marker for cerebral blood flow and should be maintained ≥40 ml/kg/min. Prolonged decreases in SVC flow are associated with impaired neurodevelopmental outcomes in very preterm neonates. In the absence of FE to monitor SVC flow, a capillary refill time of >4 seconds combined with a serum lactate concentration of >4 mmol/L has a specificity of 97% for identifying VLBW infants with a low SVC flow state on the first day of life. NIRS can be used to monitor end-organ perfusion non-invasively and is often used in neonates with congenital heart disease. A combination of FE and NIRS, in conjunction with traditional measures (MAP, peripheral oxygen saturation, capillary refill and urine output) as well as intermittent laboratory evaluations of tissue perfusion such as the potential of hydrogen (pH), mixed venous saturation, lactate, and base deficit would be ideal for monitoring severity of septic shock and response to therapy[15] **(Table 2)**.

In 2002 and 2007, the American College of Critical Care Medicine (ACCM) published 'Clinical Practice Parameters for Hemodynamic Support of Neonatal and Pediatric Shock'. These publications reported outcomes associated with the implementation of 'best clinical practices', indicating mortality rates of 0–5% in previously healthy children and 10% in children with chronic illnesses in septic shock **(Flowchart 1)**.[16,17]

## RECENT ADVANCES IN THE USE OF VASOPRESSORS AND INOTROPES IN CRITICALLY ILL INFANTS

The management fundamentals in critically ill infants encompass prompt recognition, appropriate inotropes, vasopressors and antibiotics in sepsis.

**TABLE 2:** Suggested strategies for treating circulatory compromise in the very preterm baby.

| *Subjects, cause and likely haemodynamics* | *Monitoring strategy and intervention threshold* | *Treatment* | *Comment* |
|---|---|---|---|
| • Preterm babies <24 hours<br>• Large PDA shunt<br>• Positive pressure<br>• Ventilation<br>• Low SBF<br>• Normal or low MBP | *Blood pressure*: Intervene if MBP < gestational age | • *General*: N-saline 10–20 mL/kg<br>• Consider closing the large PDA<br>• *First:* Dobutamine<br>• *Second:* Dopamine<br>• *Third:* Adrenaline and/or hydrocortisone 1–2 mg/kg | Titrate to a minimum acceptable MBP, and wean the infusion rate quickly if the MBP overshoots |
| • Preterm babies > 24 hours<br>• Large PDA shunt<br>• Sepsis Adrenocortical insufficiency<br>• Normal or high SBF<br>• Low MBP | *Blood pressure:* Intervene if MBP < gestational age | • *General:* N-saline 10-20 mL/kg<br>• Consider closing large PDA<br>• *First:* Dopamine<br>• *Second:* Adrenaline and/or hydrocortisone 1–2 mg/kg<br>• If MBP persistently low | If higher dose of dopamine or adrenaline required, ensure SBF |

(PDA: patent ductus arteriosus; MBP: mean blood pressure; SBF: systemic blood flow; N-saline: normal saline)

Haemodynamic monitoring and therapeutic support for malfunctioning organs are pivotal.

The ACCM recommends a target cardiac index (CI) of 3.3–6.0 L/min/m$^2$ for children with catecholamine-resistant septic shock.[18] Low CI, in comparison to SVR, is a leading cause of mortality in neonates. Septic shock typically manifests as vasodilatory shock during the neonatal period; however, cold shock can also occur. The American guidelines recommend dopamine for refractory shock that does not respond to fluids.

The current paediatric guidelines suggest initiating pharmacological drugs possessing inotropic effects; dopamine/epinephrine, due to the prevalence of 'cold shock in children.'[19] However, norepinephrine can be used as a vasopressor agent to increase SVR in warm shock. Albeit fluid resuscitation should be initiated before initiating vasopressors.

Dobutamine is considered the optimal choice, although it is less commonly used in premature neonates with immature myocardial contractility. Also, new burgeoning evidence is evolving to direct the treatment of hypotension

**Flowchart 1:** ACCCM consensus guidelines for treatment of shock in term infants and suggested modifications for preterm infants.

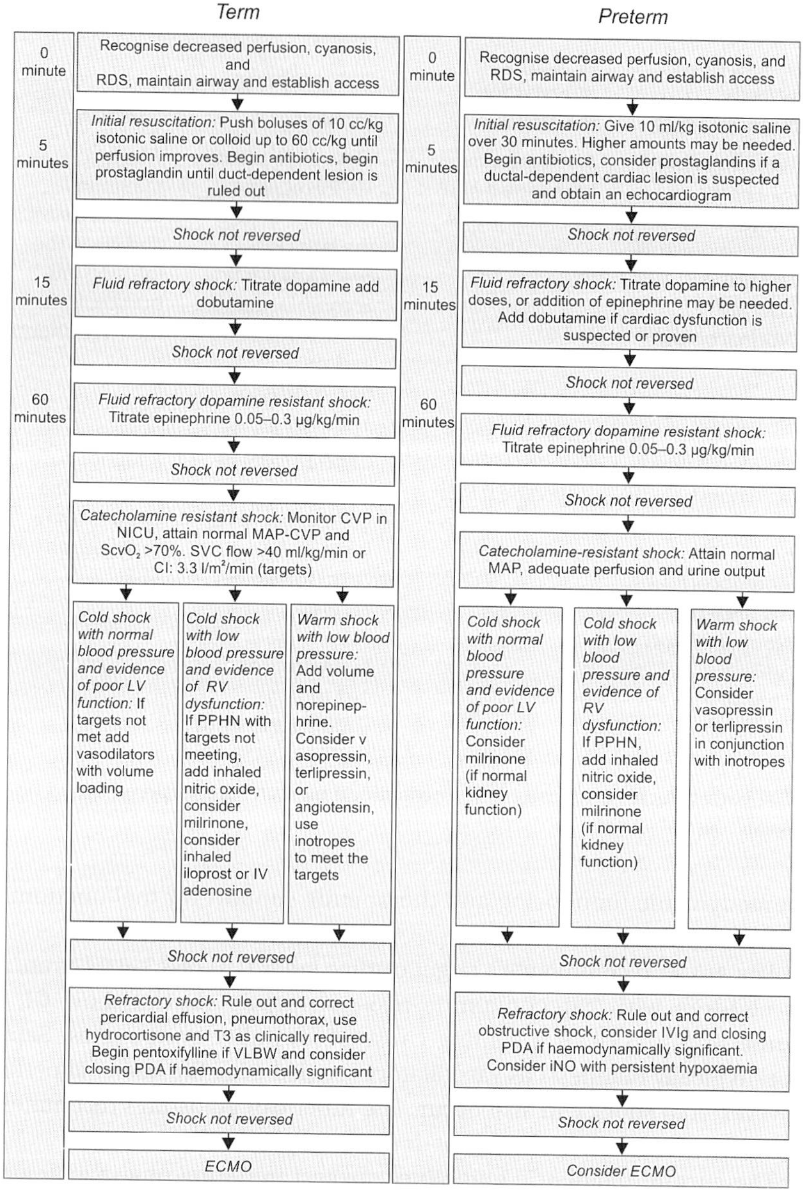


(ACCCM: American College of Critical Care Medicine; CVP: central venous pressure; LV: left ventricle; iNO: inhaled nitric oxide; IVIG: intravenous immunoglobulin; IV: intravenous; MAP: mean arterial pressure; NICU: neonatal intensive care unit; PDA: patent ductus arteriosus; PPHN: persistent pulmonary hypertension; RDS: respiratory distress syndrome; RV: right ventricle; SVC: superior venacava; $ScvO_2$: central venous oxygen saturation; T3-Triiodothyronine; VLBW: very low birth weight)

*Source:* De Waal K, Seri I. Assessment and Management of Septic Shock and Hypovolemia. In: Neonatal Clinical Management, 1st edition. Elsevier; 2019. p. 489-501.

in the background of persistent pulmonary hypertension and sepsis. Data suggests increased evidence of milrinone, norepinephrine and vasopressin in persistent pulmonary hypertension.[16]

Phosphodiesterase inhibitors such as milrinone cause vasodilatation by improving contractility and thereby improving CO without causing worrying hypertension in a few trials on septic children. The management principles include early recognition, fluid resuscitation, appropriate inotropes, antibiotic therapy in sepsis, supportive therapy for organ dysfunction, and regular haemodynamic monitoring.[20]

### Newer Inotropic Agents

#### *Levosimendan*

Levosimendan is a calcium-sensitising agent. Its inotropic actions are produced by sensitisation of myocardial troponin C to calcium and exertion of vasodilator action by stimulation of the adenosine triphosphate-sensitive potassium channels of pulmonary, systemic and coronary vascular smooth muscle cells.[18] The first use of levosimendan in the paediatric subset was reported in 2004. In a retrospective study, the authors defined levosimendan as safe and effective in paediatrics with severe myocardial dysfunction.[21]

Noteworthy clinical reports in children with low cardiac output syndrome have been published recently.[22] All this research involved premature neonates and young infants in the postoperative period.

The vasoactive-inotropic score (VIS) is an enhanced version of the Inotropic Score[23] designed to quantify the level of cardiovascular support infants require during the postoperative period. It includes using dopamine, dobutamine, epinephrine, milrinone, vasopressin, and norepinephrine. This scoring was composed to predict the haemodynamic requirement of paediatric patients precisely.

#### *Calcium*

Ionised calcium is crucial for enhancing contractility and increasing vascular tone. Addressing hypocalcaemia may be particularly beneficial in younger paediatric patients with sepsis.

Ionised calcium can play the key role in improving contractility and increasing vascular tone. Treating low ionised calcium levels may prove beneficial, especially in younger paediatric subsets with sepsis.

## DOPAMINE OR EPINEPHRINE: BEST INITIAL INOTROPE IN SEPTIC SHOCK?

The recent ACCM/Paediatric Advanced Life Support guidelines recommend using a peripheral infusion of epinephrine 0.05–0.3 μg/kg/min as the first-line inotrope in fluid-refractory shock on a recent evidence basis.[24]

The latest evidence suggests that short-term, vasoactive infusion through a peripheral cannula can be used as a bridge before commencing central venous access.[25]

Dopamine is a time-tested inotrope that can be administered from a peripheral line in a resource-limited centre. It continues to be the first inotrope used in daily clinical practice. There is great scope for research in the identification of patients not responding to inotropes and further inotropic choice.

## KEY CONSIDERATIONS IN PAEDIATRIC SHOCK MANAGEMENT

- *High mortality and morbidity:* Shock in children, particularly in resource-limited settings, is associated with significant mortality and morbidity.
- *Essential management strategies:* Early recognition, fluid resuscitation, appropriate inotropes, organ support and continuous haemodynamic monitoring are crucial.
- *Uncertainty in first-line vasoactive agents:* Epinephrine may reduce mortality compared to dopamine; however, no direct comparison exists between epinephrine and norepinephrine.
- *Peripheral vasopressor use:* Safe for temporary use until central access is secured.
- *Refractory septic shock:* Defined by high lactate levels (>8 mmol/L) and high vasoinotrope doses (VIS >200 µg/kg/min).
- *Importance of identifying reversible causes:* Essential before considering extracorporeal support.
- *Steroid supplementation:* Hydrocortisone helps maintain catecholamine sensitivity and is recommended for worsening conditions or increasing inotrope doses. Recent National Institute of Health and Care Excellence guidelines support low-dose corticosteroids for shock unresponsive to vasoactive agents.[26]

## CONCLUSION

In conclusion, managing paediatric shock, particularly in resource-limited settings, requires early recognition, fluid resuscitation, and appropriate inotropic support. Epinephrine may offer a mortality benefit over dopamine, though no direct comparison with norepinephrine exists. Peripheral vasopressor use is safe until central access is achieved. Identifying reversible causes is essential for refractory septic shock, and steroid supplementation, including hydrocortisone, can enhance catecholamine sensitivity. Recent guidelines recommend low-dose corticosteroid therapy for children unresponsive to vasoactive agents, providing valuable support in critical cases.

## REFERENCES

1. Fisher JD, Nelson DG, Beyersdorf H, Satkowiak LJ. Clinical spectrum of shock in the pediatric emergency department. Pediatr Emerg Care. 2010;26(9):622-5.
2. Wooldridge G, Hitayezu J, Venkatasubbu P. Paediatric cardiogenic shock. Update Anaesth. 2023;37:15-22.
3. Pasman EA, Watson CM. (2024). Shock in Pediatrics. [Online] Available from https://emedicine.medscape.com (Last accessed June, 2025).
4. Joynt C, Cheung P-Y. Treating hypotension in preterm neonates with vasoactive medications. Front Pediatr. 2018;6:86.
5. Patwardhan K. Inotropes in neonates. Infant. 2009;5(1):12-7.
6. Nieminen MS, Fruhwald S, Heunks LMA, Suominen PK, Gordon AC, Kivikko M, et al. Levosimendan: current data, clinical use and future development. Heart Lung Vessels. 2013;5(4):227-45.
7. Noori S, Seri I. Evidence-based versus pathophysiology-based approach to diagnosis and treatment of neonatal cardiovascular compromise. Semin Fetal Neonatal Med. 2015;20(4):238-45.
8. Nuntnarumit P, Yang W, Bada-Ellzey HS. Blood pressure measurements in the newborn. Clin Perinatol. 1999;26(4):981-96.
9. Munro MJ, Walker AM, Barfield CP. Hypotensive extremely low birth weight infants have reduced cerebral blood flow. Pediatrics. 2004;114(6):1591-6.
10. Osborn D, Evans N, Kluckow M. Randomized trial of dobutamine versus dopamine in preterm infants with low systemic blood flow. J Pediatr. 2002;140(2):183-91.
11. Stranak Z, Semberova J, Barrington K, O'Donnell C, Marlow N, Naulaers G, et al. International survey on diagnosis and management of hypotension in extremely preterm babies. Eur J Pediatr. 2014;173(6):793-8.
12. Durrmeyer X, Marchand-Martin L, Porcher R, Gascoin G, Roze JC, Storme L, et al. Abstention or intervention for isolated hypotension in the first 3 days of life in extremely preterm infants: association with short-term outcomes in the EPIPAGE 2 cohort study. Arch Dis Child Fetal Neonatal Ed. 2017;102(6):490-6.
13. Henderson KK, Byron KL. Vasopressin-induced vasoconstriction: two concentration-dependent signaling pathways. J Appl Physiol (1985). 2007; 102(4):1402-9.
14. Al-Aweel I, Pursley DM, Rubin LP, Shah B, Weisberger S, Richardson DK. Variations in prevalence of hypotension, hypertension, and vasopressor use in NICUs. J Perinatol. 2001;21(5):272e8.
15. Lasky T, Greenspan J, Ernst FR, Gonzalez L. Dopamine and dobutamine use in preterm or low birth weight neonates in the premier 2008 database. Clin Ther. 2011;33(12):2082-e8.
16. Davis AL, Carcillo JA, Aneja RK, Deyman AJ, Lin JC, Nguyen TC, et al. American College of Critical Care Medicine Clinical Practice Parameters for Hemodynamic Support of Pediatric and Neonatal Septic Shock. Crit Care Med. 2017;45(6):1061-93.
17. De Waal K, Seri I. Assessment and management of septic shock and hypovolemia. In: De Waal K, Seri I (Eds). Neonatal Clinical Management, 1st edition. Amsterdam: Elsevier; 2019. pp. 489-501.
18. Brierley J, Carcillo JA, Choong K, Cornell T, Decaen A, Deymann A, et al. Clinical practice parameters for hemodynamic support of pediatric and neonatal septic

shock: 2007 update from the American College of Critical Care Medicine. Crit Care Med. 2009;37(2):666-88.

19. Turanlahti M, Boldt T, Palkama T, Antila S, Lehtonen L, Pesonen E, et al. Pharmacokinetics of levosimendan in pediatric patients evaluated for cardiac surgery. Pediatr Crit Care Med. 2004;5(5):457-62.
20. Gold J, Cullinane S, Chen J, Seo S, Oz MC, Oliver JA, et al. Vasopressin in the treatment of milrinone-induced hypotension in severe heart failure. Am J Cardiol. 2000;85(4):506-8, A11.
21. Dündar MA, Yılmaz M, Argun M. Levosimendan: efficacy and safety in pediatric heart failure treatment. Rev Assoc Med Bras (1992). 2024;70(7):e20240257.
22. Namachivayam P, Crossland DS, Butt WW, Shekerdemian LS. Early experience with levosimendan in children with ventricular dysfunction. Pediatr Crit Care Med. 2006;7(5):445-8.
23. Gaies MG, Gurney JG, Yen AH, Napoli ML, Gajarski RJ, Ohye RG, et al. Vasoactive-inotropic score as a predictor of morbidity and mortality in infants after cardiopulmonary bypass. Pediatr Crit Care Med 2010;11:234-8.
24. Ramaswamy KN, Singhi S, Jayashree M, Bansal A, Nallasamy K. Double-blind randomized clinical trial comparing dopamine and epinephrine in pediatric fluid-refractory hypotensive septic shock. Pediatr Crit Care Med. 2016;17(11):e502-12.
25. Takeshita J, Kawaguchi A, Kawasaki T, Ishihara T, Shime N. Local adverse events associated with peripheral vasoactive infusion in children: a systematic review with meta-analysis. J Cardiothorac Vasc Anesth. 2024;38(12):3215-23.
26. Visintin C, Mugglestone MA, Fields EJ, Jacklin P, Murphy MS, Pollard AJ, et al. Management of bacterial meningitis and meningococcal septicaemia in children and young people: summary of NICE guidance. BMJ. 2010;340:c3209.

CHAPTER 11

# Common Paediatric Perioperative Emergencies and Their Management: Learn How to Handle Them Like a Pro!

*Ruchi Gupta, Anju Gupta, Priyanka Pavithran, Shelly Rana*

## ABSTRACT

Paediatric patients undergoing surgical procedures are especially vulnerable due to their unique anatomical, physiological, and emotional characteristics. Anaesthetising this unique population requires specialised knowledge and training to reduce anaesthetic risks. Perioperative paediatric emergencies are life-threatening scenarios which can arise during the pre-operative phase or can be encountered during induction, maintenance, or extubation. Cardiovascular and respiratory events are the prime causes of cardiac arrest during paediatric anaesthesia. Careful pre-operative assessment is vital for identifying potential risks and ensuring optimal pre-operative preparation. The majority of critical perioperative emergencies are amenable to therapeutic measures and can be promptly reversed if detected in a timely manner. Hence, it is of utmost importance for paediatric anaesthesiologists to be able to diagnose and manage these scenarios effectively for optimal outcomes. Following established protocols, building effective teamwork and proper communication are the pillars which can significantly reduce the morbidity and mortality when faced with such emergency situations in paediatric surgeries.

***Keywords:*** Airway extubation, Child, Critical illness, Emergencies, Morbidity, Respiratory system.

## INTRODUCTION

Paediatric patients undergoing surgical procedures are especially vulnerable due to their unique anatomical, physiological, and emotional characteristics. Hence, early identification and prompt management of perioperative emergencies in this population are essential to improve outcomes and reduce morbidity and mortality. Also, paediatric patients differ significantly from adults with respect to their smaller size, faster metabolism, and different organ functions. These variations require specialised knowledge and training to reduce risks.

Timely detection and management of life-threatening concerns in the airway, breathing, circulation, and acute neurological conditions are essential. These situations can arise during the pre-operative phase, such as while inducing a critically ill child, or can be encountered during induction, maintenance, or extubation.

## ESSENTIAL PRE-OPERATIVE ASSESSMENT AND RISK STRATIFICATION

A comprehensive pre-operative assessment is vital for identifying potential risks and ensuring optimal preparation for the surgery. This includes a thorough history, physical examination and, when indicated, targeted investigations such as blood tests, echocardiograms, or pulmonary function tests, especially in children with known comorbidities like congenital heart defects or asthma. Evidence from the Pediatric Perioperative Cardiac Arrest (POCA) registry and American Society of Anesthesiologists (ASA) closed claims indicates that cardiovascular and respiratory events are the primary causes of cardiac arrest during paediatric anaesthesia.[1]

### Pre-operative Optimisation of Critically Ill Child

#### *Managing Critically Ill Child Pre-operatively*

The child who is in a critical state may rapidly deteriorate to develop respiratory or cardiac arrest or severe neurological complications, if not recognised and treated promptly. Rapidly identifying and managing such a child can minimise the risk of permanent damage. Hence, alertness towards deteriorating vital signs, increasing oxygen demands or worsening investigations can save the situation. The treatment includes providing an open and patent airway, adequate ventilation and oxygenation along with respiratory monitoring. Airway adjuncts may be necessary to secure a definitive airway. Securing an intravenous (IV) access is an important step; invasive monitoring and giving fluid boluses may be helpful in this situation.

## AIRWAY AND RESPIRATORY EMERGENCIES

### Perioperative Respiratory Events

Factors such as recent respiratory infections, young age, type of surgery, and passive smoke exposure increase children's susceptibility to perioperative respiratory events (PRAE). The decision to wait or proceed with surgery for the group of children suffering from upper respiratory infection (URI) can be made based on the scoring system called COLDS (current signs/symptoms, onset, lung disease, airway device and surgery) **(Table 1)**.[2] Respiratory events contribute to 27% of cardiac arrests in paediatric anaesthesia, highlighting the importance of proactive management.[3]

#### *Apnoea of Prematurity*

Pre-terms are prone to apnoea up to post-conceptional age (PCA) of 48 weeks; however, the risk remains till PCA of 56 weeks.[4] Apnoea of prematurity is defined as a cessation of breathing of >15–20 seconds, or accompanied by oxygen desaturation [peripheral oxygen saturation ($SpO_2$) ≤ 80% for ≥4

**TABLE 1:** COLDS score.[2]

| *Category* | *1* | *2* | *3* |
|---|---|---|---|
| Current signs and symptoms | None | Mild (Parent confirms URI and/or congestion, rhinorrhoea, sore throat, sneezing, low fever and dry cough) | Moderate/severe (Purulence, wet cough, abnormal lung sounds, lethargy, toxic appearance or high fever) |
| Onset of symptoms | >4 weeks ago | 2–4 weeks ago | <2 weeks ago |
| Presence of lung disease | None | Mild (History of respiratory syncytial virus/mild intermittent asthma/loud snoring, bronchopulmonary dysplasia if >1 year old, or a passive smoker) | Moderate/severe (Moderate persistent asthma, infant with bronchopulmonary dysplasia, obstructive sleep apnoea or pulmonary hypertension) |
| Airway device | None or a facemask | Laryngeal mask airway/ supraglottic airway | Endotracheal tube |
| Surgery | Other | Minor airway (adenotonsillectomy, nasolacrimal duct probing, flexible bronchoscopy and dental extraction) | Major airway (Cleft palate, rigid bronchoscopy and maxillofacial surgery) |

(COLDS: current signs/symptoms, onset, lung disease, airway device and surgery; URI: upper respiratory infection)

*Source:* Lee LK, Bernardo MKL, Grogan TR, Elashoff DA, Ren WHP. Perioperative respiratory adverse event risk assessment in children with upper respiratory tract infection: Validation of the COLDS score. Paediatr Anaesth. 2018;28(11):1007-14.

seconds) and bradycardia [heart rate (HR) <2/3 of baseline for >4 seconds] in infants born at <37 weeks of gestation. This is due to an immature respiratory musculature, central control mechanism, and unstable elastic rib cage, which makes them prone to upper airway obstruction, and the lower airways to collapse. Risk factors that increase the chances of apnoea are hypothermia and anaemia. IV caffeine (10 mg/kg) is effective in treating it. If the child has this problem, regional blocks without sedation or general anaesthesia can decrease the incidence of apnoea.[5] These children need to be monitored for at least 24 hours after surgery in the high dependency area or the intensive care unit.

### *Upper Airway Obstruction*

Patients with macroglossia or micrognathia as such or in association with syndromes, e.g. with Pierre Robin Sequence (PRS) and Treacher Collins syndromes or syndromic children (e.g. Goldenhar syndrome) associated with facial asymmetry, ear abnormalities, are at a higher risk of obstruction. The reliability of the Mallampati score in predicting a difficult airway in the paediatric population is questionable, and some clinicians prefer the reliable Colorado Pediatric Airway Score (COPUR).[1,2] Hydrocephalus, meningomyelocoėle, enlarged tonsils, adenoids, blocked nose, foreign body in the laryngopharynx, etc. can also cause problems during induction. The management includes inducing the child with the mouth open; optimising the level of the airway by repositioning the head or the area of meningomyelocoele. Sometimes, children must be induced in the lateral position. After extubation, maintaining the child in lateral recovery position, inserting an oral or nasopharyngeal airway, or tongue stitch in PRS/severe micrognathia cases during emergence can be helpful.[6]

### *Laryngospasm*

This is a common airway complication that can occur during any stage: induction, maintenance(without endotracheal tube), or extubation. It is a common perioperative emergency characterised by sustained closure of the vocal cords that results in the partial or complete loss of the patient's airway. It is normally triggered by a peri-glottic stimulus mediated via the vagus nerve.

Pre-operative risk factors include reactive airways, otorhinolaryngological procedures, airway anomalies such as subglottic stenosis, cleft palate, PRS, and laryngomalacia, passive exposure to smoke, patient or family history of asthma or atopy, <1 year (three times higher in infants), and ex-premature infants.[1,7,8] Perioperative respiratory adverse effects can be predicted by using the COLDS score. The minimum score is 5, and the maximum score is 15. A higher COLDS score would suggest more perioperative risk.

In the immediate post-operative period, blood or secretions irritating the vocal cords or inadequate anaesthetic depth during airway manipulation or instrumentation may induce laryngospasm. Strategies to reduce risk include delaying surgery in children with significant URI and avoiding airway manipulation intraoperatively during periods of inadequate anaesthetic depth.[6] No difference has been observed in the incidence of laryngospasm between extubation in the deep or light planes of anaesthesia. Laryngospasm can be complete or partial. In partial laryngospasm, the vocal cords will be adducted but with a small gap posteriorly. Presentation would be inspiratory stridor, suprasternal and supraclavicular retractions and flailing of lower ribs. In complete laryngospasm, there would be no air entry, no breath sounds, paradoxical chest motion, along with hypoxia and bradycardia.

### *Management of Laryngospasm*

Removal of irritant stimulus, jaw thrust, Larson's manoeuvre (application of bilateral digital pressure on the styloid process behind the ramus of mandible in the laryngospasm notch), 100% oxygen and with continuous positive airway pressure up to 10 cm water are the first steps in the management of laryngospasm.[9] A subhypnotic dose of propofol (0.8 mg/kg) can be administered intravenously if the initial manoeuvres fail to restore airway patency. IV suxamethonium in the dose of 0.1–1 mg/kg, together with atropine 0.02 mg/kg, when associated with bradycardia or rocuronium 1.2 mg/kg IV can be administered. If IV access is not available, suxamethonium intramuscular 4 mg/kg or sublingual 2 mg/kg can be used.[1,8]

The management of recurrent laryngospasm is challenging. The use of a bilateral superior laryngeal block will interrupt the reflex arc. It also causes dissipation of the stimuli that are causing the laryngospasm. In severe recurrent post-operative laryngospasm, fibreoptic pharyngeal and laryngeal examination should be done to rule out any pathology.[9] The management of laryngospasm is summarised in **Flowchart 1**.

## *Bronchospasm*

It is a moderately common occurrence during general anaesthesia and is reported to occur in around 0.3–3.2% of children as per the APRICOT

**Flowchart 1:** Management of laryngospasm.

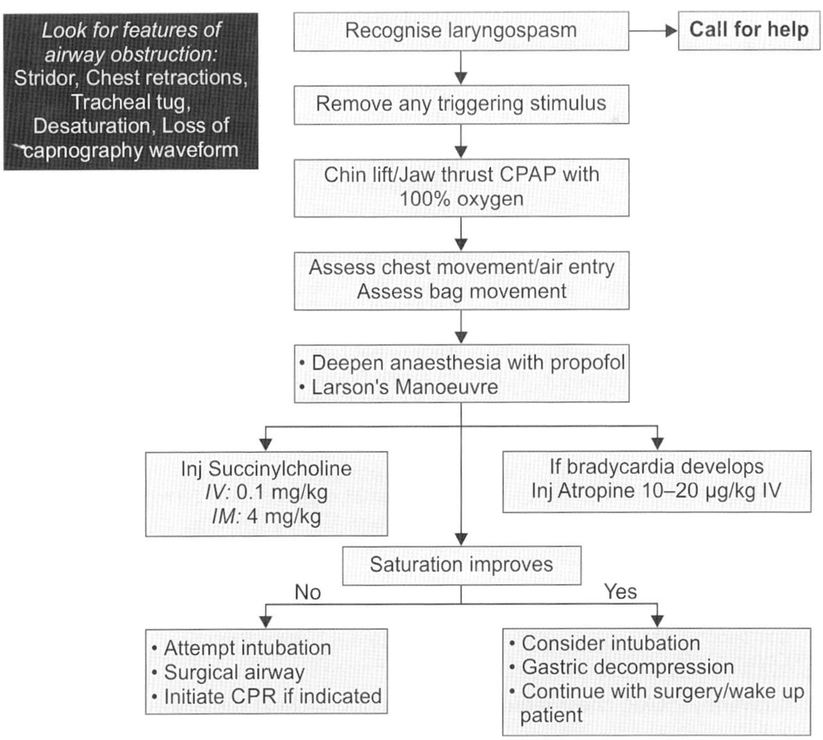


(IV: intravenous, IM: intramuscular, CPAP: continuous positive airway pressure, CPR: cardiopulmonary resuscitation)

(Anaesthesia PRactice In Children Observational Trial) study.[7] The incidence is highest in asthmatic patients (6%), but life-threatening bronchospasm can still occur in healthy patients without any underlying lung pathology.[1,2] It is often triggered by airway irritation during intubation under light plane of anaesthesia, reactive airway diseases, recent URI, history of smoke exposure and atopy. It may also be triggered by drugs like beta blockers and histamine-releasing drugs or anaphylaxis. It presents with desaturation, increased airway pressures and a shark fin pattern on the capnogram.[10] Bronchospasm can occur on emergence in light planes of anaesthesia with the endotracheal tube in situ. A risk prediction tool for the occurrence of PRAEs, including bronchospasm in the intraoperative period was validated by Subramanyam et al., and it identified five risk factors including age ≤3 years (versus >3 years), ASA physical status II and III (versus ASA physical status I), morbid obesity, preexisting pulmonary disorder, and surgery (versus radiology) for PRAE.[11]

The management of bronchospasm is summarised in **Flowchart 2**.

**Flowchart 2:** Management of bronchospasm.[10]

Suspected bronchospasm

↓ **Call for help**

- Ventilate with 100% oxygen
- Stop stimulation
- Suspecting anaphylaxis—stop any drug/blood product

↓

- Deepen anaesthesia
- Recheck ETT position
- Rule out kinking/obstruction
- If before intubation—consider laryngospasm or aspiration
- Drug therapy

↓

- Optimise ventilation
- Reconsider anaphylaxis
- Consider pulmonary oedema, embolus, pneumothorax if not responding
- Obtain CXR

**Drug therapy**

**Salbutamol**
- MDI 6–8 puffs
- Nebulised <5 years 2.5 mg, >5 years 2.5–5 mg
- IV–4 µg/kg slow IV then 0.1–1µg/kg/min

**Adrenaline**
- IV–0.1–1.0 µg/kg
- Nebulised 0.5 mL/kg of 1:1000 (max 5 millilitres)

**Ipratropium Bromide**
- Nebulised (2–12 years) 0.25 mg 6 hourly

**Magnesium sulphate**-50 mg/kg IV over 20 minutes

**Ketamine:** Infusion: 1–3 mg/kg/h

**Aminophylline**
- 5 mg/kg IV over 20 minutes then 1 mg/kg/h (< 9 years), 0.8 mg/kg/h (9–16 years) infusion
- Omit loading dose if taking theophylline

**Hydrocortisone**
- < 1 year 25 mg, 1–5 years 50 mg, 6–12 years 100 mg 6 hourly

**Chlorpheniramine**
- <6 months 250 µg/kg IV, 6 months–6 yrs 2.5 mg IV, 6 years–12 years 5 mg IV

(IV: intravenous; CXR: chest radiogram, ETT: endotracheal tube; MDI: metered dose inhaler)

*Source:* Looseley A. Management of bronchospasm during general anaesthesia. Update Anaesth. 2011;27:17-21.

### *Tight Bag Situation*

A tight bag is a condition with a disproportionate pressure increase (airway pressure that exceeds 25 cm water) in a reservoir bag in an intubated patient, leading to unsatisfactory ventilation. This condition can occur due to factors, both extrinsic and intrinsic, to the patients. The diagnosis of extrinsic causes is made on the basis of the ability to ventilate with a reservoir bag. In such a scenario, causes extrinsic to the patient, such as equipment failure and tube obstruction, need to be ruled out. The intrinsic causes occurring due to problems with the chest, such as bronchospasm, asthma exacerbation, light planes of anaesthesia, pulmonary aspiration, endobronchial intubation, pneumothorax, foreign body or anaphylaxis, can be detected by the ability to pass a suction catheter through an endotracheal tube but inability to ventilate.[12] Management principles in such a case have been highlighted in **Flowchart 3**.

### *Perioperative Aspiration*

Aspiration, though rare (0.006% incidence), poses a potentially *serious* complication. Risk factors include emergency procedures, higher ASA status, inadequate fasting, airway stimulation under suboptimal anaesthetic depth, and gastrointestinal disorders.[7,13] The signs of aspiration in a child include vomiting during anaesthesia with observation of gastric contents in the airway, reduced saturation, increased respiratory rate, coughing or wheezing after surgery. Controlled rapid sequence intubation with a 20° head-up tilt, continuous gastric aspiration, and gentle bag-mask ventilation without cricoid pressure is advised in children at risk.[14] In the event of aspiration, immediate interventions include patient positioning (head-down, lateral decubitus), airway suctioning, 100% oxygen administration and prompt management of bronchospasm.[13]

## CARDIOVASCULAR EMERGENCIES

### Bradycardia

In children, fluctuations in blood pressure and arrhythmias are less commonly seen. Bradycardia is usually a response to hypoxia or to medications such as fentanyl or neuromuscular block-reversing agents. It may also result from increased intracranial pressure (ICP) (hydrocephalus or intracranial space-occupying lesion), warranting the need for urgent intervention. Finding and treating the cause can reverse it.

As the cardiac output in children is dependent on the HR, early management is required to prevent a precipitous fall in the cardiac output. The measures include ensuring adequate oxygenation, administering IV atropine (0.02 mg/kg), IV epinephrine (0.01 mg/kg) and if necessary, performing cardiopulmonary resuscitation.

**Flowchart 3:** Management of a tight bag situation.

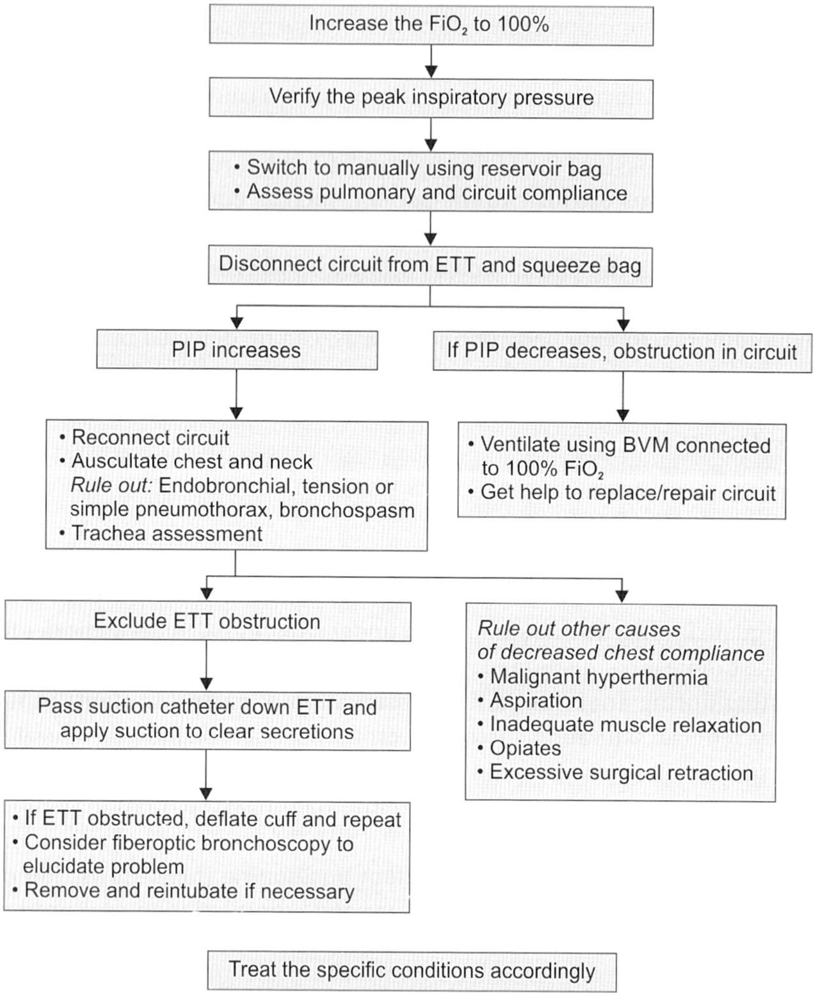


(ETT: endotracheal tube; $FiO_2$: fraction of inspired oxygen; BVM: bag-mask ventilation; PIP: peak inspiratory pressure)

## *Tachycardia/Tachyarrhythmias*

Tachycardia could be due to anxiety, pain or fluid deficit. The commonest arrhythmias in children include sinus arrhythmia, sinus bradycardia and supraventricular tachycardia (SVT). SVT is a common arrhythmia in children, the incidence varying from 26 to 43% in different age groups. 90% of paediatric dysrhythmias are SVTs.[15] If the child is haemodynamically stable, vagal manoeuvres, cold compresses, IV adenosine 0.1 mg/kg bolus, increasing to a maximum of 0.25 mg/kg/dose (maximum 12 mg) can be given.[15,16] However, if there is haemodynamic instability, the child is subjected to unstable synchronised cardioversion with 0.5-1 J/kg. If it persists, the dose is increased to 2 J/kg.

### Hypotension

Hypovolaemia and inadequate perfusion occur with inadequate correction of blood loss or hydration status. The Pediatric Advanced Life Support (PALS)/ Advanced Trauma Life Support (ATLS) define hypotension in children as systolic blood pressure below the fifth percentile for age. Hypotension is a late sign in a child with hypovolaemia. Deficit fluid therapy refers to the management of fluid and electrolyte losses that occur prior to presentation for surgery. It has three components: (1) Estimation of the severity of dehydration, (2) determination of the type of fluid deficit and (3) deficit repair. Severity of dehydration is usually estimated from the history and clinical evaluation and laboratory parameters. Pharmacological measures include the use of ionotropes, such as norepinephrine, epinephrine, phenylephrine and ephedrine.[16,17]

### Perioperative Cardiac Arrest

*Paediatric perioperative cardiac arrest (PPOCA):* The incidence ranges from 2.7 to 22.9 per 10,000 anaesthetics, out of which approximately 65% occur during the intraoperative period and 35% in the post-operative period. Young age, prematurity, and congenital heart disease in neonates and children <1 year of age are risk factors for PPOCA.[18] Moreover, paediatric patients with sepsis and those admitted through the emergency room have been found to be at the highest risk for cardiac arrest in the perioperative period.[19]

The commonest causes of cardiac arrest during anaesthesia are cardiovascular (80.5%), airway and respiratory (59.1%), or hyperkalaemia associated with the rapid administration of blood or blood products.[19,20] Various risk factors are age, ASA status, hypovolaemia, bradycardia, hypoxaemia and the experience of the anaesthesia provider. Hypoxia, aspiration, cannot intubate cannot ventilate (CICV) scenario, displaced tracheostomy/tracheal tubes, drug errors, anaesthetic agent overdose, local anaesthetic (LA) toxicity and anaphylaxis are the important causes of morbidity and mortality in children.[21,22] Cardiac arrest has been seen during the transfer of children to and from the operating room. The paediatric cardiac arrest algorithm has been provided by the American Heart Association. The causes contributed by 7 H's and 5 T's need to be considered **(Table 2)**. One has to call for help and the crash cart. The administration of potentially deleterious substances has to be stopped. 100% oxygen is administered. A leader and roles are assigned to the team members, and resuscitation is started. One has to consider giving the Trendelenburg position and rapid IV fluids if the child is hypotensive.[22] The management of POCA is summed up in **Flowchart 4**.

**TABLE 2:** The reversible causes of pulseless electrical activity.

| *H* | *T* |
|---|---|
| • Hypovolaemia<br>• Hypoxia<br>• Hydrogen ion excess (acidosis)<br>• Hypoglycaemia<br>• Hypokalaemia<br>• Hyperkalaemia<br>• Hypothermia | • Tension pneumothorax<br>• Tamponade – Cardiac<br>• Toxins<br>• Thrombosis (pulmonary embolus)<br>• Thrombosis (myocardial infarction) |

## ANAPHYLAXIS

It is a severe, potentially life-threatening systemic hypersensitivity reaction, characterised by respiratory or circulatory problems, and is usually, but not always, associated with skin, mucosal, or gastrointestinal tract involvement.

Early recognition of the signs and symptoms and prompt management are crucial as the majority of symptoms occur within minutes of induction, and are mainly due to agents administered intravenously, such as neuromuscular blocking agents, antibiotics, opioids, LAs, colloids, latex, chlorhexidine, dyes and protamine.

### Management

The injection or infusion which could have caused the anaphylaxis is stopped, and anaesthesia is maintained if necessary, with a minimal inhalational agent. The ABC (airway, breathing, and circulation) approach can be used. IV adrenaline can be administered for moderate hypotension or bronchospasm in the dose of 1–5 μg/kg (0.1–0.5 ml/kg of 1:100,000 solution) and in the dose of 5–10 μg/kg (0.5–1 ml/kg of 1:100,000 solution) for severe hypotension or bronchospasm.[16,18] An infusion of 0.1–5 μg/kg/min is started if repeated doses are required. One can also consider noradrenaline infusion—0.1 μg/kg/min and anti-histaminics, such as chlorpheniramine maleate. Once the patient is stabilised, steroids can be considered as a part of post-crisis management.

## LOCAL ANAESTHETIC SYSTEMIC TOXICITY

Seven cases of local anaesthetic systemic toxicity (LAST) in over 100,000 regional blocks with an estimated risk of severe LAST of 0.08/1,000 [95% confidence interval (CI): 0.3–1.6] were observed in the Pediatric Regional Anesthesia Network (PRAN) registry.[22] Infants have a greater risk of LA toxicity due to the immaturity of the organs that metabolise and excrete the LAs. Moreover, the lower level of LA-binding proteins (e.g. alpha-1-acid glycoprotein and albumin) leads to an increased fraction of unbound LA levels. A majority of paediatric patients are under general anaesthesia when LAs are administered. LAST manifests frequently with electrocardiographic signs of QRS complex and T-wave changes, leading to cardiac arrest.[23] Overall, the episodes of LAST

**Flowchart 4:** Management of perioperative cardiac arrest (POCA).[16]

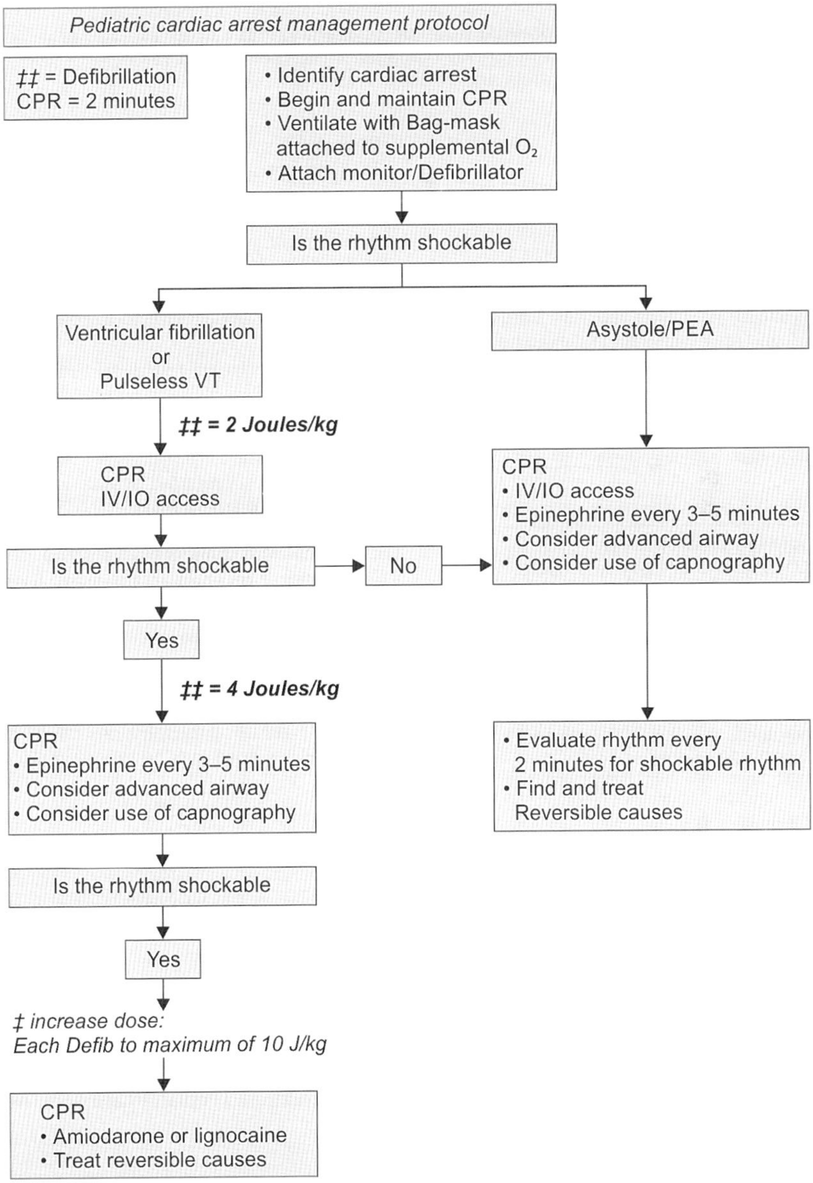


(CPR: cardiopulmonary resuscitation; $O_2$: oxygen; VT: ventricular tachycardia, PEA: pulseless electrical activity; IV: intravenous; IO: intraosseous; Defib: defibrillation)
*Source:* American Heart Association. Handbook of Emergency Cardiovascular Care for Healthcare Providers, 1st edition. Texas: Amer Heart Assn Inc; 2015.

in children are commonly related to bupivacaine (67%). Nevertheless, they can occur with all other LAs.[24] In most cases, the manifestations can occur within 5 minutes of bolus administration (81%), indicating inadvertent intravascular injection.[25] In situations where LAST occurs, intralipid therapy

**Flowchart 5:** Management of local anaesthetic toxicity.[26]

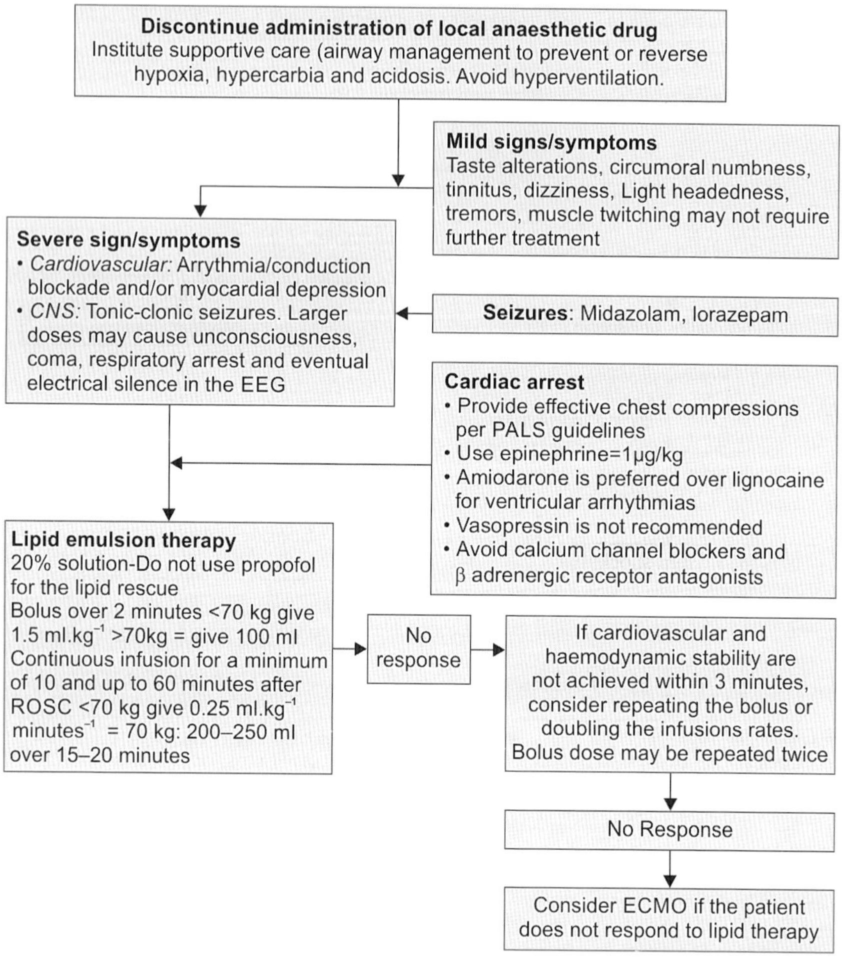


(CNS: central nervous system; ECMO: extracorporeal membrane oxygenation; PALS: paediatric advanced life support; ROSC: return of spontaneous circulation; EEG: electroencephalogram)

*Source:* Dontukurthy S, Tobias JD. Update on local anesthetic toxicity, prevention and treatment during regional anaesthesia in infants and children. J Pediatr Pharmacol Ther. 2021;26(5):445-54.

can be used.[26] The management of LAST has been depicted in an algorithm in **Flowchart 5.**[26]

## HAEMATOLOGIC EMERGENCIES

### Intraoperative and Post-operative Bleeding Emergencies

Major perioperative haemorrhage is rare in routine paediatric surgeries but can occur in trauma, liver transplant, cardiac surgery, major spinal surgery, cranial vault surgery, neurosurgical procedures, and minimally invasive (robotic/laparoscopic) procedures where direct haemorrhage control is difficult. The risk of haemorrhage is high in patients with inherited bleeding disorders such as Von Willebrand's disease and haemophilia, or acquired coagulopathy such as dilutional coagulopathy. A high level of vigilance for perioperative bleeding should be maintained in patients with these risk factors. Perioperative management of bleeding disorders includes minimising trauma, preventing coagulopathy, use of adjunctive care strategies including anti-fibrinolytics, using desmopressin for von Willebrand disease, and preparing for transfusions of platelets or clotting factors.

### Post-tonsillectomy Bleeding

Post-tonsillectomy bleeding is rare nowadays but requires immediate attention due to the risk of aspiration from swallowed blood. Management includes surgical ligation of the bleeding vessel along with volume replacement and blood transfusion. The availability of functioning suction machines, laryngoscopes, and different-sized endotracheal tubes has to be ensured. IV ketamine (2 mg/kg) or etomidate (0.2–0.3 mg/kg) are typically used for induction; however, in properly resuscitated cases, propofol can also be used. Modified or controlled rapid sequence induction with IV suxamethonium (2 mg/kg) or rocuronium (1.2 mg/kg) is preferred.[27]

### Massive Blood Transfusion

Intraoperatively, children may need transfusions exceeding 50% of total blood volume (TBV) in 3 hours or 100% TBV in 24 hours.[28] Problems associated with massive transfusion in children are: IV access, hypothermia, citrate toxicity and hyperkalaemia.[29,30] Paediatric massive transfusion protocols should be activated with packed red blood cells:fresh frozen plasma in a ratio of 1:1.[28,30] The management of massive bleeding using a massive transfusion protocol has been highlighted in **Flowchart 6**.[31] This is associated with higher survival rates in paediatric trauma cases.

## ELECTROLYTE IMBALANCE

Pre-operative assessment of electrolytes, especially in dehydrated children, is important. These need to be corrected early by establishing peripheral IV access. Hyperkalaemia occurs during massive transfusion due to the higher potassium concentration in stored blood. Potassium levels have to be monitored during rapid transfusions. Management includes larger bore peripheral IV catheters, calcium, glucose-insulin infusions, frusemide, correcting acidosis and preferring fresh red blood cells with an infusion rate of 0.5 ml/kg/min to avoid hyperkalaemia, especially in infants.[28-30] Transfusion-associated hyperkalaemia-induced cardiac arrest can occur.

**Flowchart 6:** Massive transfusion protocol.[31]

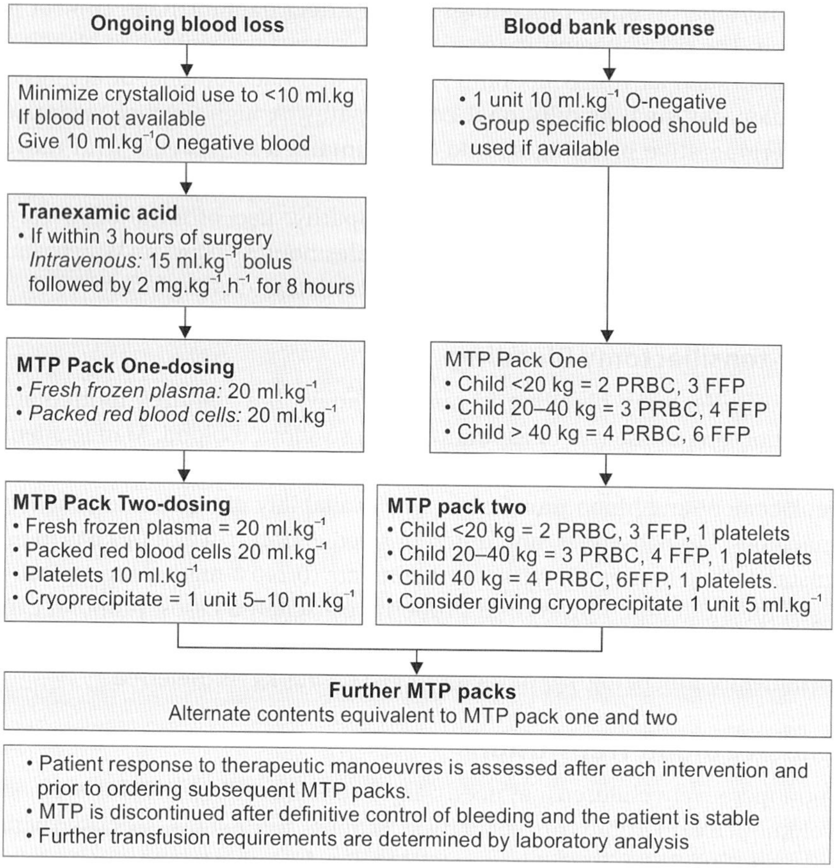


(MTP: massive transfusion protocol; PRBC: packed red blood cells; FFP: fresh frozen plasma; Neg: NEGATIVE)

*Source:* Blain S, Paterson N. Pediatric massive transfusion BJA Educ. 2016;16(8):269-75.

## GASTROINTESTINAL EMERGENCIES

### Post-operative Nausea and Vomiting

Post-operative nausea and vomiting (PONV) can significantly affect surgical recovery. The major risk factors include age > 3 years, surgery lasting > 30 minutes and strabismus or tonsillectomy surgery. Family or previous history of motion sickness are also associated with increased risk of PONV. Opioids or inhalational agents can cause PONV.[32] Vomiting in Children score (POVOC) and the vomiting in the postoperative period score (VPOP) can be used for risk stratification. The management of PONV includes reducing modifiable risk factors and avoiding general anaesthesia wherever possible, minimising fasting duration and ensuring ample hydration. Ondansetron and dexamethasone are commonly used. Metoclopramide and prochlorperazine are alternatives for PONV, but they can be associated with extrapyramidal side effects, sedation and neuroleptic malignant syndrome.[33]

### Paralytic Ileus

Post-operative ileus may be caused by wound infections or anastomotic leaks. Symptoms include abdominal pain and distension, vomiting, nausea and intolerance to feeds. Restricting IV fluids, avoiding drains and tubes and encouraging early ambulation and oral intake can prevent ileus. Strategies such as carbohydrate loading, regional anaesthesia and prophylactic antiemetics have been effective.

## METABOLIC AND ENDOCRINE EMERGENCIES

### Hypoglycaemia

A plasma glucose level of <30 mg/dl in the first 24 hours of life and <45 mg/dl thereafter constitutes hypoglycaemia in the newborn. In children, a blood glucose value of less than 40 mg/dl represents hypoglycaemia. Severe symptomatic hypoglycaemia should be corrected with an IV 10% dextrose bolus of 2 ml/kg or intramuscular glucagon. The dose of glucagon for a neonate is 0.03–0.1 mg/kg (maximum 1 mg); for <25 kg is 0.5 mg, and for ≥25 kg is 1.0 mg. Some infants of diabetic mothers may require up to 0.3 mg/kg to a maximum dose of 1 mg. The child should start to feed, and blood glucose should be rechecked within 15 minutes. Blood glucose should return to the normal range within 10–15 minutes and remain so for 1 hour. If blood glucose is still found to be low, then maintenance fluids with dextrose should be initiated (for neonates, 10% dextrose should be initiated at 60 ml/kg/day and for older children, 0.9% saline with 5% dextrose at maintenance rates). If another blood sugar reading in 30 minutes is found to be low, maintenance fluids should be increased to 10% dextrose. Persistent hypoglycaemia should warrant consultation with an endocrinologist and/or metabolic specialist. It is a critical perioperative emergency, particularly in infants and children with metabolic disorders. Immediate treatment includes the IV administration of glucose and monitoring of blood sugar levels.

### Adrenal Crisis

Adrenal crisis manifests as acute deterioration of general status along with haemodynamic disturbances and electrolyte imbalance, and is a life-threatening emergency. Treatment includes IV hydrocortisone and correction of electrolyte and fluid deficits.[34] Patients with suspected adrenal crisis should receive immediate treatment with IV injection of 100 mg (50 mg/m$^2$ for young children) hydrocortisone, following which appropriate fluid resuscitation should be administered, as well as 200 mg (50–100 mg/m$^2$ for children) of hydrocortisone/24 hours (by way of continuous IV therapy or 6-hourly injection). If hydrocortisone is unavailable, prednisolone may be used. Dexamethasone is least preferred, as its onset of action is slow.

## NEUROLOGICAL COMPLICATIONS IN PAEDIATRIC PATIENTS

### Seizures in the Perioperative Period

Seizures in the perioperative period can be triggered by general anaesthetics or drugs with pro-convulsant properties such as sevoflurane, isoflurane, LAs, etomidate, propofol and opioids. The patient-related factors contributing to perioperative seizures are withdrawal of anti-epileptic drugs, switching to alternative drugs, co-morbid conditions including cerebrovascular disease, fever, hypoglycaemia, systemic infections and metabolic disorders.[35] Moreover, intraoperative hyperventilation-induced electroencephalographic changes are seen in 95% of paediatric patients with a history of epilepsy as compared to 40% of adults.[36] Management includes general resuscitative measures to support the airway and cardiovascular system, along with IV administration of benzodiazepines, which is a first-line treatment. In the operating room, injection of thiopentone can be the first choice.[37] Treatment of the primary cause is essential. Furthermore, it is important to avoid hyperventilation in seizure-prone paediatric patients in whom sevoflurane is being used.[36] The recommended maintenance dose of sevoflurane is below 1.5 minimum alveolar concentration (MAC).[38] Benzodiazepine premedication is also advised for prevention.

### Increased Intracranial Pressure

Raised ICP is usually caused by any space-occupying lesion, raised intra-thoracic pressure, biting the tube or jugular vein compression. Management includes deepening the plane of anaesthesia, 30° head elevation, hyperventilation, avoiding neck and tube compression and administration of drugs such as mannitol and diuretics.[39]

## EMERGENCIES DURING THE POST-OPERATIVE PERIOD

In paediatric anaesthesia, the emergence and postoperative periods are as crucial as induction and intraoperative management. The recovery phase includes emergence from anaesthesia in the operation theatre, patient transport to the postoperative care unit (PACU) or recovery area, PACU stay, and finally, transfer to the ward or discharge. Common postoperative issues include pain, anxiety, agitation, delirium, nausea, vomiting, delayed emergence, respiratory distress/insufficiency and haemodynamic disturbances.

## Post-operative Agitation and Emergence Delirium

The terms post-operative agitation and emergence delirium (ED) are often used interchangeably for a period of behavioural dysregulation after emergence from general anaesthesia. Agitation is an 'unpleasant state of extreme arousal,' and can be a commonly observed symptom in patients suffering from pain, anxiety, fear, and more complex neurobehavioural syndromes such as delirium. Paediatric patients commonly exhibit abnormal behaviour in the setting of unfamiliar stressors; therefore, post-operative agitation alone will not always suggest delirium. ED is characterised by agitation, thrashing, incoherence, or inconsolability.[40] Prompt control is necessary to prevent self-injury, or the child may pull out IV cannulae, nasogastric tube, surgical drains, etc. Firstly, non-pharmacological means such as tender loving care, early feeding, etc. should be tried. Prophylactic use of IV propofol(1 mg/kg), ketamine(0.25 mg/kg), dexmedetomidine (0.15 μg/kg), fentanyl (1–2.5 μg/kg), and clonidine(2 μg/kg) can help prevent ED or at least reduce the severity.[41] Inhalational agents such as sevoflurane and desflurane are known to increase the incidence of ED.[40] Emergence agitation/ ED is often due to pain or urinary retention, especially after prolonged surgery or exposure to anaesthetics. Use of IV or neuraxial opioids increases the incidence of urinary retention. Intrathecal or epidural LAs act on the sacral and lumbar nerve fibres, and thereby block the transmission of afferent and efferent nervous impulses from the bladder, leading to urinary retention. Treatment of urinary retention is by catheterisation.

Post-operative pain management includes the use of oral non-steroidal anti-inflammatory drugs and paracetamol as soon as oral intake can be started. Opioid analgesics can be used for rescue analgesia after non-opioids.

## Oxygen Desaturation (Hypoxia)

In children, arterial oxygen saturation ($SpO_2 < 93\%$) post-operatively is a cause for concern. Causes include bleeding, retained throat packs, hypoventilation due to airway obstruction, inadequate reversal, respiratory depression, or the effect of residual anaesthetics.[42] The child can present with paradoxical see-saw breathing pattern, intercostal indrawing, subcostal retractions, sternal recession and tracheal tug. Adequate reversal needs to be assessed through clinical signs and neuromuscular monitoring. However, if it is due to opioid overdose (characterised by low respiratory rate, breathing on stimulation), it can be reversed with naloxone [(1) Neonates: Initial dose: 0.01 mg/kg IV, intramuscular, or subcutaneously; repeat dose every 2–3 minutes as needed. (2) Children: Initial dose: 0.01 mg/kg IV; if desired response not obtained, give 0.1 mg/kg IV]. The management includes treating the cause, nursing the child in the recovery position (left lateral position with neck extended), airway manoeuvres, improving ventilation, and oxygen therapy. High-frequency nasal oxygenation may be employed for short-term therapy for post-operative hypoxia due to pulmonary atelectasis.

## Post-intubation Croup

Croup presents as stridor or a 'barky' cough, and respiratory distress due to tracheal mucosal oedema, which can be a result of PRAE. Treatment involves nursing the child in the recovery position, nebulised epinephrine (up to 0.5 ml/kg of L-epinephrine 1:1,000 up to 5 ml) and dexamethasone 0.6 mg/kg IV (maximum 10 mg).[42]

## Post-obstructive Pulmonary Oedema

It is usually observed after relieving airway obstruction. It results from high negative intrathoracic pressures. Management includes administration of continuous positive airway pressure (5–10 cm water) with a high concentration of oxygen, diuretics and fluid restriction. Severe cases can require intubation and mechanical ventilation with positive end-expiratory pressure.[43]

## Peri-operative Hypothermia

Hypothermia is defined as a core temperature below 36.5°C or 36.0°C in children up to 5 years of age and children older than 5 years, respectively.[44,45] In paediatrics, a higher risk of perioperative hypothermia (PH) is correlated with low birth weight neonates, infants and sick children.[46] PH can lead to cardiac events, wound infections, and coagulopathies. Preventive measures are crucial, as shown in the algorithm **(Flowchart 7)**.[47]

**Flowchart 7:** Preventive measures for perioperative hypothermia.[12]

**Intraoperative Period**

- Maintain **ambient OT at >23°C** during induction/recovery
- Infants: maintain **ambient OT > 25°C**
- Full-term, premature newborn: **27°C, 29°C** ***when patient is not draped***

*For any of these surgeries:*
- Arthroscopic knee surgeries
- Bronchoscopy
- Mastoidectomy
- Neurosurgery
- Thoracic surgeries
- Squint surgery

OR
- If surgery >60 minutes duration

OR
- Baby age</= 1 year

*Active warming intraoperative period:*
- Bair Hugger(with disposable blanket)
- Radiant warmer (age = years)
- Warmed irrigation fluids

±
- Core temperature monitoring

(OT: operation theatre)

*Source:* Sultana R, Allen JC, Slow YN, Bong CL, Lee SY. Development of local guidelines to prevent perioperative hypothermia in children: A prospective observational cohort study. Can J Anesth. 2022;69(11):1360-74.

## CONCLUSION

Early recognition and management of perioperative emergencies in paediatric patients are essential for positive outcomes. Adhering to established protocols, fostering teamwork, and proper communication can significantly reduce the risks associated with emergency situations in paediatric surgeries. Prevention always remains the best strategy for successful outcomes.

## REFERENCES


1. Whitten CE. 10 common pediatric airway problems-and their solutions. [Online] Available from https://www.anesthesiologynews.com/Review-Articles/Article/08-19/10-Common-Pediatric-Airway-Problems-And-Their-Solutions/55657 [Last accessed June, 2025].
2. Lee LK, Bernardo MKL, Grogan TR, Elashoff DA, Ren WHP. Perioperative respiratory adverse event risk assessment in children with upper respiratory tract infection: Validation of the COLDS score. Paediatr Anaesth. 2018;28(11): 1007-14.
3. Bhananker SM, Ramamoorthy C, Geiduschek JM, Posner KL, Domino KB, Haberkern CM, et al. Anesthesia-related cardiac arrest in children: update from the Pediatric Perioperative Cardiac Arrest Registry. Anesth Analg. 2007;105(2):344-50.
4. Malviya S, Swartz J, Lerman J. Are all preterm infants younger than 60 weeks postconceptual age at risk for postanesthetic apnea? Anesthesiology. 1993;78(6):1076-81.
5. Henderson-Smart DJ, Steer P. Postoperative caffeine for preventing apnea in preterm infants. Cochrane Database Syst Rev. 2000;2001(2):CD000048.
6. Oosthuizen A. Paediatric airway emergencies. SAAJA. 2021;27(6 Suppl 1):S42-52.
7. Habre W, Disma N, Virag K, Becke K, Hansen TG, Jöhr M, et al. Incidence of severe critical events in paediatric anaesthesia (APRICOT): a prospective multicentre observational study in 261 hospitals in Europe. Lancet Respir Med. 2017;5(5):412-25. Erratum in: Lancet Respir Med. 2017;5(5):e19. Erratum in: Lancet Respir Med. 2017;5(6):e22.
8. Gil Gavel, Walker RWM, Laryngospasm in anaesthesia. Continuing Educ Anaesth, Critic Care Pain. 2014;14(2):47-51.
9. Stehling LC. Management of the Airway. In: Barash PG, Cullen BF, Stoelting RK (Eds). Clinical Anesthesia. Philadelphia: JB Lippincott; 1992. pp. 685-709.
10. Looseley A. Management of bronchospasm during general anaesthesia. Update Anaesth. 2011;27:17-21.
11. Subramanyam R, Yeramaneni S, Hossain MM, Anneken AM, Varughese AM. Perioperative respiratory adverse events in pediatric ambulatory anesthesia: Development and validation of a risk prediction tool. Anesth Analg. 2016;122(5):1578-85.
12. Parthasarathy S, Ravishankar M. Tight bag. Indian J Anaesth. 2010;54(3):193-8.
13. Engelhardt T, Virag K, Veyckemans F, Habre W; APRICOT Group of the European Society of Anaesthesiology Clinical Trial Network. Airway management in paediatric anaesthesia in Europe-insights from APRICOT (Anaesthesia Practice In Children Observational Trial): a prospective multicentre observational study in 261 hospitals in Europe. Br J Anaesth. 2018;121(1):66-75.

14. R Newton, H Hack. Place of rapid sequence induction in paediatric anaesthesia. BJA Educ. 2016;16(4):120-3.
15. Kafalı HC, Ergül Y. Common supraventricular and ventricular arrhythmias in children. Turk Arch Pediatr. 2022;57(5):476-88.
16. American Heart Association. Handbook of Emergency Cardiovascular Care for Healthcare Providers, 1st edition. Texas: Amer Heart Assn Inc; 2015.
17. de Graaff JC, Frykholm P. Ephedrine to treat intraoperative hypotension in infants: what is the target? Br J Anaesth. 2023;130(5):510-5.
18. Mehra B, Gupta S. Common pediatric medical emergencies in office practice. Indian J Pediatr. 2018;85(1):35-43.
19. Foz C, Staffa SJ, Brown ML, DiNardo JA, Nasr VJ. Predictors and outcomes of perioperative cardiac arrest in children undergoing noncardiac surgery. BJA Open. 2023;8:100244.
20. Gong CL, Hu JP, Qiu ZL, Zhu QQ, Hei ZQ, Zhou SL, et al. A study of anaesthesia-related cardiac arrest from a Chinese tertiary hospital. BMC Anesthesiol. 2018;18(1):127.
21. Arpa SR, Chaikittisilpa N, Srikongrak S, Udomnak S, Aroonpruksakul N, Kiatchai T. Incidences and outcomes of intra-operative vs. postoperative paediatric cardiac arrest: A retrospective cohort study of 42 776 anaesthetics in children who underwent noncardiac surgery in a Thai tertiary care hospital. Eur J Anaesthesiol. 2023;40(7):483-94.
22. Walker BJ, Long JB, Sathyamoorthy M, Birstler J, Wolf C, Bosenberg AT, et al. Complications in pediatric regional anesthesia: an analysis of more than 100,000 blocks from the pediatric regional anesthesia network. Anesthesiology. 2018;129(4):721-32.
23. Ramesh AS, Boretsky K. Local anesthetic systemic toxicity in children: a review of recent case reports and current literature. Reg Anesth Pain Med. 2021;46(10):909-14.
24. Groban L. Central nervous system and cardiac effects from long-acting amide local anesthetic toxicity in the intact animal model. Reg Anesth Pain Med. 2003;28(1):3-11.
25. Gitman M, Barrington MJ. Local anesthetic systemic toxicity: a review of recent case reports and registries. Reg Anesth Pain Med. 2018;43(2):124-30.
26. Dontukurthy S, Tobias JD. Update on local anesthetic toxicity, prevention and treatment during regional anesthesia in infants and children. J Pediatr Pharmacol Ther. 2021;26(5):445-54.
27. Lee AC, Haché M. Pediatric Anesthesia management for post-tonsillectomy bleed: Current status and future directions. Int J Gen Med. 2022;15:63-9.
28. Goobie SM, Haas T. Perioperative bleeding management in pediatric patients. Curr Opin Anaesthesiol. 2016;29(3):352-8.
29. Diab Y, Wong E, Luban N. Massive transfusion in children and neonates. Br J Haematol. 2013;161(1):15-6.
30. Noland DK, Apelt N, Greenwell C, Tweed J, Notrica DM, Garcia NM, et al. Massive transfusion in pediatric trauma: an ATOMAC perspective. J Pediatr Surg. 2019;54(2):345-9.
31. Blain S, Paterson N. Pediatric massive transfusion. BJA Educ. 2016;16(8):269-75.
32. Martin S, Baines D, Holtby H, Carr A. Guidelines on the prevention of post-operative vomiting in children. London: The Association of Paediatric Anaesthetists of Great Britain & Ireland; 2016.

33. Morrison C, Wilmshurst S. Postoperative vomiting in children. BJA Educ. 2019;19(10):329-33.
34. Mushtaq T, Ali SR, Boulos N, Boyle R, Cheetham T, Davies JH, et al. Developed by the Paediatric Adrenal Insufficiency Group on behalf of the British Society for Paediatric Endocrinology and Diabetes (BSPED). Emergency and perioperative management of adrenal insufficiency in children and young people: British Society for Paediatric Endocrinology and Diabetes consensus guidance. Arch Dis Child. 2023;108(11):871-8.
35. Murdoch D. Mechanisms of status epilepticus: an evidence-based review. Curr Opin Neurol. 2007;20(2):213-6.
36. Perks A, Cheema S, Mohanraj R. Anaesthesia and epilepsy. Br J Anaesth. 2012;108(4):562-71.
37. Constant I, Seeman R, Murat I. Sevoflurane and epileptiform EEG changes. Paediatr Anaesth. 2005;15(4):266-74.
38. Akeson J, Didriksson I. Convulsions on anaesthetic induction with sevoflurane in young children. Acta Anaesthesiol Scand. 2004;48(4):405-7.
39. Kukreti V, Mohseni-Bod H, Drake J. Management of raised intracranial pressure in children with traumatic brain injury. J Pediatr Neurosci. 2014;9(3):207-15.
40. Kararmaz A, Kaya S, Turhanoglu S, Ozyilmaz MA. Oral ketamine premedication can prevent emergence agitation in children after desflurane anaesthesia. Pediatr Anesth. 2004;14(6):477-82.
41. Chen J, Li W, Hu X, Wang D. Emergence agitation after cataract surgery in children: A comparison of midazolam, propofol and ketamine. Pediatr Anesth. 2010;20(9):873-9.
42. Pawar D. Common post-operative complications in children. Indian J Anaesth. 2012;56(5):496-501.
43. Bolaji BO, Oyedepo OO, Dunmade AD, Afolabi OA. Negative pressure pulmonary oedema following adenoidectomy under general anaesthesia: A case series. West Afr J Med. 2011;30(2):121-4.
44. Bajwa SJS, Swati. Perioperative Hypothermia in pediatric patients: diagnosis, prevention and management. Anaesth Pain Intens Care. 2014;18(2014):97-100.
45. Nemeth M, Miller C, Bräuer A. Perioperative hypothermia in children. Int J Environ Res Public Health. 2021;18(14):7541.
46. Tander B, Baris S, Karakaya D, Ariturk E, Rizalar R, Bernay F. Risk factors influencing inadvertent hypothermia in infants and neonates during anesthesia. Paediatr Anaesth. 2005;15(7):574-9.
47. Sultana R, Allen JC, Slow YN, Bong CL, Lee SY. Development of local guidelines to prevent perioperative hypothermia in children: A prospective observational cohort study. Can J Anesth. 2022;69(11):1360-74.

CHAPTER 12

# Updates on Massive Blood Transfusion Protocol: Ensure You are Up to Date on This Critical Procedure

*Geeta Kamal, Mridul Dhar, Neeru Sahni*

## ABSTRACT

Adult protocols for blood loss and massive transfusion management cannot be extrapolated to the paediatric age group due to a large difference in physiological reserve and the body's response to haemorrhagic insult. Definitions of massive blood transfusion as well as activation triggers vary in the absence of robust data in children. Preventive strategies such as damage control resuscitation and perioperative blood conservation strategies can help mitigate the risk of massive blood transfusion. Point-of-care diagnostic modalities such as thromboelastography may have an increasing use in children and help in providing targeted blood product therapy. Existing massive blood transfusion protocols in hospitals must be audited for quality improvement through multidisciplinary coordination and proper documentation of transfusion metrics as well as adverse events. Future scope includes more use of whole blood, synthetic blood replacements, and use of artificial intelligence to better predict patient outcomes in paediatric patients.

***Keywords:*** Blood coagulation factors, Blood transfusion, Haemorrhage, Haemostasis, Thromboelastography.

## INTRODUCTION

Blood loss and strategies to manage the same have been sparsely studied in the paediatric population, and the protocols framed for adults cannot be followed due to significant differences between the adult and paediatric populations. Moreover, generalised management strategies cannot be applied to children in all age groups as smaller children have a different physiology from that of 10- to 12-year-olds.

Developmentally, the haemostatic system is underdeveloped at birth, the levels of anticoagulant and procoagulant proteins are low and the platelets are qualitatively dysfunctional. All these reach maturity by about 6 months of age. Still, due to a large physiological reserve, children tolerate a relatively larger volume of blood loss. Based on the evidence, over time, the practice of massive blood transfusion has evolved to improve outcomes.[1]

## DEFINITION OF MASSIVE BLOOD TRANSFUSION

Due to changes in blood volume with age, it is a difficult task to define massive transfusion in the paediatric population. It has been defined as a

**BOX 1:** Definitions of massive blood transfusion in paediatrics.

- Transfusion of 50% of total blood volume in 3 hours
- Transfusion of 100% of total blood volume in 24 hours
- 100 ml/kg for premature neonates
- 90 ml/kg for mature neonates
- 80 ml/kg for infants
- 70–80 ml/kg for older children
- 40 ml/kg within the first 24 hours
- >37 ml/kg every 4-hourly time point

transfusion of 50% of total blood volume in 3 hours or a transfusion of 100% of total blood volume in 24 hours. The blood volume conversion factors need to be considered which are 100 ml/kg for premature neonates, 90 ml/kg for mature neonates, 80 ml/kg for infants and 70–80 ml/kg for older children.

An alternative definition of massive transfusion is the administration of 40 ml/kg of blood within the first 24 hours. Although this criterion shows high sensitivity and specificity for identifying children at risk of mortality beyond 24 hours, it is inherently affected by survival bias, as not all patients survive long enough to meet this threshold. In the Trauma Quality Improvement Project (TQIP), it has been suggested to define massive transfusion as >37 ml/kg every 4-hourly time point **(Box 1)**. Another issue is the limitation of applying these definitions in perioperative settings. The clinical settings are not the same as research settings, making the identification of patients developing massive blood loss unpredictable.[2,3]

## PATHOPHYSIOLOGY OF MASSIVE BLOOD LOSS

Massive blood loss can either disrupt the vessel structure or derange the coagulation cascade. Due to decreasing blood volume, there is a fall in cardiac output as well as oxygen delivery, resulting in a mismatch of oxygen consumption and delivery. In the initial phase, the oxygen extraction might increase, but over a prolonged course, this oxygen consumption occurring in response to tissue acidosis and hypoxia also starts decreasing. This will affect the organs such as the brain and intestine that are less tolerant to hypoxia.[4]

Trauma patients are at an increased risk of shock and coagulopathy. A decrease in pre-load reduces cardiac output and oxygen delivery, leading to shock. An alteration in blood redox potential and increase in adrenergic mediators and lactic acidosis occurs. Shock, along with injury, results in endothelial damage leading to inflammation as well as haemostatic dysfunction. Reduced oxygen delivery with endothelial cell damage and impaired haemostatic function ultimately precipitates 'trauma-induced blood failure'. The blood failure is characterised by coagulopathy, endotheliopathy and immune dysfunction **(Flowchart 1)**. The ongoing

**Flowchart 1:** Pathophysiology of massive blood loss.

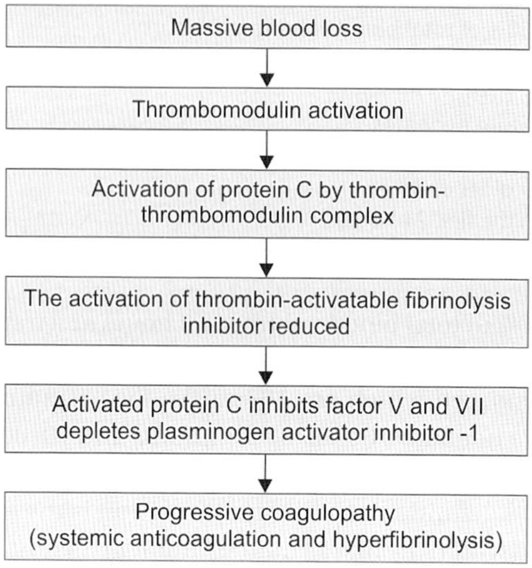


dilution of plasma and consumption of coagulation factors and platelets, in addition to acidosis and hypothermia, further exacerbate the blood failure.[2]

# CONSIDERATIONS DURING MASSIVE BLOOD TRANSFUSION PROTOCOL

## Blood Product Ratios and Variation in Practice

The evidence for an optimum blood product ratio usage in paediatric massive blood transfusion is sparse. Cannon et al. did not find survival benefits with the use of high fresh frozen plasma (FFP) to packed red blood cell (PRBC) ratio (>1:2), but Cunningham et al. found high survival in the high ratio group, i.e. (≥1:1) FFP to PRBC ratios.[5,6] In another study, Noland et al. also found a survival benefit with a 1:1 PRBC:FFP ratio in paediatric patients requiring massive transfusion.[7]

The TQIP database which is a large database reported a 51% decrease in mortality following resuscitation using high (>1:1 FFP:PRBC) ratios with an adjusted relative risk of 0.49 and 95% confidence interval of 0.27–0.87. Thus, it may be apt to use at least 1:1 FFP:RBC ratios in paediatric massive transfusion protocols (MTPs), especially if there is a non-availability of viscoelastic haemostatic assays.[2]

FFP transfusion can be considered in the dose of 10–20 ml/kg up to a maximal single dose of four units in paediatric massive blood loss.

Additionally, the inventory of O negative blood group should be made available which helps in immediate resuscitation in patients with massive blood loss, especially in trauma.

## Haemostatic Adjuncts

Tranexamic acid (TXA) is a lysine analogue that inhibits plasminogen activation and fibrinolysis. By preventing plasmin development and fibrin breakdown, it prevents the disruption of clots. The PED-TRAX study data and that from adult studies support the use of TXA in paediatric massive blood transfusion. Evidence from the Cochrane review suggests that the use of TXA in paediatrics significantly reduces the transfusion requirement in children undergoing surgery without causing any adverse effects.

On the contrary, the evidence so far does not support the incorporation of recombinant factor VIIa (rFVIIa) into paediatric massive blood transfusion. Even in the adult population, it may not be used for patients other than those with bleeding diathesis such as haemophilia.[2,3]

The use of prothrombin complex concentrate (PCC) in the setting of massive transfusion is one of its off-label uses, and there is no definite evidence for the same. It must be remembered that PCC lacks factor V; hence, it is not beneficial as a single agent. FFP will need to be given along with it.

## Activation Triggers

Since the arrangement and transfusion of a blood product is very regulated as well as an intensively laborious process, one should be able to predict when to activate an MTP. Currently available scoring systems in paediatric patients can predict mortality but cannot be used to predict which patient will require a blood transfusion, leaving the decision to the discretion of the clinician. Many a times, there can be issues of either inconsistent utilisation or ineffective transfusion or both due to this. There is a centre-wise difference in practices with some centres practising the release of the first packet (including PRBC, plasma and platelets) at every trauma activation and other centres emphasising initial crystalloid resuscitation followed by partial activation of MTP.[2,3]

Clinically, the failure to respond to initial crystalloid transfusion is considered as a decision point for activation of MTP. Some authors suggest that every high-acuity trauma be considered an activation trigger for MTP in paediatrics. In the absence of any scoring system, the clinician's discretion using clinical signs such as tachycardia, reduced capillary filling, cold extremities, pallor and decreased urine output in the clinical setting of haemorrhage may be considered an activation trigger for MTP.[2]

The communication of MTP activation is an area for simulation training. A designated person to call the blood bank, an MTP card from the operating room or emergency room with specific blood and blood product requirements and a closed-loop communication are needed.

### Diagnostic Adjuncts

Point-of-care coagulation tests such as thromboelastography (TEG) and rotational thromboelastometry (ROTEM) have evidence-based practice potential to guide the administration of blood products. These two viscoelastic haemostatic assays are useful in patients who require massive transfusion because the traditional laboratory tests (haemogram and coagulogram) cannot keep pace with such clinical situations where a patient is bleeding heavily. TEG and ROTEM provide immediate feedback and can guide specific blood component therapy, mitigating potential complications. TEG and ROTEM parameters are available for paediatric patients, but their use is yet not a main component of any of the paediatric MTPs.[2,3]

## PREVENTIVE STRATEGIES FOR MASSIVE BLOOD LOSS

### Damage Control Resuscitation

Damage control resuscitation (DCR) has classically been described for trauma patients. Similar principles can also be applied to perioperative surgical trauma and haemorrhagic shock as well, especially in paediatric patients. The core aim of DCR is to prevent hypothermia, acidosis and coagulopathy. The broad principles of DCR include the following:

- *Early and appropriate venous access:* The largest possible catheter or venous access should be obtained early. Pressure bags are useful for the rapid delivery of fluids in children as compared to commercial rapid infusers.[8] Intraosseous access or central access can be obtained early if intravenous (IV) access is difficult to secure, especially in trauma cases or loss of IV access in surgical cases.[9]
- *Rapid and early bleeding control:* Non-surgical means include mechanical pressure and the use of tourniquets.[8] Urgent surgical control of bleeding is also a priority in both perioperative and trauma cases. In rare cases, embolisation of bleeding sources also has a role in DCR when surgical control fails.
- *Avoidance of over-resuscitation with crystalloids:* Prevent haemodilution and avoid overcorrecting the losses till bleeding is controlled, with the aim to maintain vital organ perfusion. Hypotensive resuscitation or permissive hypotension is to be done with caution in children and may be useful if the source of bleeding is arterial.[8,10] Excess crystalloid use has been found to increase the odds of mechanical ventilation as well as longer hospital stays in paediatric trauma.[11]
- *Appropriate blood use:* Use of balanced blood product ratios to prevent coagulopathy or early administration of whole blood if available.[11] The availability of pedipacks of blood and blood components prevents wastage of blood products, especially in smaller children, infants and

neonates. Details about patient blood management have been discussed in previous sections.

- *Use of adjuncts:* Topical haemostatic agents such as fibrin/thrombin or TXA-impregnated gauze pieces can be applied over the bleeding source for wound packing during trauma or surgery.
- *Prevent hypothermia and treat acidosis:* Warm IV fluids and blood products are to be given, in addition to active warming of the patient. In operative cases, pre-induction warming and intraoperative maintenance of normothermia are essential. Ideally, equipment such as blood warmers, in-line fluid warmers, surface warmers and continuous core temperature monitors should be available.

## Blood Conservation Strategies

The basic principle of patient blood management is to optimise red cell mass with interventions starting from the pre-operative to the post-operative period so that the risks of transfusion-related complications can be minimised.[10,12] The various techniques are as follows:

- *Pre-operative diagnosis and treatment of anaemia*: Pre-operative anaemia is associated with poor outcomes in non-cardiac surgical paediatric and neonatal patients. Iron deficiency anaemia is one of the most common causes. Treatment options include oral/parenteral iron, erythropoietin, folate and vitamin B12. IV iron preparations have been found to be safer and more effective than oral iron in children. Erythropoietin use has concerns of thrombosis, but no clear evidence has been demonstrated in the current data. A combination of all the above measures has been found to produce a significant reduction in perioperative transfusions.[10,12]
- *Treatment of pre-existing coagulopathy/disorders of haemostasis:* This includes diseases such as von Willebrand disease and Haemophilias.[9]
- *Prevent iatrogenic anaemia:* Minimal essential blood sample volume should be drawn for investigations, especially from younger patients with lower absolute blood volumes.[10]
- *Antifibrinolytics:* These have been recommended in high-risk paediatric surgery such as cardiac, craniofacial and spine surgeries.[10,13] TXA and epsilon aminocaproic acid (EACA) have been found to increase survival[3] and reduce intraoperative blood loss as well as requirements of blood transfusions in paediatric patients. Doses recommended for TXA range from 10 to 30 mg/kg loading dose (lower range in children < 1 year of age), followed by an infusion of 5–10 mg/kg/h, to maintain a plasma concentration of 20–70 μg/ml. For EACA, a loading dose of 40 mg/kg followed by 30 mg/kg/h has been recommended. In the above doses, no major side effects have been observed in the current data.[10,12,14]
- *Haemodilution:* Both acute normovolaemic haemodilution and hypervolaemic haemodilution have been found to be beneficial compared

to no conservation strategy in cranial vault and spine surgery.[10,14] These also require careful monitoring of coagulopathy using point-of-care tests and assays. Subjects should be considered based on their age, pre-operative haemoglobin and type of surgery.[14]

- *Induced or deliberate hypotension:* They should be used with caution in paediatric patients as they have variable physiology and limited clinical vital signs for assessment. Their use should be avoided in combination with reduction in haematocrit and congenital heart disease.[10] Limited data is available on children with trauma and for surgery.[10,13]
- *Pre-operative vessel embolisation:* It is useful in specific situations such as arteriovenous malformation or highly vascular tumours. Anaesthesia may be required for the embolisation procedure.[9]
- *Surgical interventions:* Surgical techniques should be aimed to minimise bleeding, and staged operations are planned to limit losses in a single sitting.
- *Cell salvage:* Initial data shows a trend towards fewer post-operative transfusions and coagulation factor replacement.[10] It has also been shown to be cost-effective in addition to a decreased incidence of thrombosis and mechanical ventilation days. The use of smaller bowls has led to earlier and faster processing of salvaged blood with a decrease in the incidence of transfusion-related hyperkalaemia and acidosis.[10,13] The technique is useful in cases of blood loss > 20–40% of blood volume.[9,13] Caution should be exercised with the use of this technique in cases of malignancy and sepsis.[9,14]
- *Restrictive transfusion strategy and thresholds:* There is a large variation in data regarding appropriate transfusion thresholds in a largely variable paediatric age group. But excluding neonates and those with congenital heart disease, a restrictive trigger of 7 g/dl has been found to be beneficial in avoiding the complications of excessive product transfusion.[10,12]

## MONITORING AND TERMINATION OF MASSIVE TRANSFUSION PROTOCOLS

### Monitoring During Massive Transfusion Protocol

- Clinical and haemodynamic monitoring (blood pressure, heart rate, temperature, urine output, pulse oximetry, near-infrared spectroscopy and echocardiography)
- Blood gas monitoring (lactate, base deficit and mixed venous saturation)
- Viscoelastic point-of-care testing (TEG, ROTEM)
- Biochemical laboratory testing (haemoglobin, platelet count, potassium, calcium, magnesium, glucose and coagulation factors if available)
- Monitoring and documentation of blood products given and any adverse events during MTP activation and before it[9,14]
- The group of blood components compatible with the patient's blood group can be identified and transfused in case of non-availability of the same blood group components.

### Termination of Massive Transfusion Protocol

Timely recognition and termination of a MTP is equally essential as its activation, in order to prevent the complications of overtransfusion to the patient and the unnecessary issue of and wastage of blood products.

- Broadly, a MTP should formally be terminated when the bleeding is definitively controlled and the haemodynamic parameters are stable with minimal or reduced vasopressor support and transfusion rate.[14] Goal-directed targeted therapy is ideal for making these clinical decisions using the above-mentioned monitoring modalities.
- TEG or ROTEM can help in guiding real time which specific blood products are required and can be stopped after achieving normalisation of the values.[9]
- Specific treatment targets include a fibrinogen level of >150 mg/dl (>200 mg/dl in cardiac surgery), a platelet count of >50,000/μL (>100,000/μL in intracranial haemorrhage) and an international normalised ratio of <1.8.[14] Haemoglobin levels may not accurately reflect post-massive transfusion, and other markers of adequate tissue oxygen delivery (e.g. lactate < 2 mmol/L, an adequate urine output > 1 ml/kg/h) should also be considered to target a haemoglobin of 7–9 g/dl.[9,13,14]

## LIMITATIONS AND CHALLENGES OF MASSIVE TRANSFUSION PROTOCOLS

Barriers and challenges in the uniform implementation and standardisation of MTP include the following:

- A relatively small sample of patients is available, with a lack of large multicentre studies.
- There is ambiguity in the actual adherence or fulfilment of MTP criteria or blood product ratios due to the unique challenges of venous access in the paediatric age group.
- Often, there is a lag or difference in availability of packed cells versus plasma or platelets or the time it takes to deliver each component.
- Lack of infrastructure and a well-established blood bank
- Lack of monitoring of complications and documentation and reporting of MTP events, especially in the middle of a crisis scenario[15]
- Lack of point-of-care monitoring for better titration of product transfusion
- Due to the lack of set protocols in this paediatric subset of patients, there may be overactivation or unnecessary activation of MTP, which may lead to wastage of blood products and complications of overtransfusion, which are more detrimental in the paediatric age group[15]

## COMPLICATIONS OF MASSIVE BLOOD TRANSFUSION

The complications arising from a massive blood transfusion in paediatric haemorrhage are dependent on the number of units transfused, rate of transfusion and patient factors.

A brief overview of these is as follows:

- *Immunological reactions*: These include allergic, haemolytic and febrile non-haemolytic reactions. It is better to use leucoreduced and phenotypically matched blood to prevent alloimmunisation. Transfusion-related acute lung injury, transfusion-related immunomodulation and graft-versus-host disease may also be seen.[9]
- *Metabolic derangements*: The most common metabolic derangements are hypocalcaemia (due to citrate preservatives in packed cells) and hyperkalaemia (old stored packed cells). Neonates are at a higher risk of hypocalcaemia due to the inability to metabolise citrate and may require IV calcium supplementation. Hyperkalaemia can be prevented by using freshly packed or washed blood cells.[9,13] Hypomagnesaemia and hypokalaemia may also be observed.
- *Coagulopathy and hypothermia*: Trauma-related activation of protein C leads to inhibition of factors V and VIII, contributing to coagulopathy, in addition to transfusion-related dilutional coaguloapthy. Hypothermia is common if large volumes of cold blood products are administered rapidly which further decreases coagulation factor activity. Severe hypocalcaemia also hampers coagulation activation.[13]
- *Other systemic complications*: Infection/sepsis, transfusion-related circulatory overload and air embolism in rare cases of use of rapid fluid infusers[13]

## MASSIVE TRANSFUSION PROTOCOL AS A HOSPITAL POLICY AND PATIENT OUTCOMES

Hospitals catering to paediatric trauma and paediatric surgery should aim to develop standardised protocols and processes for the efficient implementation of massive blood transfusion protocols in these subgroups of patients. Recent reviews have analysed the limited available literature on the efficacy of the implementation of MTP in paediatric centres.[3,16,17] Widely cited retrospective studies by Chidester et al. and Hendrickson et al. found no significant advantage of MTP activation in terms of mortality compared to traditional non-MTP groups, with a clinical trend of a worse outcome with MTP implementation.[18-20] However, in the above-mentioned as well as other similar studies, the time to first transfusion was significantly shorter in the MTP-implemented patients. In addition, the incidence of thromboembolic events was lower in the MTP group.[3,19] As already suggested, at least 1:1 FFP:RBC ratios in paediatric MTPs have a mortality benefit, especially in the absence of viscoelastic haemostatic assays.[2,21] The limitation of this analysis is that due to a lack of standardised protocols, different institutes had variable definitions and triggers, as well as management guidelines for MTP, including the ratios of blood products used. Another issue was the ambiguity regarding the actual complete implementation of the MTP.[15]

To summarise, till further concrete data is available, it is prudent to try and set up a formal MTP and use more physiologically balanced blood product ratios.

## QUALITY IMPROVEMENT OF MASSIVE TRANSFUSION PROTOCOLS

Multidisciplinary coordination between a motivated group of stakeholders is essential for the success of a MTP policy.[16] Training using simulation is a great tool to establish practices of clear communication as well as assignment of roles in a crisis scenario. Perioperative crisis simulation training of anaesthesiology trainees as well as physicians should try to incorporate multidisciplinary exercises which can include surgeons and blood bank personnel as well.[11] Team briefing during the time-out period before surgery should include a detailed discussion of blood management strategy in cases at high risk of massive haemorrhage, especially in paediatric cases, where the margins of error are minimal. Allocation of roles for blood product handling, labelling and documentation should also be done.[13]

*Quality assessment and improvement:* The quality and success of an existing MTP of a hospital must be assessed at regular intervals. The various metrics that can be used for this include the following:

- Time taken from activation of MTP to deliver the blood products and time taken to recognise the need for activation of MTP by physicians
- Clinical outcomes such as morbidity and mortality
- Transfusion metrics such as the ability to achieve balanced ratio transfusion or as per hospital protocol and the number of total products administered within a time frame
- Adverse event documentation such as allergic reactions, transfusion-related circulatory overload and lung injury
- Resource utilisation and cost-benefit analysis, to avoid wastage of blood products
- Feedback from all stakeholder departments

Audit of the MTP should be followed by quality improvement initiatives. There should be a regular review and refinement of the MTP based on clinical experiences and multidisciplinary discussions.[11]

## FUTURE DIRECTIONS

- *Whole blood:* It is mostly used in paediatric patients in military setups. It is conventionally not used frequently in civilian setups due to issues with storage, shelf life and difficulty in processing, in addition to the fact that paediatric massive transfusion as an event is low in general.[16] Theoretically, whole blood is more physiological and less coagulopathic and avoids the extra volume of anticoagulants infused with each component of a balanced transfusion. Low-titre group O blood with platelet-specific filters has been developed to avoid the risk of transfusion reactions and haemolysis. Initial data on the use of whole blood in paediatric trauma has established its safety with no major complications, including concerns of platelet dysfunction.[15]

- *Need for standardisation of MTP:* There is an urgent need to generate prospective multicentre data on paediatric massive transfusion, transfusion triggers, blood product ratios and the overall efficacy of MTP in paediatric patients in terms of mortality and morbidity.
- *Use of haemoglobin-based oxygen carriers:* These are synthetic molecules which have been designed to replicate the function of haemoglobin-carrying capacity. They have the potential to have a longer shelf life and fewer compatibility issues compared to conventional blood products. Limited data is available in adults, and there is potential for research in children.[15,22,23]
- *Data management:* This includes the development of scoring systems for the early detection of the requirement for MTP activation using machine learning. This may be especially useful in paediatric patients to save precious time in a haemorrhagic emergency.[11,15]

## CONCLUSION

Massive blood transfusion is required to sustain the organ perfusion and tissue oxygenation, and thereby reduce morbidity and mortality following major surgeries and trauma in paediatric patients. Prompt recognition of the need for massive transfusion, DCR, coordination of team members, timely administration of required blood products as guided by point-of-care coagulation tests and the use of haemostatic agents can significantly reduce the mortality and morbidity in paediatric patients.

## REFERENCES


1. Cotton BA, Dossett LA, Au BK, Nunez TC, Robertson AM, Young PP. Room for (performance) improvement: provider-related factors associated with poor outcomes in massive transfusion. J Trauma. 2009;67(5):1004-12.
2. Neff LP, Beckwith MA, Russell RT, Cannon JW, Spinella PC. Massive transfusion in pediatric patients. Clin Lab Med. 2021;4:35-49.
3. Maw G, Furyk C. Pediatric massive transfusion: a systematic review. Pediatr Emerg Care. 2018;34:594-8.
4. Gonzalez KW, Desai AA, Dalton BG, Juang D. Hemorrhagic shock. J Pediatr Intensive Care. 2015;4:4-9.
5. Cannon JW, Johnson MA, Caskey RC, Borgman MA, Neff LP. High ratio plasma resuscitation does not improve survival in paediatric trauma patients. J Trauma Acute Care Surg. 2017;83:211-7.

6. Cunningham ME, Rosenfeld EH, Zhu H, Naik-Mathuria BJ, Russell RT, Vogel AM. A high ratio of plasma: RBC improves survival in massively transfused injured children. J Surg Res. 2019;233:213-20.
7. Noland DK, Apelt N, Greenwell C, Tweed J, Notrica DM, Garcia NM, et al. Massive transfusion in pediatric trauma: an ATOMAC perspective. J Pediatr Surg. 2019;54:345-9.
8. Gilley M, Beno S. Damage control resuscitation in pediatric trauma. Curr Opin Pediatr. 2018;30(3):338-43.
9. Spilka J, Goobie SM. (2020) Perioperative blood management in the pediatric patient. [online] Available from https://resources.wfsahq.org/wp-content/uploads/418_english.pdf. [Last accessed June, 2025]
10. Switzer T, Faraoni D. Blood conservation in pediatric surgical patients. Curr Anesthesiol Rep. 2020;10:289-96.
11. Russell RT, Leeper CM, Spinella PC. Damage-control resuscitation in paediatric trauma: what you need to know. J Trauma Acute Care Surg. 2023;95:472-80.
12. Downey LA. Patient blood management in pediatric anaesthesiology. Curr Anesthesiol Rep. 2021;11:477-82.
13. Blain S, Paterson N. Paediatric massive transfusion. BJA Education. 2016;16:269-75.
14. Tan GM, Murto K, Downey LA, Wilder MS, Goobie SM. Error traps in pediatric patient blood management in the perioperative period. Paediatr Anaesth. 2023;33:609-19.
15. Evangelista ME, Gaffley M, Neff LP. Massive transfusion protocols for pediatric patients: current perspectives. J Blood Med. 2020;11:163-172.
16. Kinslow K, McKenney M, Boneva D, Elkbuli A. Massive transfusion protocols in paediatric trauma population: a systematic review. Transfus Med. 2020;30:333-42.
17. Horst J, Leonard JC, Vogel A, Jacobs R, Spinella PC. A survey of US and Canadian hospitals' paediatric massive transfusion protocol policies. Transfus Med. 2016;26:49-56.
18. Hwu RS, Spinella PC, Keller MS, Baker D, Wallendorf M, Leonard JC. The effect of massive transfusion protocol implementation on pediatric trauma care. Transfusion. 2016;56:2712-9.
19. Chidester SJ, Williams N, Wang W, Groner JI. A paediatric massive transfusion protocol. J Trauma Acute Care Surg. 2012;73:1273-7.
20. Hendrickson JE, Shaz BH, Pereira G, Parker PM, Jessup P, Atwell F, et al. Implementation of a pediatric trauma massive transfusion protocol: one institution's experience. Transfusion. 2012;52:1228-36.
21. Edwards MJ, Lustik MB, Clark ME, Creamer KM, Tuggle D. The effects of balanced blood component resuscitation and crystalloid administration in pediatric trauma patients requiring transfusion in Afghanistan and Iraq, 2002 to 2012. J Trauma Acute Care Surg. 2015;78:330-5.
22. Chen L, Yang Z, Liu H. Haemoglobin-based oxygen carriers: where are we now in 2023? Medicina (Kaunas). 2023;59:396.
23. Pusateri AE, Glassberg E, Weiskopf RB. Reassessment of the need for an oxygen carrier for the treatment of traumatic hemorrhage when blood is not an option. Shock. 2019;52:55-9.

CHAPTER 13

# Challenges and Newer Modalities in Non-operating Room Anaesthesia in Children: Overcome Challenges and Provide the Best Care!

*B Vishnu Mahesh Babu, Ranju Singh, Dinesh Gunasekaran, Shwethashri K*

## ABSTRACT

Non-operating room anaesthesia (NORA) describes anaesthesia delivered outside a traditional operating room setting. Sedation or providing anaesthesia to children in an unfamiliar environment, with the lack of support staff and non-availability of choice of medication and equipment, is often challenging. Studies have shown an increased risk of airway-related adverse events, complications, and even death outside the operating room locations. It is crucial to be familiar with the anatomical and physiological variations in children, be well-versed with the difficult airway algorithm and have support from the main operating room at any point in time. The most common event in NORA claims was inadequate oxygenation/ventilation, which is preventable with vigilant monitoring. With the advent of new anaesthetic drugs with rapid onset and rapid recovery, along with the recent monitoring devices, there has been a significant decline in untoward incidents and NORA in children has become as safe as in the operating room. This article gives an idea of the various aspects of NORA, such as sedation guidelines, monitoring standards, procedure-specific risks and complications of NORA in children.

***Keywords:*** Non-operating room anaesthesia, Paediatric, Procedural sedation, Sedation.

## INTRODUCTION

The administration of sedation/anaesthesia to patients undergoing painful or uncomfortable procedures at off-site locations is referred to as non-operating room anaesthesia (NORA). NORA is an expanding area of paediatric anaesthesia practice. Locations include diagnostic and interventional radiology, dental clinics, gastroenterology and pulmonary suites, radiation oncology locations, and the cardiac catheterisation laboratory, among others. The trend towards more outfield procedures, which is seen in both adult and paediatric anaesthesia, is driven by many factors. These include evolving technology with an increasing range of treatment options, availability of non-portable equipment such as magnetic resonance imaging (MRI) scanners, linear accelerators, and radiation sources, as well as increasing caseload in the operating rooms, which, however, has not decreased despite increases in NORA cases. The anaesthesiologist working in these off-site locations must understand the unique environmental, logistical and perioperative considerations to minimise risk in each remote location.

With an integrative approach focusing on these challenges, anaesthesia and procedural teams can coordinate to deliver consistent, safe, high-quality care. Modern practice has seen the role of the anaesthesiologist expand beyond the walls of the operating room (OR) complex. Whilst the ORs have experienced staff, adequate equipment and monitors, providing anaesthesia outside the operation theatre complex is challenging and requires expertise, skill and patience.

## DEMOGRAPHIC TRENDS

There has been a steady growth in the number of anaesthesia cases outside the OR. From 2010 to 2014, a review of the National Anesthesia Outcomes Registry (NACOR) revealed an increase from 28 to 36% of all anaesthesia cases classified as NORA.[1] Should current trends continue, within the next decade, NORA will constitute 50% of all anaesthesia encounters. Although adults require anaesthesia primarily for painful, invasive procedures, such as cardiac catheterisation and endoscopy, the largest category of cases for which children require anaesthesia is diagnostic radiologic imaging, illustrating that many children cannot cooperate with procedures tolerated by awake adults.

Cardiopulmonary resuscitation has been reported to be required in two cases and pulmonary aspiration in 4 cases in over 49,000 paediatric patients subjected to propofol sedation.[2] One in 70 cases required interventions to rescue the airway. This depicts the importance of skilled and competent anaesthesiologists during sedation or anaesthesia procedures in NORA, along with trained staff to assist in major catastrophic events.

## LOCATIONS FOR NON-OPERATING ROOM ANAESTHESIA

These may include several areas in the hospital other than the OR **(Box 1)**.

**BOX 1:** Locations for NORA.

- Radiology suites for CT scan, MRI and interventional radiology
- Cardiac catheterisation laboratory
- Burns unit
- Dental clinic
- Psychiatry unit for modified electroconvulsive therapy
- Endoscopy suites
- Radiotherapy and chemotherapy units

(CT: computed tomography; MRI: magnetic resonance imaging; NORA: non-operating room anaesthesia

## REQUIREMENTS FOR NON-OPERATING ROOM ANAESTHESIA

Joint Commission on Accreditation of Health Care Organizations (JCAHO), along with the American Society of Anesthesiologists (ASA), has set forth multiple requirements for NORA:

- Pre-procedure assessment
- Continuous physiological monitoring
- Credentialing of individuals providing different levels of sedation
- Post-sedation recovery and discharge
- Maintenance of institution-wide standards of care and quality assurance for all levels of care

## ANAESTHETIC CONSIDERATIONS AND CHALLENGES FOR NON-OPERATING ROOM ANAESTHESIA

Possible challenges must be anticipated and prepared for. If adequate preparation is not ensured, critical incidents may occur in a remote location where appropriate help and intervention may not be readily available. Factors related to the patient, staff, procedure and equipment should be considered and optimised to ensure a safe and quality outcome.

### Patient-related Considerations

Pre-procedure assessment should include:

- *Medical history:* Review the patient's medical history, including previous anaesthesia experiences, allergies, and current medications.
- *Physical examination:* Conduct a comprehensive physical exam, focusing on the airway, cardiovascular, and respiratory systems.
- *Fasting status:* Ensure adherence to fasting guidelines to minimise the risk of aspiration. Typically, this involves fasting for 2 hours for clear liquids, 4 hours for breast milk, and 6 hours for solid food and non-clear liquids. The likelihood of prolonged fasting with its attendant challenges of dehydration, restlessness and haemodynamic disturbance should be anticipated and prevented. Plans should be made to make venous cannulation as bearable as possible by taking measures such as application of eutectic mixture of local anaesthetics (EMLA) cream (2.5% prilocaine and 2.5% lignocaine) at least 1 hour before cannulation.
- *Airway assessment:* Pre-anaesthetic evaluation should emphasise on a complete airway evaluation to anticipate any airway difficulty, and all the equipment required for the difficult airway management should be kept ready. An experienced anaesthesiologist, well-versed with paediatric airway management, should take up these cases. The Mallampati score can be used for older children who are cooperative. The anaesthetist may need some ingenuity to achieve these assessments in a small,

uncooperative child. The other parameters that should be assessed and inspected include the following:

- Mouth opening.
- Range of neck movement.
- Mandibular hypoplasia—micrognathia makes intubation difficult. Assess the airway by observing the child inside view rather than from the front.
- Mandibular hyperplasia—ameloblastoma may cause jaw protrusion and can make laryngoscopy and intubation difficult.
- Oral cavity (e.g. for intraoral masses).

The Colorado Pediatric Airway Score (COPUR) Score:[3] It was developed to assess the airway in syndromic babies with an anticipated difficult airway.

- *Parental consent:* Informed consent should be obtained from the parents or guardians, discussing the risks and benefits of anaesthesia for the planned procedure.
- *Risk Stratification:* Patients are assessed and classified based on their ASA physical status:
  - *ASA I:* Healthy patients without systemic disease.
  - *ASA II:* Patients with mild systemic disease.
  - *ASA III:* Patients with severe systemic disease that is not incapacitating.
  - *ASA IV:* Patients with incapacitating systemic disease that is a constant threat to life.
  - *ASA V:* Moribund patients not expected to survive without the operation.

## Staff-related Considerations

### *American Society of Anesthesiologists Guidelines for Sedation and Anaesthesia by Non-anaesthesiologists*

- Children must be evaluated before the procedure by qualified personnel to ensure that they are not compromised by co-existing medical conditions.
- Appropriate nil per oral (NPO) status.
- Take informed consent from the parents.
- During the procedure, the level of consciousness, ventilation, oxygenation and haemodynamics are to be evaluated with standard monitors by a designated individual who should be trained to recognise complications of analgesia and sedation.
- At least one individual trained in basic life support should be present continuously when moderate or deep sedation is used.

### *American Society of Anesthesiologists Guidelines for Sedation and Anaesthesia by Anaesthesiologists*

Procedures in remote areas have been associated with increased morbidity and critical incidents largely due to human error, inability to recognise impending crisis, inability to manage emergencies and the lack of a trained, skilled assistant.[4,5]

Adequate skills in airway management and the ability to intervene when required are a prerequisite for anaesthesia providers delivering NORA. All personnel involved in NORA should be trained in paediatric anaesthesia and resuscitation techniques. A means of reliable two-way communication with the main OR complex is needed to request for assistance. Continuous education and simulation training are recommended to maintain high proficiency levels.

## PROCEDURE-RELATED CONSIDERATIONS

### *Emergency Protocols*

As per ASA, a lead anaesthesiologist for each area should be involved in writing policies and standard operating procedures, including different aspects of care. Patient safety must be replicated in NORA locations as implemented in the ORs. Emergency response protocol should be developed and regularly practised. These should include:

- *Rapid access to advanced life support:* Ensure the ability to initiate paediatric advanced life support measures promptly.
- *Transfer plans:* Establish clear plans for transferring patients to a fully equipped OR or intensive care unit (ICU) in case of emergencies.

When in doubt, communicating with the surgeon or proceduralist involved is crucial for effective pre-anaesthetic preparation. The required information should include, but not be limited to, the following:

- Nature of the procedure and any special requirements that will influence anaesthesia
- Position
- How long the procedure is anticipated to take
- Associated pain
- Possible side effects
- Equipment and devices to be used

## Equipment-related Considerations

### *American Society of Anesthesiologists Guidelines for Minimal Equipment Requirements for Non-operating Room Anaesthesia*

*Equipment checklist for anaesthesia or sedation in a remote location:*

*Acronym: SOAP ME (S:* Suction; *O:* Oxygen; A: Airway equipment; *P:* Pharmacy (drugs); *M:* Monitors; *E:* Equipment)

- *Reliable source of oxygen with backup:* Oxygen should be piped from a central source that meets applicable codes. It is recommended to have a backup system that includes at least the equivalent of one full E-type cylinder, and it should be capable of administering at least 90% oxygen as a means to deliver positive pressure ventilation.

- Suction apparatus
- Waste gas scavenging unit
- Standard monitoring equipment, which includes
  - Pulse oximetry with an audible pulse tone and a low threshold alarm
  - Capnography
  - Blood pressure monitoring
  - Temperature monitoring
  - Electrocardiography
- Electrical outlet
- Adequate illumination of the patient and anaesthesia workstation.
- Emergency cart with self-inflating bag, emergency drugs, anaesthesia drugs, defibrillator.
- Venous cannulae of different sizes meant for paediatric usage.
- Intravenous pumps/drip stands
- Transport capability
  - Oxygen delivery
  - Oxygen tanks
  - Portable monitors
- Specific equipment as per location, e.g. for MRI suite **(Table 1[6] and Fig. 1)**

## SEDATION/ANAESTHESIA TECHNIQUES AND DRUGS USED IN NON-OPERATING ROOM ANAESTHESIA

The depth of sedation to be targeted and the drugs used **(Table 2[7])** depend upon the procedure performed, the degree of pain anticipated, allowable patient movement, duration of the procedure, and other patient factors such as last oral intake, comorbidities (e.g. upper respiratory infection), prior sedation experience, and urgency of the procedure.

### Choice of Anaesthetic Technique

- Monitored anaesthesia care
- Sedation
- Regional anaesthesia
- Total intravenous anaesthesia (TIVA)
- General anaesthesia (GA) and controlled ventilation

### Levels of Sedation

(Defined by ASA on 13th October, 1999)

- *Minimal sedation (anxiolysis):* Patient responds to commands, no change in ventilation/cardiovascular status, cognitive/motor function impaired.

**TABLE 1:** Specific equipment required for the MRI suite.[6]

| *Equipment* | *Description* |
|---|---|
| ECG | High impedance graphite electrodes and leads (thermal injury has been reported) |
| Blood pressure monitor | Oscillometer with nonferrous gauge |
| Respiratory gas analyser | Side-stream sampling with a long sampling line |
| Pulse oximeter | Non-ferromagnetic with fibreoptic signals |
| Laryngoscope | Plastic scopes with paper or aluminium covered lithium cells |
| Temperature probe | Skin temperature sensing strips with radiofrequency filters |
| Stylet | Copper stylets to be used |
| Endotracheal tubes | Spring within the cuff valve may distort images; a nonmagnetic version needs to be used |
| Supraglottic devices | Spring within the cuff valve may distort images; reinforced LMA (Proseal) cannot be used |
| Infusion pumps | Not permitted inside the MRI suite. Extensions are needed |
| Self-inflating bag | Needs to be valveless with no ferromagnetic parts |
| Suction apparatus | Wall mounted with a 10 m tubing |
| Anaesthesia workstation | Non-magnetic machine, aluminium cylinders required |
| Defibrillator | Not permitted into the MRI suite. Resuscitation is usually carried out outside a magnetic field |

(ECG: electrocardiogram; LMA: laryngeal mask airway; MRI: magnetic resonance imaging;)

- *Moderate sedation/analgesia:* Patient responds purposefully to commands alone or with light tactile stimulation, maintains spontaneous ventilation, and cardiovascular status is maintained. This was known as conscious sedation in the past.
- *Deep sedation/analgesia:* Patient not easily arousable, responds to pain, may need assistance with airway and ventilation, cardiovascular function is usually maintained. Paediatric sedation state scale (PSSS), developed by Cravero et al.,[8] is a measure of quality and effectiveness of procedural sedation in children and can be used for assessment of sedation.
- *General anaesthesia:* No response/reflex withdrawal; patients often require assistance in maintaining a patent airway, and positive pressure ventilation may be required because of depressed spontaneous ventilation or drug-induced depression of neuromuscular function. Cardiovascular function may be impaired.

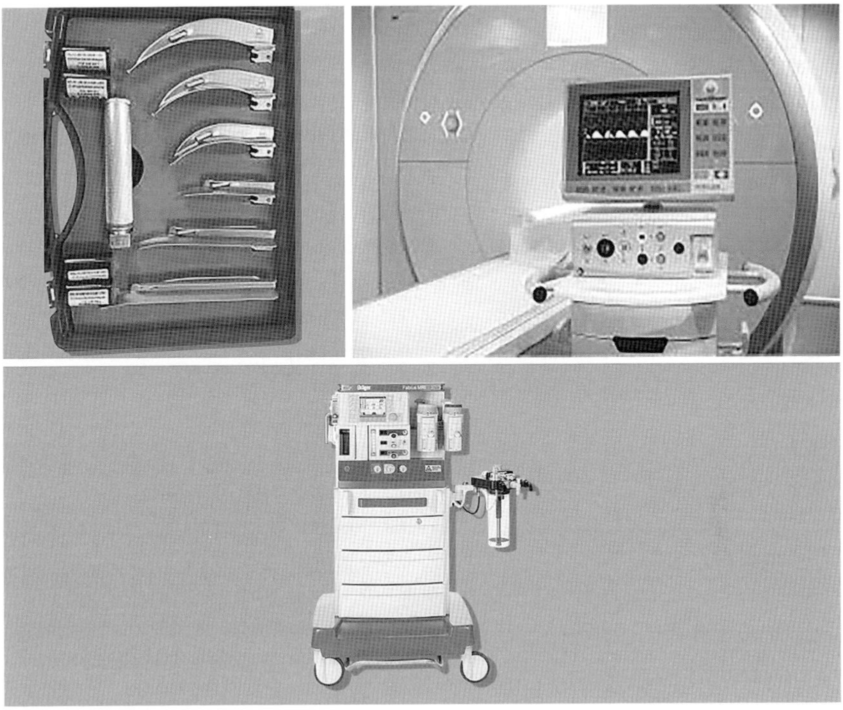

**Fig. 1:** Magnetic resonance imaging (MRI) compatible laryngoscope with blades, MRI compatible pulse oximeter and workstation. *(For color version, see Plate 9)*

## PROCEDURE-SPECIFIC CONCERNS IN NON-OPERATING ROOM ANAESTHESIA

### Non-operating Room Anaesthesia for Neurointerventional Radiology

Most common procedures include embolisation of cerebral and dural arteriovenous malformations, coiling of cerebral aneurysms, thrombolysis, and balloon dilatation of vessels.[9] GA with controlled ventilation is usually preferred for better maintenance of cerebral perfusion pressure and control of intracranial pressure. Haemodynamic variations are to be tackled with vigilant monitoring. During the procedures, haemorrhage, thromboembolic phenomenon, coil occlusion and cerebral vasospasm are the major complications encountered, and this can further worsen hypotension and compromise haemodynamics.

Anaesthetic equipment should comprise working laryngoscopes, appropriately sized endotracheal tubes and supraglottic airway devices such as laryngeal mask airways (LMAs) and i-gel. Proseal LMAs are also available in the market for paediatric usage. The LMA Gastro™ is not available for paediatric usage.

**TABLE 2:** Drug dosages for sedation/anaesthesia in children.

| *Drug* | *Route of administration* | *Dose* |
|---|---|---|
| Midazolam | IV<br>IM<br>Per rectal<br>Oral<br>Intranasal | 0.02–0.1 mg/kg<br>0.1–0.15 mg/kg<br>0.3–1 mg/kg<br>0.3–1 mg/kg<br>0.2 mg/kg |
| Propofol | IV<br>IV infusion | 2–3.5 mg/kg<br>125–150 µg/kg/min |
| Ketamine | IV (sedation)<br>IV (analgesic)<br>IM | 0.5–2 mg/kg<br>0.1 mg/kg<br>2–5 mg/kg |
| Etomidate | IV | 0.1–0.3 mg/kg |
| Dexmedetomidine | IV infusion | 0.5–1 µg /kg over 10 minutes, then 0.5–1 µg/kg/h |
| Fentanyl<br>Remifentanil | IV<br>IV infusion | 0.5–2 µg/kg<br>0.025–0.5 µg/kg/min |

*Source:* adapted from Aaron O, Gathuya Z. Paediatric anaesthesia outside the operating room in children. Update Anaesth. [Online] Available from www.wfsahq.org/resources/update-in-anaesthesia [Last accessed June, 2025].[7]
(IV: Intravenous; IM: intramuscular)

### *Special Circumstances: Magnetic Resonance Imaging Suite*

All equipment that is taken into the MRI suite should be MRI compatible **(Table 2 and Fig. 1)**. If any emergency occurs, it is better to take the patient out of the MRI room and perform resuscitation.

## Non-operating Room Anaesthesia in the Interventional Gastroenterology Suite

Diagnostic endoscopy may be done under moderate sedation. However, advanced endoscopic procedures such as dilatation and stenting of stricture oesophagus, endoscopic retrograde cholangiopancreatography (ERCP) and treatment of oesophageal varices may require deep sedation or preferably GA. Patients with achalasia cardia, gastro-oesophageal reflux are at high risk of aspiration, and their trachea must be intubated to protect against aspiration. ERCP is an uncomfortable procedure requiring deep sedation or preferably GA. Deep sedation may compromise the airway, and desaturation can occur. The prone position may further limit timely airway intervention. GA with target-controlled infusion with propofol and fentanyl has shown shorter extubation time, better respiratory and haemodynamic stability. As a part of deep sedation for

ERCP, an intravenous loading dose of 0.7 μg/kg dexmedetomidine can be administered over 10 minutes, followed by a maintenance infusion of 0.5 μg/kg/h. Just prior to the procedure, intravenous 0.5 mg/kg ketamine and 0.5 μg/kg fentanyl are administered. The child can be kept on spontaneous breathing with oxygen supplementation via nasal prongs. The procedure can be controlled with minimal haemodynamic changes without any spells of desaturation.[10] A target-controlled propofol infusion with 50% effective concentration of propofol between 2.8 and 3.7 μg/ml, and a remifentanil infusion of 0.025 μg/kg/min have been found to be effective starting doses in children undergoing oesophagogastroduodenoscopy. Increasing the rate of the remifentanil infusion might increase the risk of opioid-related side effects.[11]

## Non-operating Room Anaesthesia for Interventional Cardiology

Common cardiac interventional procedures performed include placement of occlusion devices for congenital heart diseases such as atrial septal defect/ ventricular septal defect and patent ductus arteriosus, balloon dilatation/ valvuloplasty for pulmonary and mitral stenosis, electrophysiological studies and permanent pacemaker insertion.

A detailed pre-anaesthetic checkup eliciting a history of cyanosis, shortness of breath, signs/symptoms of congestive cardiac failure, history of previous surgical or cardiological interventions, anticoagulant therapy and other cardiac medications is necessary.[12] Sedation/GA must be titrated depending on the degree of cardiac dysfunction and the cardiac defect. Adequate perfusion of systemic and pulmonary circulation, filling pressures, heart rate, and coronary perfusion pressures need to be maintained. Invasive monitoring and blood gas analysis may be needed. GA with endotracheal intubation may be required for transoesophageal echocardiography (TEE), as most children may not tolerate the TEE probe under sedation.

## Non-operating Room Anaesthesia for Electroconvulsive Therapy (ECT)

Not commonly performed in children

*Absolute contraindications for ECT are:*

- Raised intracranial tension.
- Phaeochromocytoma.
- Recent myocardial infarction <3 months
- Severe angina, congestive heart failure
- Aneurysm of major vessels
- Severe respiratory failure

*Relative contraindications for ECT are:*
- Pregnancy
- Cardiac dysrhythmia
- Thyrotoxicosis
- Glaucoma
- Retinal detachment

The principle of anaesthesia for ECT is to provide ultrabrief, light GA with a moderate degree of muscular relaxation. Pre-procedural evaluation should include a detailed inquiry about the psychotropic medications taken by the patient. Tricyclic antidepressants may cause significant hypertension and dysrhythmia during ECT. Monoamine oxidase inhibitors also impose the risk of hypertension. In addition to standard respiratory and haemodynamic monitoring, electromyography and electroencephalography are used to monitor seizure activity.

### Non-operating Room Anaesthesia for Burns Dressings

Sedation with ketamine is usually administered for frequent burn dressings in children. Propofol with fentanyl with or without midazolam can also be used. In children without intravenous access, oral transmucosal fentanyl citrate can be used.

## COMPLICATIONS OF NON-OPERATING ROOM ANAESTHESIA

- *Respiratory complications:* Respiratory depression is more frequent during NORA. The most common event in NORA claims was inadequate oxygenation/ventilation, which is preventable with vigilant monitoring using pulse oximetry and capnography.[13]
- *Hypothermia:* Lower temperatures are usually maintained in diagnostic suites to prevent equipment overheating. Children are vulnerable to hypothermia, and although bleeding is uncommon in the setting of NORA, even mild hypothermia is known to increase surgical blood loss and thereby increase the risk of transfusion. Hypothermia also delays recovery and increases oxygen consumption. Active warming measures, such as body and fluid warmers, need to be used.
- *Aspiration and postoperative nausea and vomiting (PONV):* Fasting guidelines should be strictly followed. Prophylactic antiemetic agents are to be administered to prevent PONV. Postoperative vomiting in children (POVOC) score developed by Eberhart et al can be used to predict the incidence of PONV.[14]

  Major risk factors for PONV in children (POVOC score) **(Table 3)**:
  - Age >3 years
  - Duration of surgery is >30 minutes

**TABLE 3:** Predicting postoperative nausea and vomiting (POVOC) score.

| *Risk factors* | *Predict postoperative nausea and vomiting (PONV)* |
|---|---|
| 0 (None) | 9% |
| 1 | 10% |
| 2 | 30% |
| 3 | 55% |
| 4 | 70% |

- Type of surgery
- Strabismus surgery
- Positive history of PONV in the child or an immediate family member with a history of PONV

- *Antiemetic prophylaxis:*
  - *Serotonin 5HT-3 receptor antagonists*: Ondansetron (50–100μg/kg), granisetron (40 μg/kg), dolasetron (350 μg/kg) and tropisetron (0.1 μg/kg up to 2 mg)
  - Dexamethasone 150 μg/kg up to 5 mg
  - Perphenazine 75 μg/kg up to 5 mg
  - Droperidol 75 μg/kg
  - A combination of two to three drugs is much preferred
- *Hypovolaemia and hypoglycaemia:* Prolonged fasting can predispose to dehydration, hypovolaemia, and hypoglycaemia. Maintenance of a sufficient volume status before the procedure by prehydration and maintenance fluid administration can prevent these complications.

## POST-PROCEDURE CARE

A designated area for post-anaesthesia care, with equipment for emergency resuscitation, should be available. The post-sedation period requires thorough monitoring of peripheral oxygen saturation and blood pressure, and watching for complications like shivering and PONV. It is imperative to ensure that adequate staff is available to monitor the child, and the child is discharged after satisfying the Modified Aldrete score.

## CONCLUSION

The anatomical and physiological variations in infants and children and the unfamiliar and non-conventional environment of NORA pose challenges to anaesthetic management. There is an increasing need to provide anaesthesia for children undergoing procedures outside the familiar OR environment. It is, therefore, important to establish systematic guidelines and to follow the American Society of Anesthesiologists' protocols to enhance safety and quality of care. Guidelines on patient selection, improved monitoring and management of common complications are essential to minimise the potential adverse outcomes. Good communication among care providers involved in NORA procedures and good commitment and support of the institution are required for safe and successful outcomes.

## REFERENCES

1. Gross WL. Non-operating room anaesthesia. In: Miller RD (Ed). Miller's Anaesthesia, 8th edition. Philadelphia: Elsevier; 2015. pp. 2646-73.
2. Cravero JP, Beach ML, Blike GT, Gallagher SM, Hertzog JH. Pediatric Sedation Research Consortium. The incidence and nature of adverse events during pediatric sedation/anesthesia with propofol for procedures outside the operating room: a report from the Pediatric Sedation Research Consortium. Anesth Analg. 2009;108(3):795-804.
3. Lane G. Intubation techniques. Operative Techniques in Otolaryngology-Head and Neck Surgery. 2005;16(3):166-70.
4. Melloni C. Morbidity and mortality related to anesthesia outside the operating room. Minerva Anestesiol. 2005;71(6):325-34.
5. Epstein BS. The American Society of Anesthesiologist's efforts in developing guidelines for sedation and analgesia for nonanesthesiologists: the 40th Rovenstine Lecture. Anesthesiology. 2003;98(5):1261-8.
6. Melloni C. Anesthesia and sedation outside the operating room: how to present risk and maintain good quality. Curr Opin Anaesthesiol. 2007;20(6):513-9.
7. Aaron O, Gathuya Z. Paediatric anaesthesia outside the operating room in children. Update Anaesth. [Online] Available from www.wfsahq.org/resources/update-in-anaesthesia [Last accessed June, 2025].
8. Cravero JP, Askins N, Sriswasdi P, Tsze DS, Zurakowski D, Sinnott S. Validation of the pediatric sedation state scale. Pediatrics. 2017;139(2):e20162897.
9. Varma MK, Price K, Jayakrishnan V, Manickam B, Kessell G. Anaesthetic considerations for interventional neuroradiology. Br J Anaesth. 2007;99(1):75-85.
10. Ko BJ, Jang JH, Park JW, Lee SC, Choi SR. Procedural sedation with dexmedetomidine for pediatric endoscopic retrograde cholangiopancreatography guided stone retraction. Korean J Anaesthesiol. 2012;63(6):567-8.
11. Drover DR, Litalien C, Wellis V, Shafer SL, Hammer GB. Determination of the pharmacodynamic interaction of propofol and remifentanil during esophagogastroduodenoscopy in children. Anesthesiology. 2004;100(6):1382-6.
12. Reddy K, Jaggar S, Gillbe C. The anaesthetist and the cardiac catheterisation laboratory. Anaesthesia. 2006;61(12):1175-86.
13. Robbertze R, Posner KL, Domino KB. Closed claims review of anesthesia for procedures outside the operating room. Curr Opin Anaesthesiol. 2006; 9(4):436-42.
14. Eberhart LHJ, Geldner G, Kranke P, Morin AM, Schäuffelen A, Treiber H, et al. The development and validation of a risk score to predict the probability of postoperative vomiting in pediatric patients. Anesth Analg. 2004;99(6):1630-37.

CHAPTER 14

# Toxicity of Local Anaesthesia in Paediatric Patients: Stay Aware of Risks and Take Appropriate Measures

*Sanjeev Palta, Sapna Bathla, Pratheeba Natarajan, Aditi Jain, Khushboo Mehta*

## OBJECTIVES

- To understand why children are more susceptible to local anaesthetic systemic toxicity than adults
- To attain knowledge about the common procedures and drugs involved in paediatric care
- To gain information on the prevention and management of paediatric local anaesthetic systemic toxicity

## ABSTRACT

Regional anaesthesia in children has gained popularity worldwide in the last few years. The incidence of local anaesthetic systemic toxicity (LAST) in paediatric patients has been reported to be about 8 in 100,000 blocks because certain physiological factors put them at a higher risk than their adult counterparts which have been highlighted in the chapter. Along with being used for regional anaesthesia, topical local anaesthetic agents are also commonly used in this age-group to make minor interventions such as venipuncture painless. This chapter includes a discussion on local anaesthetic agents and their safe doses. The presentation of LAST in children is different from that in adults because a block in a child is usually given after the administration of general anaesthesia and unlike adults, children cannot express prodromal symptoms. Hence, preparation and monitoring play a vital role in the prevention of LAST in paediatrics. Immediate recognition, airway control, cardiovascular support, seizure management and intralipid therapy followed by post-recovery care form the keystones of management of LAST in children.

***Keywords:*** Local anaesthesia, Paediatric, Systemic, Toxicity.

## INTRODUCTION

Local anaesthetic (LA) agents have become an indispensable part of modern-day regional anaesthetic practise. Regional anaesthesia (RA) in children has gained popularity worldwide in the last few years, especially with the development of the enhanced recovery after surgery in paediatrics, due to its notable advantages such as reduced opioid consumption, reduced incidence of post-operative nausea and vomiting and superior analgesia with reduced incidence of respiratory complications.[1,2] The advent of ultrasonography has revolutionised the domain of RA and perioperative pain management.

LA agents work by blocking the propagation of action potentials in nerves by their action on voltage-gated sodium channels. Their wide variety of applications ranges from simple infiltration around the wound to complex fascial plane blocks. Both ester and amide LA agents can have adverse reactions and the extent to which these can occur depends on multiple factors. Moreover, patients at the extremes of age (neonates, infants and elderly) are at a much higher risk of developing adverse manifestations to LAs.

The incidence of local anaesthetic systemic toxicity (LAST) in paediatric patients has been reported to be about 8 in 100,000 blocks.[3] It is a life-threatening adverse event occurring due to the systemic absorption of LAs, predominantly presenting with central nervous system (CNS) and cardiovascular system (CVS) toxicity. The effects may range from perioral numbness and tingling to loss of consciousness, seizures, respiratory arrest, arrhythmias, coma and death.

## WHY ARE CHILDREN MORE SUSCEPTIBLE TO LOCAL ANAESTHETIC SYSTEMIC TOXICITY?

Certain physiological changes in paediatric patients put them at a higher risk of developing LAST. These include the following:

- Lower lean muscle mass
- Decreased protein binding: At birth, the concentration of alpha-1 acid glycoprotein is 20–50% than that in adults, thus increasing the free fraction. Children below 6 months of age have decreased protein binding which may further be exacerbated by hypoxia, hypercarbia and acidosis. However, the low levels of albumin do not seem to have a major effect on protein binding due to the significantly lower affinity of LAs for albumin.[4]
- Immature hepatic metabolism: Most commonly used amide LAs are metabolised by the cytochrome P450 enzymes in the liver, which are not fully developed in infancy, contributing to accumulation of LAs.[5]
- Immature plasma esterase: Plasma esterases are involved in the metabolism of ester LAs which may also accumulate.[5]
- Greater systemic absorption of LA can occur due to increased cardiac output.
- *Site of injection:* Certain routes of LA administration have been associated with a much higher risk of systemic toxicity.
- *Difference in anatomy at the neuronal level:* Incomplete myelination at birth, lasting till 12 years of age, may result in a rapid onset of block even with dilute LA. However, the duration of action is also reduced owing to the greater systemic absorption and decreased trapping of LA in the immature sheath.[5]
- An immature blood–brain barrier coupled with greater systemic absorption, results in a higher possibility of CNS toxicity. Since most blocks in children are performed under either sedation or general anaesthesia (GA), the timely identification of CNS toxicity by the LA may be difficult.[6]

## PROCEDURES INVOLVING THE USE OF LOCAL ANAESTHETIC AGENTS IN CHILDREN

LA agents are used in a wide variety of procedures in paediatric patients:

- *Central neuraxial blocks (caudal/epidural/subarachnoid block):* LAs are most commonly used for these procedures to provide surgical anaesthesia/analgesia for a wide variety of abdominal, thoracic and lower limb procedures. For children, the total cerebrospinal fluid is 4 ml/kg body weight as compared to 2 ml/kg in adults, primarily located in the spinal column. Along with unmyelinated nerve fibres and high cardiac output, children are likely to respond to lower concentrations of LA at a fast rate. Hence, though not 100% sensitive, a test dose is usually given, preceding the actual epidural dose to rule out accidental intrathecal/intravascular placement. Usual doses include 0.1 ml/kg of LA with 1:200,000 epinephrine and a rise in heart rate ≥10 beats/min or systolic blood pressure ≥15 mmHg above baseline within 90 seconds of injection, or >25% change in T wave or ST segment size indicates intravascular injection. However, under GA, the sensitivity and specificity of this method may go further down, and the epidural test dose may itself result in LAST in children.[7] Hence, following slow incremental doses after repeated negative aspiration is the safest way to practise.
- *Peripheral nerve blocks*: The administration of peripheral nerve blocks has been extended for use in emergency and critical care set-ups which is primarily due to the use of ultrasound beyond the arena of elective surgical procedures. Examples of the commonly performed peripheral nerve blocks are supraclavicular/infraclavicular and axillary blocks for upper limb procedures and femoral/sciatic/popliteal nerve blocks for lower limb procedures.
- *Fascial plane blocks*: These blocks predominantly involve the use of high volumes of dilute LA agents. Common examples include the transversus abdominis plane block, rectus sheath block, erector spinae plane block and quadratus lumborum block. These form a part of the multimodal analgesia protocol for major surgeries, but themselves are not sufficient to provide surgical anaesthesia.
- *Local wound site infiltration*: Apart from providing analgesia for minor surgical procedures, wound infiltration may be used as an adjunct along with GA, e.g. port-site infiltration in laparoscopic surgeries.
- *Topical and RA for awake fibreoptic intubation*: Nebulised lignocaine along with blocks of glossopharyngeal, superior and recurrent laryngeal nerves may be used to facilitate awake fibreoptic intubation in cases with a difficult airway.
- *Continuous infiltration of LA*: Infiltration of LA around the incision site as a single dose carries the disadvantage of a short duration of action, 4–8 hours for bupivacaine. However, placement of a catheter by the

surgeon into the wound, especially in cases where the amount of visceral pain is expected to be high, can be done for better post-operative analgesia. Combined with an elastomeric/spring-powered/electronic infusion pump, a preset amount of LA can be delivered to the wound site.[8]

## MONITORING AFTER ADMINISTRATION OF PAEDIATRIC REGIONAL ANAESTHESIA

All children receiving LA agents must be monitored adequately in the intraoperative period, extending to the post-operative period, till after the infusion has been stopped (depending on the type of drug used and its duration of action), as LAST may have delayed presentations also. All children should be monitored in an area fully equipped for emergency resuscitation. Standard monitors, oxygen supply, suction apparatus, defibrillator, emergency drugs, inotropes, antiepileptics and airway equipment should be readily available. Apart from this, 20% intralipid emulsion should be available at all times with its expiry date checked, and the person administering the block should be aware of where the intralipid is kept. Preferably, charts displaying the dosing guidelines for intralipid emulsion and other emergency drugs should be clearly displayed to help in emergency situations. The staff responsible should be thoroughly aware of all the danger signs of LAST and be trained enough to react timely.

All children should be monitored for signs of CNS and CVS toxicity from systemic absorption of LA. CNS toxicity can clinically manifest as perioral numbness, twitching, agitation, confusion, dizziness, dysarthria, dysphoria, seizures, respiratory arrest and coma. Clinical manifestations of CVS toxicity include hypotension, bradyarrhythmias, chest pain, changes on electrocardiography (ECG) such as ST-segment changes, ventricular ectopy/tachycardia/fibrillation and asystole. Monitoring should thus, include heart rate, non-invasive blood pressure, ECG, oxygen saturation and mentation.

## MOST COMMONLY USED LOCAL ANAESTHETIC DRUGS AND THEIR SIDE EFFECTS

### Drugs for Topical Application

#### *Eutectic Mixture of Local Anaesthetics—2.5% Lidocaine and 2.5% Prilocaine[9]*

It is a topical agent commonly used to numb the skin before procedures such as intravenous cannulations and lumbar punctures. It is generally applied with an occlusive dressing 45–60 minutes prior to intervention. The effect lasts for 1–2 hours after removal of cream and can even last until 4 hours.

*Side effects:* One of its constituents, prilocaine, is contraindicated in children with congenital methemoglobinemia or in children having predisposition to the same such as glucose-6-phosphate dehydrogenase deficiency and in those who are taking medications such as dapsone, sulfonamides, nitrates, nitrites, primaquine, chloroquine, etc. which may make them susceptible to methemoglobinemia. There is also a higher chance of systemic absorption in children having skin conditions such as atopic dermatitis.

### *Liposomal Lidocaine*[10]

It is a composition of lidocaine encapsulated in liposomes. It is available as 4–5% in 5, 15 or 30 g tubes. 1–2.5 g can be applied on 6.25 $cm^2$ area of skin in children >1 month of age. These liposomes prevent the drug from being rapidly metabolised. It can be applied 30 minutes prior to intervention and does not need an occlusive dressing.

*Side effects:* It should not be applied on skin regions that have a rash or are broken, as it can lead to systemic absorption and subsequent lignocaine toxicity if it is applied on large areas of skin.

### *Tetracaine Gel*[11]

Tetracaine gel contains 40 mg of tetracaine per 1 g of gel. It is applied 30–40 minutes prior to intervention with an occlusive dressing. Its effect lasts for 4–6 hours. 1 g is to be applied over 6.25 $cm^2$ area of skin.

*Side effects:* Skin erythema is common as it leads to capillary dilatation. It is contraindicated in premature infants and neonates.

### *Heated Lidocaine–Tetracaine Patch*[12]

Heated lidocaine–tetracaine patch is available as a 70 mg lignocaine and 70 g tetracaine self-heating patch. It should be applied 20–30 minutes prior to intervention.

*Side effects:* It should not be used for children with sensitivity to its components. It needs to be removed before magnetic resonance imaging, as it contains iron.

### *Needle-free Lidocaine Administration*[13]

This is a device which propels 2–2.5 mg of lignocaine using carbon dioxide propellant. It has a rapid onset of action—1–3 minutes.

*Side effects:* It has a higher rate of systemic absorption but has low chances of systemic toxicity due to its low dose.

## Chloroprocaine[14]

Chloroprocaine is an ultra-short-acting LA which has recently been brought back in use in RA. It is available as 1, 2 and 3% solution. Controversy had surrounded it in the early 1980s when there were reported cases of cauda equina syndrome and backache with its use. It was later found that these were most probably due to the addition of sodium bisulphite, a preservative. Since then, preservative-free chloroprocaine has been used for clinical purposes. Continuous infusion of chloroprocaine has been used for surgical anaesthesia via caudal route as well as via epidurals and continuous catheters in peripheral blocks for supplemental intraoperative and post-operative analgesia. It is an attractive alternative to its amide counterparts because it has low chances of toxicity due to its rapid plasma-based metabolism and wide therapeutic window. Its maximum recommended dose is 11 and 14 mg/kg without and with epinephrine, respectively.

## Bupivacaine[15-17]

Bupivacaine is one of the most common agents used for RA. In the paediatric population, it is used for spinal anaesthesia, epidurals and peripheral nerve blocks. It is associated with a longer clearance time because of the low hepatic extraction, reduced protein binding and cytochrome P450 activity in children. Its maximum dose should not be exceeded and should be decreased in children with increased susceptibility to seizures.

## Ropivacaine[15-17]

Ropivacaine is another long-acting amide LA, but it has lesser potential for CNS and CVS toxicity. It also shows age-related clearance changes but has been seen to have a lower rate of systemic absorption from the caudal space.

## Lidocaine[15-17]

Lidocaine is a short-acting amide anaesthetic with a high hepatic extraction ratio. It is most commonly used as a local infiltrate in paediatric dentistry as well as plastic surgery. It is also used in combination with longer-acting agents for blocks.

## Adjuncts[15-17]

Several drugs such as opioids, alpha agonists and neostigmine have been used to prolong and improve the quality of blocks alongside LAs. Other than clonidine and preservative-free morphine, none of the other adjuncts are approved for use in neuraxial block.[12] Clonidine in the dose of 1–2 μg/kg and morphine in the dose of 10–30 μg/kg can be used to prolong the effect of spinal anaesthesia as well as caudal analgesia. S-ketamine and racemic ketamine have also been used but are not recommended in infants and neonates due to concerns regarding neurotoxicity. Dexmedetomidine has also been used as an off-label adjunct to prolong neuraxial blocks. Though fentanyl is widely used in the adult population, there is lack of evidence for its beneficial use in paediatrics. Each of these adjuncts has its own pharmacological profile and offers benefits such as prolongation of block, decreasing general anaesthetic dosage and allowing smoother recovery. However, due to limited data on toxicity in paediatrics, they should be used cautiously after their intended benefits are weighed.

## SAFE DOSES OF LOCAL ANAESTHETIC DRUGS

Systemic toxicity can occur from the administration of LAs, and this occurs with rising serum concentrations of the LA as it is absorbed into the circulation of the patient. The LA dose, site and method of administration affect this concentration and the resultant systemic toxicity. Hence, knowledge of the safe dose of LA drugs injected by different routes is important for the anaesthesiologist **(Table 1)**.[10,16,17]

**TABLE 1:** Safe doses of local anaesthetic drugs in children.[10,16,17]

| *Local anaesthetic drug* | *Route of administration* | *Dose* |
|---|---|---|
| EMLA | Topical | 1–2 g per 10 cm$^2$ in children >3 months or 5 kg |
| Liposomal lignocaine | Topical | 1–2.5 g of 4% lignocaine can be applied on 6.25 cm$^2$ in children older than 1 month of age |
| Tetracaine | Topical | 1 g per 6.25 cm$^2$ in children >1 month of age |
| | Spinal | 1 mg/kg in <4 kg and 0.5 mg/kg in >4 kg |
| Bupivacaine | Spinal | 1 mg/kg in <5 kg, 0.4 mg/kg in 5–15 kg and 0.3 mg/kg in >15 kg |
| | Maximum allowable single dose | 3 mg/kg |
| | Continuous infusion rate | 0.4–0.5 mg/kg/h, <6 months: 0.2–0.25 mg/kg/h |
| Ropivacaine | Maximum allowable single dose | 3 mg/kg |
| | Continuous infusion rate | 0.4–0.5 mg/kg/h, <6 months: 0.2–0.25 mg/kg/h |
| Lidocaine | Maximum allowable single dose | 5 mg/kg, with epinephrine (5 µg/ml) 7 mg/kg |
| | Continuous infusion rate | 1.6 mg/kg/h; <6 months 0.8 mg/kg/h |
| Chloroprocaine | Maximum allowable single dose | 11 mg/kg in children >3 years of age |

(EMLA: eutectic mixture of local anaesthetics)

## SIGNS AND SYMPTOMS OF LOCAL ANAESTHETIC SYSTEMIC TOXICITY IN PAEDIATRICS

In paediatric practice, GA and RA are administered concurrently; hence, the first clinical presentation is different from that in adults. In patients receiving GA and in young children, prodromal signs cannot be trusted. Children who have been anaesthetised frequently have cardiac symptoms, since GA either masks or suppresses CNS symptoms. CNS symptoms are more likely to be present in awake people. Apnoea, convulsions and altered consciousness are amongst the CNS signs of paediatric LAST that have been documented in case reports. Cardiovascular symptoms that have been reported include bradycardia, asystole, ventricular tachycardia, hypotension and cardiac arrest. ECG changes include enlargement of the QRS complex, changes in the ST segment and peaked or inverted T waves.

## MANAGEMENT OF PAEDIATRIC LOCAL ANAESTHETIC SYSTEMIC TOXICITY

### Preparation

Following established procedures and having quick access to resuscitation, equipment and drugs are essential. It is recommended to always calculate the LA dosages pre-emptively. Oxygen via face mask and routine monitoring should be implemented. Identification of delayed presentations of complications can be averted by continuing to monitor for at least 30 minutes after completion of injection.[18,19]

### Immediate Management

#### *Maintain Airway, Oxygenation and Ventilation*

The first and foremost step in the management of LAST is to cease administering LA injections, call for help and start basic life support. The airway, breathing and circulation have to be taken care of. Early airway management and 100% oxygen administration should be an anaesthesiologist's priority in order to prevent hypoxia, hypercapnia or acidosis, which could accentuate LAST. Positive-pressure ventilation is the most important step in the management of LA overdose. Since respiratory alkalosis is deleterious to patients, caution should be exercised to avoid hyperventilation.

#### *Cardiovascular Support*

One has to remember that the concurrent administration of GA may obscure early warning signs and symptoms of toxicity in the paediatric age range. Cardiovascular collapse or arrhythmia will occur without any warning symptoms. In case of cardiac arrest, paediatric advanced cardiac life support

(PALS) guidelines need to be followed for resuscitation. Since cardiac arrhythmias are refractory most of the time, all resuscitation efforts should be carried out for a respectably long time. Prompt defibrillation and treatment of both bradyarrhythmias and tachyarrhythmias are mandatory for successful resuscitation efforts. Extracorporeal membrane oxygenation (ECMO) should be considered for circulatory support when advanced life support measures and intravenous lipid emulsion therapy are not followed by a rapid recovery. Recent evidence shows a good prognosis with the use of ECMO since LAST in paediatrics is mainly due to cardiovascular collapse. Also, the dose of epinephrine should be reduced to 1 μg/kg as per the American Society of Regional Anesthesia and Pain Medicine (ASRA) guidelines rather than the routine 10 μg/kg dose in paediatric cardiac arrest. It is hypothesised that higher doses of adrenaline can potentiate/aggravate life-threatening arrhythmias.

### *Seizure Management*

Prevention and termination of seizure activity is very essential as it may exacerbate metabolic acidosis. Benzodiazepines are considered as the first drugs of choice for the management of seizures. In cases where all attempts (securing airway, administration of antiseizure medications, correction of acidosis, correction of hypoxia and hypercarbia) to stop the seizures are unsuccessful, low-dose neuromuscular blockade (atracurium 0.3–0.5 mg/kg) may be an option to lessen metabolic acidosis and hypoxia caused by continuous muscle contraction. If the patient is haemodynamically unstable, it is prudent to avoid propofol for the control of seizures.

## Intravenous Lipid Emulsion Therapy

Lipid emulsion therapy has been used to treat LAST, and recent developments and a number of authors have documented its mechanism of action. Research suggests that lipid emulsion works through a multimodal setting comprising the following mechanisms:

- Lipid shuttles move the drugs from high-flow organs such as cardiac tissue and brain to muscles where they are stored and to the liver where their metabolism leads to detoxification.[20]
- Improving myocardial contractility, cardiac output, blood flow and blood pressure through actions on the vasculature and heart
- Activating cardioprotective pathways and providing a post-conditioning benefit

It has been observed that the early administration of 20% intravenous lipid emulsion therapy right after airway control is advantageous. The ASRA and the Association of Anaesthetists of Great Britain and Ireland have established recommendations for the management of LAST.[13,14] A continuous infusion of 20% lipid emulsion (0.25 ml/kg/min) is recommended after the first bolus dose of 20% lipid emulsion (1.5 ml/kg) over a period of 2–3 minutes, as per the established procedure.[21] The maximal cumulative dose of lipid emulsion in the paediatric population should not exceed 12 ml/kg.

A 100% long-chain fatty acid, intralipid is most frequently utilised to treat LAST.[22,23] When intralipid is not available, LAST is treated with alternative intravenous lipid injectable emulsions such as SMOFlipid® (soy, medium-chain triglyceride, olive and fish oil lipid), lipofundin medium-/long-chain triglyceride and ClinOleic,[24] but propofol cannot act as a replacement for intralipid.

### Post-Event Management

Children who endure LAST may benefit greatly from lipid emulsion therapy. Patients should be observed for a minimum of 6 hours after an episode of LAST with CVS characteristics and for at least 2 hours after an episode with isolated and fast terminating CNS abnormalities. It is advisable that cases should be reported to the registry at www.lipidrescue.org.[25,26]

## CONCLUSION

Children have increased susceptibility to LAST because of their developing physiology. Hence, monitoring is imperative whenever LAs are used in this age group. Special attention should be paid to avoid overdosing. As they are generally administered after the induction of general anaesthesia, and initial symptoms can be masked, one should be vigilant. Immediate management should focus on the maintenance of oxygenation and circulatory stability. Administration of intralipid emulsion therapy should be initiated as early as possible as it is the definitive therapy for the same.

## REFERENCES

1. Roberts K, Brindle M, McLuckie D. Enhanced recovery after surgery in paediatrics: a review of the literature. BJA Educ. 2020;20(7):235-41.
2. Merella F, Canchi-Murali N, Mossetti V. General principles of regional anaesthesia in children. BJA Educ. 2019;19(10):342-8.
3. Ramesh AS, Boretsky K. Local anesthetic systemic toxicity in children: a review of recent case reports and current literature. Reg Anesth Pain Med. 2021;46(10):909-14.
4. Oda Y. Pharmacokinetics and systemic toxicity of local anesthetics in children. J Anesth. 2016;30(4):547-50.
5. Feehan T, Packiasabapathy S. Pediatric Regional Anesthesia. Treasure Island (FL): StatPearls Publishing; 2024.
6. Walker BJ, Long JB, Sathyamoorthy M, Birstler J, Wolf C, Bosenberg AT, et al. Complications in Pediatric regional anesthesia: an analysis of more than 100,000 blocks from the pediatric regional anesthesia network. Anesthesiology. 2018;129(4):721-32.

7. Patel D. Epidural analgesia for children. Contin Educ Anaesth Crit Care Pain. 2006;6(2):63-6.
8. Whiteman A, Bajaj S, Hasan M. Novel techniques of local anaesthetic infiltration. Contin Educ Anaesth Crit Care Pain. 2011;11(5):167-71.
9. Steward DJ. Eutectic mixture of local anesthetics (EMLA): what is it? What does it do? J Pediatr. 1993;122:S21.
10. Maulidi H, McNair C, Seller N, Kirsh J, Bradley TJ, Greenway SC, et al. Arrhythmia associated with tetracaine in an extremely low birth weight premature infant. Pediatrics. 2012;130(6):e1704-7.
11. Zempsky WT. Pharmacologic approaches for reducing venous access pain in children. Pediatrics. 2008;122 Suppl 3:S140-53.
12. Veneziano G, Tobias JD. Chloroprocaine for epidural anesthesia in infants and children. Pediatric Anesthesia. 2017;27:581-90.
13. Suresh S, Ecoffey C, Bosenberg A, Lonnqvist PA, de Oliveira GS Jr, de Leon Casasola O, et al. The European Society of Regional Anaesthesia and Pain Therapy/American Society of Regional Anesthesia and Pain Medicine recommendations on local anesthetics and adjuvants dosage in pediatric regional anesthesia. Reg Anesth Pain Med. 2018;43:211-6.
14. Brull R, Macfarlane AJR, Chan VWS. Spinal, epidural and caudal anesthesia. In: Gropper MA, Eriksson LI, Fleisher LA, Wiener-Kronish JP, Cohen NH, Leslie K (Eds). Miller's anesthesia, 9th edition. Philadelphia: Elsevier Health Sciences; 2020. pp. 1695-717.
15. Bosenberg AT. Local anaesthetic agents. In: Davis PJ, Cladis FP (Eds). Smith's Anesthesia for Infants and Children, 8th edition. Philadelphia: Elsevier Health Sciences; 2016. pp. 2014-18.
16. El-Boghdadly K, Pawa A, Chin KJ. Local anesthetic systemic toxicity: current perspectives. Local Reg Anesth. 2018:8;11:35-44.
17. Neal JM, Barrington MJ, Fettiplace MR, Gitman M, Memtsoudis SG, Mörwald EE, et al. The third American Society of Regional Anesthesia and Pain Medicine practice advisory on local anesthetic systemic toxicity: executive summary 2017. Reg Anesth Pain Med. 2018;43(2):113-23.
18. Risk Management Analysis Committee of the French Society for Anesthesia and Critical Care (SFAR), French Society for Clinical Pharmacy (SFPC). Preventing medication errors in anesthesia and critical care (abbreviated version). Anaesth Crit Care Pain Med. 2017;36(4):253-8.
19. Gitman M, Barrington MJ. Local anesthetic systemic toxicity: a review of recent case reports and registries. Reg Anesth Pain Med. 2018;43(2):124-30.
20. Mochizuki T, Sato S. Hypocapnia prolongs bradycardia induced by bupivacaine or levobupivacaine in isolated rat hearts. Can J Anaesth. 2008;55(12):836-46.
21. Association of Anaesthetists of Great Britain and Ireland. (2010). AAGBI Safety Guideline: Management of Severe Local Anaesthetic Toxicity. [online] Available from https://anaesthetists.org/Home/Resources-publications/Guidelines/Archived-guidelines/Management-of-severe-local-anaesthetic-toxicity [Last accessed June, 2025].
22. Lee SH, Sohn JT. Mechanisms underlying lipid emulsion resuscitation for drug toxicity: a narrative review. Korean J Anesthesiol. 2023;76:171-82.
23. Wanten GJ, Calder PC. Immune modulation by parenteral lipid emulsions. Am J Clin Nutr. 2007;85:1171-84.

24. Hippalgaonkar K, Majumdar S, Kansara V. Injectable lipid emulsions-advancements, opportunities and challenges. AAPS PharmSciTech. 2010;11:1526-40.
25. Hoegberg LC, Bania TC, Lavergne V, Bailey B, Turgeon AF, Thomas SH, et al. Systematic review of the effect of intravenous lipid emulsion therapy for local anesthetic toxicity. Clin Toxicol (Phila). 2016;54:167-93.
26. Weinberg G. (2012). LipidRescue™ resuscitation: 20% lipid emulsion for rescue from drug toxicity. [online] Available from http://www.lipidrescue.org. [Last accessed June, 2025].

CHAPTER 15

# Enhanced Recovery after Surgery in Paediatrics: Optimise Outcomes for Your Patients!

*Sukhminder Jit Singh Bajwa, Madhuri Kurdi, Geeta Singariya, Smriti Anand*

## ABSTRACT

Paediatric surgery has lagged behind its adult counterpart in enhanced recovery after anaesthesia (ERAS) guideline creation and implementation. There are several differences between ERAS protocols in children and adults. ERAS guidelines have been developed for adolescents and neonates. In paediatric surgery, ERAS has successfully been employed across almost all disciplines from congenital cardiac surgery to colorectal surgery. There are various challenges in the implementation of ERAS in children. However, the interest in ERAS in paediatric surgery is growing rapidly. Evidence on ERAS protocols including pre-operative, intra-operative and post-operative interventions, and their implementation in children is gradually building up. Robust data support ERAS as a tool to promote quality and patient safety. Researchers from various countries have begun carrying out studies to implement ERAS protocols from available evidence and recommendations. Nevertheless, the differences between ERAS protocols in children and adults, the evidence for common ERAS interventions in paediatric surgery, the challenges and barriers in ERAS implementation in children and the ways to counter these hurdles are discussed in this chapter.

***Keywords:*** Enhanced recovery after surgery, Interventions, Intra-operative, Paediatric, Post-operative, Pre-operative, Protocols.

## INTRODUCTION

Enhanced recovery after surgery (ERAS) is a multimodal, cross-disciplinary, patient-centric, evidence-based peri-operative strategy that includes elements that cover pre-operative, intra-operative, and post-operative care and is aimed at improving post-operative results. It was originally developed as fast-track surgery in the 1990s for adult patients undergoing sigmoid colon resection and has steadily evolved over the years.[1] However, the widespread adoption of ERAS in paediatric surgery has been slow.[2]

Since 2016, there has been a growing number of groups worldwide involved in the creation and adoption of ERAS guidelines for various paediatric surgeries. There have been several important developments over the last 5 years, including the publication of the first ERAS® Society guideline in neonatal intestinal surgery and the formation of the paediatric ERAS® Society.[3] A paediatric appendicitis ERAS® guideline is currently being considered.[4]

## HOW IS PAEDIATRIC ENHANCED RECOVERY AFTER SURGERY DIFFERENT FROM ADULT ENHANCED RECOVERY AFTER SURGERY?

Paediatric surgery is considered to be distinctive with regards to ERAS protocol implementation because it embraces variable age groups ranging from neonates, infants, children, to adolescents with unique physiologies. The surgical stress response is complicated by physiological considerations based on a child's developmental stage.[5] Physiologically, neonates encounter considerable challenges when exposed to operative stress; their immune systems are immature, their circulation is transitioning from the intrauterine to the extra-uterine state, their thermoregulation is depressed and their respiratory systems may be under developed, among numerous other physiologic challenges.[6] In addition, the energy requirements for growth and neurodevelopment must compete with those of healing, making nutritional management complex.[7] Paediatric surgical care is also complex sociologically, with evolving patient participation. Eighty per cent of all paediatric surgeries are outpatient, with an unanticipated admission rate of <1%. Moreover, the key role of parents or caregivers as advocates and decision-makers is very pivotal for paediatric ERAS implementation.[8]

## ENHANCED RECOVERY AFTER SURGERY PROTOCOLS IN PAEDIATRICS

Enhanced recovery after surgery protocols in children cover all the aspects of the pre-operative, intra-operative and post-operative period as in adults. Currently, there are no ERAS society paediatric guidelines.

However, for the adolescent population undergoing elective intestinal surgery, 19 elements of the ERAS protocol, with the exclusion of mechanical bowel preparation (MBP) and insulin administration to treat hyperglycaemia, have been aptly explicated **(Table 1)**.[9]

Neonates represent a separate subset of the paediatric population requiring special approaches for care. Gibb et al. have been the pioneers in developing ERAS protocols for neonatal abdominal surgeries.[6] Similarly, Brindle et al. have presented evidence-based 17 ERAS recommendations for neonates undergoing intestinal resection surgeries **(Table 2)**.[3]

Though the adolescent and adult ERAS protocols are quite reproducible, the same cannot be implied for the neonates. Additionally, the paediatric ERAS protocols in outpatients are considerably variable from those applied in urology or surgeries for correction of congenital aberrations.

## EVIDENCE FOR COMMON ENHANCED RECOVERY AFTER SURGERY INTERVENTIONS IN PAEDIATRIC SURGERY

Clinical outcomes, patient and family happiness, and healthcare costs have been shown to significantly improve with enhanced recovery pathways in the

**TABLE 1:** ERAS protocols for adolescents undergoing elective intestinal surgery.[9]

| *Pre-operative* | *Intra-operative* | *Post-operative* |
|---|---|---|
| Parents, family and adolescent counselling | Antimicrobial prophylaxis | Avoidance of routine peritoneal drainage or early removal if warranted |
| Remediation of medical conditions | Multimodal antiemetic prophylaxis | Early enteral feeding |
| Minimising prolonged fasting | Use of laparoscopy or minimally invasive surgical techniques | Early ambulation |
| Use of multimodal opioid-sparing analgesia | Evasion or early removal of surgical drains or nasogastric tubes | Avoidance or early removal of the urinary catheter |
| Minimising the use of hyperosmolar mechanical bowel preparation | Implementation of protocols for hypothermia prevention | Avoidance of post-operative ileus |
| | Use of regional anaesthesia as an adjunct to standard anaesthesia techniques | Judicious use of fluids with the use of goal-directed fluid therapy or the zero fluid balance model |
| | Prophylaxis for venous thromboembolism | Scrutiny of protocol adherence and outcomes |

(ERAS: enhanced recovery after surgery)

paediatric population.[10] Nevertheless, the existing literature on paediatric ERAS is limited.

## Pre-operative Interventions

### *Pre-operative Education and Planning*

The theme of the pre-operative phase is 'education and optimisation.'[11] This should include a multidisciplinary, virtual pre-operative clinic visit involving surgeons, anaesthesiologists, psychologists, and nurses to provide age-appropriate, robust and comprehensive education, educational reading material and promote active involvement of older children and adolescents in order to aid their post-operative recovery.[2,5] At the initial clinic visit, the surgeon meets the patient and family to introduce the ERAS programme. This includes explaining to the child and the family that they will take an active role in recovery, including early nutrition and ambulation. Also, the parents are educated regarding their role in post-operative pain control, especially at home and monitoring for complications. The multimodal analgesia plan is explained, and the family is given a handout that emphasises the information discussed during the clinic visit and asked to watch a short video that takes the child through the entire ERAS experience. The risk for opioid misuse

**TABLE 2:** ERAS recommendations for neonatal intestinal surgery.[3]

| *Pre-operative* | *Intra-operative* | *Post-operative* |
|---|---|---|
| Early institution of prophylactic antibiotics within 60 minutes of surgical incision | Use of opioid restrictive analgesia and implementation of multimodal analgesic techniques, including regional blocks and acetaminophen | Structured multidisciplinary team communication |
| Optimisation of Hb (Target Hb ≥9 g/dl for term neonates not requiring oxygen and target Hb ≥ 11 g/dl for term neonates requiring oxygen or intubated) | Judicious peri-operative fluid administration to prevent hypovolaemia, hypervolaemia, hyperglycaemia and hyponatraemia | Use of multimodal opioid limiting analgesics, including regional anaesthesia and lingual sucrose |
| Structured multidisciplinary team communication | Monitor core temperatures and maintain normothermia | In neonates with enterostomy, use mucous fistula refeeding |
| | Prefer primary anastomosis in uncomplicated cases | Peri-operative antibiotics to be discontinued <24 hours of surgery |
| | | • Early institution of enteral feed (24–48 hours) with preferably breast milk<br>• Monitor and target in neonates with stoma urinary sodium levels >30 mmol/L and exceeding the level of urinary potassium |
| | | Individualise parental involvement to facilitate purposeful practice by parents |

(Hb: haemoglobin, ERAS: enhanced recovery after surgery)

and addiction in children and adolescents starts with the first peri-operative exposure to opioids. An education game (during pre-anaesthesia assessment or before discharge from the hospital) to educate the parents and the child regarding responsible opioid use may be very helpful.

Additionally, as chewing gum has been demonstrated to speed up the healing process of the gastrointestinal tract, children are asked to bring sugar-free gum to the hospital so that they can start chewing as soon as possible following surgery.[12]

### *Prehabilitation*

There is a paucity of data on prehabilitation in the paediatric surgical population. Those with reduced pre-operative functional capacity may benefit from additional therapies to build reserves for optimised recovery. Also, insulin resistance and inflammation are said to lead to post-operative metabolic derangements. Hence, children with proinflammatory conditions may benefit from pre-operative optimisation of these conditions.[13] Nutritional supplementation can be done, and immunonutrition can be administered in cancer surgery.[2]

### *Pre-operative Fasting and Carbohydrate Loading*

Dehydration, pain, and a catabolic state are linked to excessive pre-operative fasting. The pre-operative fasting time should be kept to a minimum. Recent guidelines have recommended that clear liquids should be allowed up to 2 hours, breast milk may be ingested up to 4 hours, and formula, solids and non-human milk up to 6 hours before general anaesthesia for an elective procedure.[11]

A clear liquid carbohydrate drink 2 hours before the induction of anaesthesia may promote a more stable peri-operative metabolic state, including less catabolism and insulin resistance, particularly for longer operations in children.[14] The results of a study showed that a pre-operative carbohydrate load may provide a more stable metabolic state at the induction of anaesthesia, but no reduction in post-operative nausea and vomiting (PONV).[15] In a randomised controlled trial comparing pre-operative carbohydrate beverage loading with standard fasting in 120 children scheduled for gastroscopy under general anaesthesia, carbohydrate loading was associated with significantly less gastric content, fewer patients experiencing post-operative nausea, with no significant difference in post-operative vomiting.[16]

### *Mechanical Bowel Preparation*

Mechanical bowel preparation (MBP) carries increased morbidity, often requiring an additional hospital day, nasogastric (NG) tube placement for administration of the preparation, additional laboratory tests and intravenous fluids to ensure adequate fluid and electrolyte balance during the preparation. Several small studies done in paediatric elective colorectal surgical patients have found no differences in the incidence of surgical site infection or other post-operative complications between paediatric patients who underwent MBP and those who did not.[17] An early retrospective study comparing outcomes and complications in children undergoing augmentation cystoplasty with versus without MBP found that those who were spared from bowel preparation had shorter median length of stay (LOS), earlier time to post-operative oral intake, and similar rates of infections and anastomotic leaks. However, the risk of shunt infections existed in patients with spina bifida with ventriculoperitoneal shunts in whom MBP was omitted.[18]

### *Pre-emptive Analgesia*

Pre-emptive analgesia includes drugs such as acetaminophen, ibuprofen, gabapentin and tramadol administered to the child to attenuate pain and the surgical inflammatory response.[11] Intravenous dexmedetomidine, ketamine and locoregional blocks such as caudal blocks and regional nerve blocks can also be used to provide pre-emptive analgesia.[19]

## Intra-operative Interventions

### *Maintenance of Normothermia*

It is a well-known fact that neonates, infants and children are more susceptible to anaesthetic-induced temperature dysregulation, which can affect recovery. The Pediatric Urology Recovery After Surgery Endeavor (PURSUE) multicentric study has incorporated maintenance of normothermia, defined as body temperature of 36–38°C during skin-to-skin time, into their revised ERAS protocol for lower urinary tract reconstruction.[20]

### *Maintenance of Euvolaemia and Fluid Management*

Aggressive use of intravenous fluids has been associated with worse outcomes in paediatric patients undergoing cardiac surgery and colorectal surgery.[5] Specifically, giving fluids >90th percentile in colonic resection overall was associated with LOS >6 days, time to first meal >4 days and supplemental oxygen requirement >24 hours.[21] Goal-directed fluid resuscitation is now commonly practised and has been shown to significantly decrease the volume of intra-operative fluids administered and reduce surgical morbidity.[22] New technologies can help assess a patient's fluid responsiveness (oesophageal Doppler, non-invasive cardiac output monitoring, plethysmography variability index, stroke volume index, transoesophageal echocardiography, aortic peak blood flow velocity). Currently, no single method has been shown to be superior.

### *Use of Regional Anaesthesia*

The use of regional anaesthesia as the prime technique/as an adjunct to general anaesthesia for the surgical procedure can help reduce/avoid the use of sedatives, including opioids, provide both intra-operative and post-operative analgesia, and thereby facilitate early recovery after the surgery. Also, exposure to general anaesthetic drugs in neonates may cause neuronal apoptosis. This can be reduced by the use of neuraxial anaesthesia, including spinal and epidural anaesthesia and regional nerve blocks. Both peripheral and fascial plane nerve blocks can be used as part of multimodal analgesia regimens.[23,24] Local anaesthetics can be used along with dexmedetomidine/clonidine/dexamethasone/fentanyl for the blocks. Peripheral nerve blocks that are administered in children include ilioinguinal/iliohypogastric nerve block, penile block, adductor canal block, femoral nerve block, popliteal block, obturator block, brachial plexus block, paravertebral block, etc. There is no convincing scientific evidence currently for the use of fascial plane blocks in children, except for rectus sheath block and quadratus lumborum block.[23] Fascial plane blocks do not appear to provide surgical anaesthesia, and it is not possible to perform surgery using only a fascial plane block.[23] They can be used as an adjunct technique for peri-operative analgesia. Blocks such as paravertebral block, transversus abdominis plane block, rectus sheath block, quadratus lumborum block, erector spinae plane block are some modalities that can be used in neonates. However, as in children, fascial plane blocks may be unpredictable and variable in neonates.[25] Nevertheless, various researchers have demonstrated several potential advantages of peripheral nerve block techniques and fascial plane blocks such as transversus abdominis plane, erector spinae plane, paravertebral, rectus sheath and quadratus lumborum blocks in paediatric patients for improving post-operative analgesia and reducing adverse effects related to opioids. Epidural, caudal epidural or combined spinal-epidural techniques are safe and may have physiological benefits in ERAS protocols in children.[26,27]

### *Use of Multimodal Analgesia*

Options for multimodal analgesia to reduce opioid requirements in children include regional nerve blocks, paracetamol, acetaminophen, midazolam, gabapentin, dexamethasone, clonidine, dexmedetomidine and non-steroidal anti-inflammatory drugs (NSAIDs) such as ibuprofen or ketorolac. Central neuraxial block, ring block with local anaesthetics, oral sucrose, non-nutritive sucking, eutectic mixture of local anaesthetics (EMLA) cream for topical anaesthesia can be used in neonates and infants. Reduction in parenteral opioid requirements potentially contributes to faster return of gut motility, reduction in length of hospital stay and oversedation. Also, the child's first exposure to opioids may be during operative pain management. Multimodal analgesia can reduce the risk of opioid misuse and addiction in children and adolescents that can result after surgery.[28] Short-acting opioids such as remifentanil, which have favourable characteristics for ERAS, such as short duration of action and rapid elimination, can be used in neonates and children.

### *Use of Nasogastric Tubes*

The older theory suggests that children swallow a lot of air when they are upset or crying. NG tubes are thought to be necessary in paediatric surgery, but evidence exists for the avoidance of routine NG tubes in paediatrics. A significant decrease in time to first feed, first stool and discharge has been found in patients without NG tubes. However, the absence of NG tube decompression can be associated with a higher incidence of post-operative vomiting. Current literature challenges the concept of NG tube placement for paralytic ileus that can accompany gastrointestinal surgeries.[29]

### *Minimising Placement of Tubes and Drains*

Current evidence suggests no association of operative drain placement and improved outcomes in many paediatric urologic procedures.[30] Several paediatric urology studies have effectively included this element in their improved recovery regimens without experiencing a rise in unfavourable outcomes.[31]

## Post-operative Interventions

### *Adequate Post-operative Analgesia*

Opioid-sparing multi-modal analgesia is the best option. Cool packs can be kept on the wound to reduce oedema and pain. Non-opioid analgesics such as acetaminophen, ibuprofen and ketorolac in parenteral form, oral suspensions or rectal suppositories aid early recovery. Transdermal patches of lappaconitine (a C18-diterpenoid alkaloid)/diclofenac can be used in older children, especially for oropharyngeal pain, e.g., post-tonsillectomy.[32] Nerve blocks and local anaesthetic wound infiltration that have been used as a part of multimodal analgesia regimens can provide post-operative analgesia.[23,24] Port site local anaesthetic infiltration can provide post-operative analgesia after laparoscopic surgery in children. Acetaminophen, NSAIDs, peripheral nerve blocks, caudal blocks and remifentanil can be used in neonates.[25]

### *Prevention of Post-operative Nausea and Vomiting*

A few ways to lower a child's risk of PONV include avoiding nitrous oxide and volatile anaesthetics. This can be done by the utilisation of propofol for induction and maintenance, use of regional anaesthesia such as transversus abdominis plane block, rectus sheath block for abdominal surgery, epidural and spinal analgesia to avoid general anaesthesia, use of multimodal analgesia to minimise intra- and post-operative opioids, and adequate hydration.[29,30] Risk scores for PONV and antiemetics such as 5-hydroxytryptamine type 3 (5-HT3) receptor antagonists, specifically intravenous ondansetron

0.1 mg/kg, dexamethasone 0.15–0.3 mg/kg and aprepitant 40 or 80 mg are commonly used for both prophylaxis and rescue treatment of PONV.[33]

### *Early Mobilisation*

Pedometers, patient diaries, corridor posters, and the lack of in-room entertainment are a few tactics that have been effective. The goal of early mobilisation necessitates a multidisciplinary strategy that includes physical therapy, encouragement from nurses, and pain management.[11]

### *Early Oral Intake*

According to studies, it is safe to begin early enteral feeding in children with intestinal anastomosis without waiting for conventional indicators of the return of bowel activity. It lowers hospital stay with no adverse effects.[34]

In a multicentric study, it was found that early oral feeding following intestinal anastomosis surgery in infants was associated with shorter duration of post-operative parenteral nutrition, shorter hospital stay, higher rates of abdominal distension and vomiting and no difference in anastomotic leakage compared to delayed oral feeding.[35]

### *Prevention of Post-operative Ileus*

This can be achieved by the use of minimally invasive surgery, use of thoracic epidural analgesia, abdominal trunk blocks and avoiding excessive intra-operative fluids. Post-operative ileus can be avoided by using multimodal techniques such as localised analgesia, opioid-sparing techniques using drugs such as gabapentin and ketorolac, and/or the use of opioid antagonists like methylnaltrexone or alvimopan.[11]

In a retrospective study including children who underwent appendectomy, pyloromyotomy, transabdominal Soave procedure, Meckel's diverticulum resection, or reduction of intussusception, the surgical outcomes were compared between children who underwent surgery under conventional peri-operative regimens and those who were treated with ERAS protocols. In comparison to the control group, the ERAS group saw considerably shorter recovery times for bowel function, post-operative intravenous nutrition times, post-operative hospital stays, and hospital expenses. There was no significant intergroup difference in the complication rate.[36]

In a prospective observational study aimed at comparing the outcomes between ERAS and conventional peri-operative care protocol in colostomy closure in children, the post-operative outcome (return of bowel movement and commencement of oral feeding) was 4.13 times better in the ERAS group than that of the conventional group. 66.7% of subjects needed only 7 days of post-operative hospital stay in the ERAS group, whereas only 16.7% of subjects showed 7 days of post-operative hospital stay.[37]

## CHALLENGES AND BARRIERS IN THE IMPLEMENTATION OF ENHANCED RECOVERY AFTER SURGERY PROTOCOLS IN PAEDIATRIC SURGERY

The following challenges and barriers have contributed to the slow adoption of paediatric ERAS even in protocol areas in which strong and high-quality evidence is available:

- The definition of recovery is not very clear in children. Assessing complete recovery in children has always been a challenge.
- The published literature in support of ERAS protocols in children has always been limited and not supported with good-quality evidence.[8]
- There have been the following arguments against the implementation of ERAS in the paediatric population: (1) As compared to adults, children have better baseline physiology and reduced morbidity and mortality associated with surgery; therefore, there is very little benefit in adopting a formal ERAS guideline for children.[38] (2) Since children have very different physiological and neurological development as compared to adults, the data obtained from adults cannot be applied to children. (3) Many surgeons believe that they are already implementing practices which improve clinical outcomes and therefore a formal ERAS guideline is not required.[39]
- Lack of support from the institute, ignorance of hospital staff and peri-operative team regarding ERAS protocols, challenges in the coordination of multidisciplinary care, and resistance to altering surgical practices out of concern for unfavourable results have been observed in many areas.[40]
- Shortage of trained medical staff and specific medical equipment, specifically in India, acts as one of the key barriers in the implementation of the ERAS programme.
- Hospitals are not willing to formulate a formal policy and allocate funds to implement ERAS protocols, and as a result, there is a lack of willingness in medical staff and departmental leaders to try new concepts.
- Surgeons have antiquated ideas and are hesitant to adopt innovative procedures, primarily due to concerns about patient safety. Some of the surgeons still believe that early discharge of the paediatric patients can result in an increased complication rate at home.
- Due to heavy patient load and lack of medical staff, information conveyed by the doctors to patients is often insufficient and unclear, which leads to incomplete following of the pre-operative and post-operative instructions given to the patients.
- The awareness about ERAS protocols among parents is still very low. Furthermore, parents are always resistant to trying new concepts in their children and continue to practice traditional methods in their children for recovery.

## FUTURE APPROACH TO IMPROVING THE IMPLEMENTATION OF PAEDIATRIC ENHANCED RECOVERY AFTER SURGERY PATHWAY AND OPTIMISING OUTCOMES

For the better implementation of ERAS guidelines, there should be large multicentric randomised controlled trials that compare traditional practice and ERAS protocols to reveal the gaps in implementation. Such studies are costly and time-consuming and require extensive cooperation from various medical specialities and nursing staff. Nevertheless, anaesthesiologists in cooperation with paediatric surgeons can carry out large-scale prospective studies, which can help in developing specific paediatric ERAS protocols.

Anaesthesiologists are already the administrators of the operating room; however, they should assume a more central role in peri-operative care too and by doing so, they can play a vital role in overcoming the challenges and barriers in the implementation of ERAS. A study conducted in South Korea on the attitudes of hepatobiliary surgeons towards ERAS protocols cited inadequate cooperation from various departments, particularly anaesthesiology, as one of the main reasons for its poor implementation.[41] There are some components of ERAS, such as pre-operative optimisation and opioid-sparing multimodal analgesia, in which anaesthesiologists can play a key role.

The identification and addressing of barriers in the adoption of ERAS among a larger proportion of paediatric surgeons is necessary. Working together with specialists in implementation science, a discipline that investigates and creates plans to encourage the integration of evidence-based treatments into clinical practice, will be necessary to accomplish this.[42]

The application of even a few elements of the ERAS pathway can increase patients' comfort and parental satisfaction and reduce hospital LOS.[5] It has been observed that improvement in results can occur with 70–80% adherence to ERAS elements.[43] A 'soft launch' strategy, in which teams choose one or two low-cost ERAS protocol components they wish to try to improve upon (e.g. early feeding, avoidance/early removal of urinary catheter), can make the process of establishing a formal ERAS programme in a hospital easier. Over time, they can choose more items in the protocol and implement them.[44] Each institution, based on the surrounding local culture, setting, and health care system, has to develop common strategies that are likely to positively influence the development and implementation of paediatric ERAS programmes. In addition to all surgeons, anaesthesiologists, nurse practitioners, nurses, research staff, and ancillary medical professionals (dieticians, physiotherapists, occupational therapists and child life specialists) who are dedicated to developing and implementing paediatric ERAS protocols, an ERAS working group can be established. This can include an ERAS nurse coordinator.[4]

## CONCLUSION

ERAS protocols have been developed and implemented in various types of paediatric surgery. However, paediatric ERAS has been slow to develop due to various barriers. Nevertheless, evidence on its implementation in children is gaining gradual momentum.

## REFERENCES

1. Ljungqvist O. Enhanced Recovery After Surgery: A Paradigm Shift in Perioperative Care. In: Ljungqvist O, Francis N, Urman R (Eds). Enhanced Recovery After Surgery. Cham, Switzerland: Springer; 2020.
2. Ha D, Harris KT, Brockel MA, Rove KO. The role of enhanced recovery after surgery (ERAS) in promoting quality improvement and patient safety in pediatric urology. Front Urol. 2023;3:1275276.
3. Brindle ME, McDiarmid C, Short K, Miller K, MacRobie A, Lam JYK, et al. Consensus guidelines for perioperative care in neonatal intestinal surgery: Enhanced Recovery After Surgery (ERAS®) society recommendations. World J Surg. 2020;44(8):2482-92.
4. Emil S, Ferriera J, Frigon C, Guadagno E, Frigon C, Guadagno E, et al. Starting on the road to pediatric enhanced recovery after surgery: strategies and themes. J Pediatr Surg Open. 2024;(6):100128.
5. Roberts K, Brindle M, McLuckie D. Enhanced recovery after surgery in paediatrics: a review of the literature. BJA Education. 2020;20(7):235-41.
6. Gibb ACN, Crosby MA, McDiarmid C, Urban D, Lam JYK, Wales PW, et al. Creation of an Enhanced Recovery After Surgery (ERAS) Guideline for neonatal intestinal surgery patients: a knowledge synthesis and consensus generation approach and protocol study. BMJ Open. 2018;8(12):e023651.
7. Velazco CS, Zurakowski D, Fullerton BS, Bechard LJ, Jaksic T, Mehta NM. Nutrient delivery in mechanically ventilated surgical patients in the pediatric critical care unit. J Pediatr Surg. 2017;52(1):145-8.
8. Leeds IL, Boss EF, George JA, Strockbine V, Wick EC, Jelin EB. Preparing enhanced recovery after surgery for implementation in pediatric populations. J Pediatr Surg. 2016;51(12):2126-9.
9. Short HL, Heiss KF, Burch K, Travers C, Edney J, Venable C, et al. Implementation of an enhanced recovery protocol in pediatric colorectal surgery. J Pediatr Surg. 2017;53(4):688-92.
10. Heiss KF, Raval MV. Patient engagement to enhance recovery for children undergoing surgery. Semin Pediatr Surg. 2018;27(2):86-91.
11. Rafeequi T, Pearson EG. Enhanced recovery after surgery in children. Transl Gastroenterol Hepatol. 2021;6:46.
12. Meyer JP, Fawcett D. The use of chewing gum for preventing postoperative ileus. BJU Int. 2008;101(1):1-2.
13. Chabot K, Gillis C, Carli F. Prehabilitation: metabolic considerations. Curr Opin Clin Nutr Metab Care. 2020;23(4):271-6.
14. Ljungqvist O. Modulating postoperative insulin resistance by preoperative carbohydrate loading. Best Pract Res Clin Anaesthesiol. 2009;23(4):401-9.
15. Laird A, Bramley L, Barnes R, Englin A, Winderlich J, Mount E, et al. Effects of a preoperative carbohydrate load on postoperative recovery in children:

A randomised, double-blind, placebo-controlled trial. J Pediatr Surg. 2023;58(9):1824-31.
16. Tudor-Drobjewski BA, Marhofer P, Kimberger O, Huber WD, Roth G, Triffterer L. Randomised controlled trial comparing preoperative carbohydrate loading with standard fasting in paediatric anaesthesia. Br J Anaesth. 2018;121(3):656-61.
17. Janssen Lok M, Miyake H, O'Connell JS, Seo S, Pierro A. The value of mechanical bowel preparation prior to pediatric colorectal surgery: a systematic review and meta-analysis. Pediatr Surg Int. 2018;34(12):1305-20.
18. Gundeti MS, Godbole PP, Wilcox DT. Is bowel preparation required before cystoplasty in children? J Urol. 2006;176(4 Pt 1):1574-6.
19. Matsota PK, Kaminioti EN, Kostopanagiotou GG. Preemptive and preventive analgesia in different paediatric surgical settings: A systematic review of prospective randomized controlled trials. Clin Surg. 2019;4:2393.
20. Rove KO, Strine AC, Wilcox DT, Vricella GJ, Welch TP, VanderBrink B, et al. Design and development of the pediatric urology recovery after surgery endeavor (Pursue) multicentre pilot and exploratory study. BMJ Open. 2020;10(11):e039035.
21. Sanford EL, Zurakowski D, Litvinova A, Zalieckas JM, Cravero JP. The association between high-volume intraoperative fluid administration and outcomes among pediatric patients undergoing large bowel resection. Paediatr Anaesth. 2019;29(4):315e21.
22. Mathew PJ, Sharma S, Bhardwaj N, Ashok V, Malik MA. Goal-directed fluid therapy guided by plethysmographic variability index (PVI) versus conventional liberal fluid administration in children during elective abdominal surgery: A randomized controlled trial. J Pediatr Surg. 2023;58(4):735-40.
23. Lonnqvist PA. Fascial plane blocks in children-Scientifically supported or not? Paediatr Anaesth. 2024;34(1):13-8.
24. Kedall MC, Alves LJC, Suh EI, McCormick ZL, De Oliveira GS. Regional anesthesia to ameliorate postoperative analgesia outcomes in pediatric surgical patients: an updated systematic review of randomized controlled trials. Local Reg Anesth. 2018;11:91-109.
25. Visoiu M. Evolving approaches in neonatal postoperative pain management. Semin Pediatr Surg. 2022;31(4):151203.
26. Phillips MR, Adamson WT, McLean SE, Hance L, Lupa MC, Pittenger SL, et al. Implementation of a pediatric enhanced recovery pathway decreases opioid utilization and shortens time to full feeding. J Pediatr Surg. 2020;55(1):101-5.
27. Pirrera B, Alagna V, Lucchi A, Berti P, Gabbianelli C, Martorelli G, et al. Transversus abdominis plane (TAP) block versus thoracic epidural analgesia (TEA) in laparoscopic colon surgery in the ERAS program. Surg Endosc. 2018;32(1):376-82.
28. Abraham O, Rosenberger CA, Birstler J, Tierney K. Examining adolescents' opioid knowledge and likelihood to utilize an educational game to promote medication safety. Res Social Adm Pharm. 2022;18(7):3191-8.
29. Peter SDS, Valusek PA, Little DC, Snyder CL, Holcomb GW, Ostlie DJ. Does routine nasogastric tube placement after an operation for perforated appendicitis make a difference? J Surg Res. 2007;143(1):66e9.
30. Neville JJ, Aldeiri B. Drain placement in paediatric complicated appendicitis: A systematic review and meta-analysis. Pediatr Surg Int. 2023;39(1):171.

31. Rickard M, Chua M, Kim JK, Keefe DT, Milford K, Hannick JH, et al. Evolving trends in peri-operative management of pediatric ureteropelvic junction obstruction: working towards quicker recovery and day surgery pyeloplasty. World J Urol. 2021;39(9):3677-84.
32. Xu J, Wu M, Duan B, Ni Y, Wang A. The analgesic effect of a transdermal lappaconitine patch combined with ibuprofen suspension for children after adenoidectomy and tonsillectomy: A randomized clinical trial. J Perianesth Nurs. 2025;40(1):126-33.
33. Urits I, Orhurhu V, Jones MR, Adamian L, Borchart M, Galasso A, et al. Postoperative nausea and vomiting in paediatric anaesthesia. Turk J Anaesthesiol Reanim. 2020;48(2):88-95.
34. Mamatha B, Alladi A. Early oral feeding in pediatric intestinal anastomosis. Indian J Surg. 2015;77(Suppl 2):S670-2.
35. Lu C, Sun X, Geng Q, Tang W. Early oral feeding following intestinal anastomosis surgery in infants: a multicenter real world study. Front Nutr. 2023;10:1185876.
36. Gao R, Yang H, Li Y, Meng L, Li Y, Sun B, et al. Enhanced recovery after surgery in pediatric gastrointestinal surgery. J Internat Med Res. 2019;47(10):4815-26.
37. Atiquzzaman TM, Hossain T, Mondal SK, Huq AU, Mahammad N, Haque N, et al. Evaluation of outcome of enhanced recovery after surgery (ERAS) versus conventional method in colostomy closure in children. Med Res Chronicles. 2022;9(5):272-82.
38. Brindle ME, Heiss K, Scott MJ, Herndon CA, Ljungqvist O, Koyle MA; on behalf Pediatric ERAS (Enhanced Recovery After Surgery) Society. Embracing change: the era for pediatric ERAS is here. Ped Surg Inter. 2019;35(6):631-4.
39. Short HL, Taylor N, Thakore M, Piper K, Baxter K, Heiss KF. et al. A survey of pediatric surgeons' practices with enhanced recovery after children's surgery. J Pediatr Surg. 2018;53(3):418-30.
40. Xie N, Xie H, Tang W. Baseline assessment of enhanced recovery after pediatric surgery in mainland China. Pediatr Surg Int. 2022;39(1):32.
41. Shin SH, Kang W, Han IW, You Y, Lee H, Kim H, et al. National survey of Korean hepatobiliary-pancreatic surgeons on attitudes about the enhanced recovery after surgery protocol. Ann Hepatobiliary Pancreat Surg. 2020;24(4):477-83.
42. Yi JA, Hakimi A, Vavra AK. Application of dissemination and implementation science frameworks to surgical research. Semin Vasc Surg. 2022;35(4):456-63.
43. Ljungqvist O, Scott M, Fearon KC. Enhanced recovery after surgery: a review. JAMA Surg. 2017;152(3):292-8.
44. Nelson G. The time is right to implement Enhanced Recovery After Surgery (ERAS) broadly across paediatric surgery. J Pediatr Sur Open. 2024;(5):100113.

CHAPTER 16

# Assessment and Management of Paediatric Trauma: Be Prepared for Any Situation!

*Kajal Jain, Jeetinder Kaur Makkar, Nidhi Bhatia*

## ABSTRACT

Trauma in paediatric patients represents a diverse population due to their unique anatomic, physiologic, and psychological characteristics, particularly in response to injury. Evaluation and management of paediatric trauma warrants protocols based on a child's weight and age, and mechanism of injury. In prehospital settings or arrival to the emergency trauma bay, the initial management of paediatric patients should prioritise the airway, breathing and circulation, with the goals being to rapidly identify the injuries, determine management priorities, and provide critical interventions at the same time. In addition, neurological assessment and temperature monitoring should be documented as part of the primary survey. Initial primary evaluation should be followed by a detailed secondary survey, ensuring complete head-to-toe physical examination along with a detailed history, followed by definitive management. In addition to managing specific injuries, pain in paediatric trauma victims also needs redressal, which is often poorly understood, under-recognised and hence inadequately treated. The pain experienced after trauma in children is a complex interplay of somatic, visceral, and neuropathic pain, compounded by psychological, social, and cultural factors, making pain evaluation particularly challenging. Literature emphasises the necessity of adequate and timely analgesic relief in paediatric patients to avoid complications of chronic pain. At all times, it is important to keep in mind that since paediatric patients have different anatomical and physiological characteristics as compared to adults, their response to trauma is different and they should be managed accordingly.

***Keywords:*** Management, Paediatric, Rescue, Resuscitation, Shock, Trauma.

## INTRODUCTION

Trauma is one of the most common causes of mortality in children. Although adult trauma systems are robust, trauma centres in low-resource settings are limited, and not every child who is injured may have easy access to a trauma centre, in contrast to Western countries. The paediatric patients represent a diverse population due to their unique anatomic, physiologic, and psychological characteristics, particularly in response to injury. The majority of paediatric traumatic injuries are unintentional (88%) and blunt in nature (>90%), occurring either at home (33.6%) or on the street (29.9%). While traumatic injuries are often referred to as "accidents", the vast majority are foreseeable and thus represent discrete opportunities for prevention.[1-3]

According to the National Trauma Database, the top three mechanisms of injury are falls (34.1%), motor vehicle collisions [(MVCs) 23.7%], and pedestrians struck by drivers (9.8%). While falls are the leading cause of injuries in children 0–14 years of age, MVCs are more common in adolescents.[4,5]

## INITIAL RESCUE

Effective prehospital triage is necessary for optimal utilisation of resources. Various triage scoring tools that emphasise physiological parameters rather than just the mechanism of injury have demonstrated greater accuracy in predicting injury severity. The most commonly used scores include Paediatric Trauma Score (PTS), Paediatric Glasgow Coma Scale (P-GCS) and paediatric age-adjusted shock index (SIPA) **(Tables 1 to 3)**.[1,6-8]

While using the Glasgow Coma Scale (GCS) for young children, obtaining accurate verbal and eye components can be difficult. Relying on the motor score alone may make it simpler for first responders as well as physicians in emergency departments (EDs) to identify paediatric patients with severe injuries who should be transferred to paediatric trauma centres. The shock index is a tool that uses physiological parameters to identify severely injured trauma patients by calculating the ratio of heart rate (HR) to systolic blood pressure (SBP). Because normal vital sign ranges differ significantly among children of various ages, SIPA was developed. It is calculated by dividing the maximum HR by the minimum SBP based on age. In resource-limited settings like India, where paediatric or trauma surgeons may not always be available, it is crucial to identify the most urgent cases for prompt

**TABLE 1:** Paediatric trauma score (PTS).

| *Assessment component* | *Score* | | |
|---|---|---|---|
| | +2 | +1 | −1 |
| Weight (kg) | >20 | 10–20 | <10 |
| Airway | Normal | Oral/nasal airway | Intubated / tracheostomy |
| Systolic Blood Pressure (mmHg) | >90, good peripheral pulses and perfusion | 50–90, carotid/ femoral pulses palpable | <50, weak/no pulses |
| Conscious Level | Awake | Obtunded/any loss of consciousness | Comatose |
| Fractures | None | Single, closed | Multiple and/or open |
| Cutaneous | Nonvisible | Contusions/abrasions/ lacerations (<7 cm, not through the fascia) | Tissue loss, penetrating wound through the fascia, burns |

**TABLE 2:** Paediatric Glasgow Coma Scale (P-GCS).

| ***Assessment component*** | ***Age (years)*** | ***Score*** | | | | | |
|---|---|---|---|---|---|---|---|
| *Eye opening* | ≤2 | 1—none | 2—to pain | 3—to speech | 4—spontaneously | | |
| | >2 | 1—none | 2—to pain | 3—to speech | 4—spontaneously | | |
| *Verbal response* | ≤2 | 1—none | 2—moans in response to pain | 3—cries in response to pain | 4—irritable/cries | 5—coos and babbles | |
| | >2 | 1—none | 2—incomprehensible sounds | 3—incomprehensible words | 4—confused | 5—oriented | |
| *Motor response* | ≤2 | 1—none | 2—abnormal extension to pain | 3—abnormal flexion to pain | 4—withdrawal to pain | 5—withdraws to touch | 6—moves spontaneously and purposefully |
| | >2 | 1—none | 2—abnormal extension to pain | 3—abnormal flexion to pain | 4—withdrawal to pain | 5—localises pain | 6—obeys commands |

**TABLE 3:** Shock index, paediatric age-adjusted (SIPA) Score Cut-off Values.

| *Age (years)* | *Heart rate (beats/min)* | *Systolic blood pressure (mmHg)* | *SIPA cut-off values* |
|---|---|---|---|
| 1–3 | 70–110 | 90–110 | 1.2 |
| 4–6 | 65–110 | 90–110 | 1.2 |
| 7–12 | 60–100 | 100–120 | 1.0 |
| >12 | 55–90 | 100–135 | 0.9 |

referral to higher-level centres. In this context, utilising available resources to calculate a screening score based on vital parameters, such as the SIPA score, can be extremely beneficial.

However, prehospital care is often suboptimal in low and middle-income countries (LMICs). Paediatric patients are most likely to be transferred from the scene of the accident by either the police personnel, an immediate family member or untrained observers. Hence, in low-resource settings, initial patient stabilisation mostly begins at the hospital. The goals of initial trauma management in children, as in adults, with minor modifications due to anatomical and physiological differences, are to rapidly assess the injuries, determine management priorities, and provide critical interventions. Achieving these goals requires a systematic and logical approach presented below in an expanded format to emphasise the importance of performing specific procedures rapidly in the ED and the crucial need to continuously reassess vital functions:[1,7]

- Primary survey (rapid primary evaluation)
- Resuscitation of vital functions (e.g. airway, breathing, circulation and mentation)
- Utilisation of adjuncts to the primary survey and resuscitation
- Secondary survey (more comprehensive secondary assessment)
- Continued post-resuscitation monitoring with further resuscitation as needed
- Utilisation of adjuncts to the secondary survey
- Transition to definitive care

## INITIAL MANAGEMENT OF TRAUMA PATIENT

The initial management of the paediatric trauma patient should prioritise the airway, breathing and circulation.

### Airway with Cervical Spine Protection

In the supine position, a child's relatively large occiput flexes the neck, which can lead to airway obstruction, especially in those with altered mental status. The small oral cavity and relatively large tongue increase the likelihood of upper airway obstruction. Additionally, the larynx is positioned more cephalad and anterior in infants and children, complicating endotracheal intubation. Other anatomical considerations include a short trachea, a relatively large and floppy epiglottis, a small distance between tracheal rings in infants, and a cricothyroid membrane that is difficult to palpate.[5-7]

The common indications for securing the airway include actual, impending, or potential airway obstruction, respiratory distress and impaired mental status (GCS ≤8). In small children requiring a surgical airway, needle cricothyroidotomy is the preferred approach and is a temporising measure while resources are gathered for a definitive tracheostomy.

### *Airway Management*[4-6]

Airway management in children differs from that in adults due to distinct anatomical characteristics, mentioned above, that must be considered before intubation. In addition, it is vital to keep in mind that:

- Oxygen saturation decreases rapidly because they have a lesser oxygen reserve, stemming from a smaller functional residual capacity and higher oxygen consumption.
- Supplemental oxygen must be administered at all times.
- *Proper positioning is crucial for intubation:* Optimal position is achieved when the child's head is positioned with the neck in a neutral or slightly extended (sniffing) position, with the ears aligned with the sternum.
- Avoid pressure on the floor of the mouth, as this can push the tongue back against the palate, causing airway obstruction.
- Infants have a more pronounced vagal response to endotracheal intubation than children and adults, often resulting in bradycardia with direct laryngeal stimulation.
- Orotracheal intubation under direct vision with restricted cervical motion is the preferred method for achieving definitive airway control.
- For intubation, cuffed endotracheal tubes are preferred even in toddlers and small children, as they improve ventilation and carbon dioxide management, enhancing cerebral blood flow. In children above the age of 2 years, the size of the tracheal tube can be calculated using these formulas:
- Uncuffed tracheal tube: 4 + (age in years/4)
- Cuffed tracheal tube: 3.5 + (age in years/4)

For children under 2 years, the appropriate cuffed tube sizes are:

- *Up to 1 year:* 3.0 mm inner diameter (ID)
- *From 1 to 2 years:* 3.5 mm ID
- To roughly estimate the endotracheal tube size for a specific patient, approximate the diameter of the child's external nares or the tip of their smallest finger and use a similarly sized tube. Length-based paediatric

resuscitation tapes, i.e. Broselow tape, also list the appropriate tube sizes. The length for tube fixation can be calculated using:

- Centimetres at mouth fixation: child's height in cm/10 + 5
- Centimetres at nose fixation: Child's height in cm/10 + 7
- Most trauma centres follow a protocol for emergency intubation known as drug-assisted or rapid sequence intubation. Clinicians must carefully consider the child's weight, vital signs (pulse and blood pressure), and level of consciousness to determine the appropriate drugs.
- Supraglottic airway devices are suitable adjuncts for infants and children, but their placement requires experience, and vigorous ventilation may distend the stomach. Oropharyngeal airway/nasopharyngeal airway (OPA/NPA) can be used as adjuncts to bag-valve-mask ventilation or temporary measures prior to endotracheal intubation (NPA is contraindicated if cribriform plate fracture is suspected). An appropriate size of OPA is measured from the mouth's angle to the patient's mandibular angle. An appropriate size guide of measurement for NPA is from the lateral aspect of the nares to the tragus of the ear on the same side. Paediatric NPA sizing may also be accomplished using a Broselow tape, a colour-coded tape measure that classifies a child into one of eight colour zones by height. The Broselow tape also contains additional guides about size selection for other airway equipment types and medications used during resuscitation.
- Surgical cricothyroidotomy is rarely indicated for infants or small children but can be performed in older children with a palpable cricothyroid membrane (usually >12 years of age).
- Restriction of cervical spine mobility must always be maintained during airway management. As appropriately sized paediatric cervical collars may be difficult to find, the head can be taped to a firm backboard using towels or saline bags as supports.

## Breathing and Ventilation[1,4,5]

Hypoxia is the primary cause of cardiac arrest in children, making adequate oxygenation and ventilation critical to maintain acid-base balance. Since infants and children have limited functional residual capacity and higher oxygen consumption, they become hypoxaemic much faster than adults. It is important to remember that the compliant paediatric chest wall predisposes children to underlying pulmonary contusion, often without rib fractures. While managing a child's breathing and ventilation, the normal respiratory rate needs to be kept in mind. Respiratory rate in children decreases with age, with an infant breathing at a rate of 30–40 breaths/min and a child having a respiratory rate of 15–20 breaths/minute. Additionally, the tidal volumes vary from 4 to 6 ml/kg in infants and children. Excessive volume/pressure during assisted ventilation should be avoided as there is a substantially increased risk of iatrogenic barotrauma due to the fragile and immature tracheobronchial tree.

## Circulation[6-10]

Early recognition of circulatory compromise in children is crucial; the first signs include tachycardia, poor skin perfusion, and diminished capillary refill. Due to their robust catecholamine-induced compensation, children can maintain blood pressure even after losing 30–45% of their total blood volume **(Table 4)**. As a result, hypotension indicating uncompensated shock is a late and sudden development, requiring immediate intervention. In infants, early-stage uncompensated shock with hypotension is marked by tachycardia, which can progress to bradycardia if blood loss continues unchecked. HR and blood pressure vary with age in the paediatric population **(Tables 5 and 6)**.

Haemorrhage control, intravenous (IV) access for administration of crystalloid or blood, and advanced procedures for persistent haemodynamic compromise constitute the primary management issues for the circulation phase of the primary survey.

**TABLE 4:** Estimated blood volume in children.

| *Age* | *Blood volume* |
|---|---|
| Premature infants | 100 cc/kg |
| <3 months | 85 cc/kg |
| Children >3 months | 75 cc/kg |
| Adolescents | 70 cc/kg |

**TABLE 5:** Normal paediatric heart rate by age.

| *Age (years)* | *Normal HR* | *Awake HR* | *Paediatric trauma HR* |
|---|---|---|---|
| 1 | <160 | 100–180 | 120–169 |
| 2–3 | <140–150 | 98–140 | 100–159 |
| 4 | <140 | 80–120 | 80–139 |
| 5–6 | <120–140 | 80–120 | 80–119 |
| 7–8 | <120 | 75–118 | 80–99 |
| 9–11 | <120 | 75–118 | 80–99 |
| 12–13 | <100–120 | 60–100 | 80–99 |
| 14 | <100 | 60–100 | 60–99 |

(HR: heart rate in beats per minute)

**TABLE 6:** Lower limit of normal paediatric systolic blood pressure by age.

| *Age (years)* | *SBP (lower limit)* (mmHg)* | *SBP (lower limit)# (mmHg)* |
|---|---|---|
| 1 | 60 | 70 |
| 2–3 | 70–75 | 74–76 |
| 4 | 75 | 78 |
| 5–6 | 75–80 | 80–82 |
| 7–8 | 80 | 84–86 |
| 9–11 | 80 | 88–90 |
| 12–13 | 80–90 | 90 |
| 14 | 90 | 90 |

*As per Advanced Trauma Life Support (ATLS®) guidelines
#As per Paediatric Advanced Life Support (PALS®) guidelines
(SBP: systolic blood pressure)

- Upon arrival in the trauma bay, two large-bore IV catheters should be promptly inserted in paediatric patients. However, this can be challenging, especially in cases of diminished circulatory volume. If two attempts at IV access fail, an intraosseous (IO) catheter should be placed. IO access can be obtained in the proximal or distal tibia, distal femur, or proximal humerus. To prepare for insertion, the leg should be stabilised (e.g. using a rolled towel under the knee) in slight external rotation. Proper site selection and preparation are crucial, whether using a mechanical device like the EZ-IO® or manual techniques. The IO needle should be inserted at a 90° angle to the bone, and the placement can be confirmed by aspirating the bone marrow or checking for fluid flow. The IO needle should not remain in place for more than 24 hours. Potential complications include bone fracture during insertion, growth plate injury, dislodgment of the IO needle, and extramedullary infusion with a risk of compartment syndrome. Close monitoring is essential, focusing on limb colour, needle position, patency and signs of extravasation.
- While percutaneous femoral vein access can be attempted, it often presents challenges. Jugular and subclavian lines should generally be avoided as initial vascular access in paediatric trauma due to the risks of vascular injury or pneumothorax. A venous cut-down on the saphenous vein is another option, but it can be time-consuming.

### *Assessment of Circulation*

- Assessment of the circulation begins with examining the level of consciousness, skin colour, HR, blood pressure, and peripheral pulses. Haemorrhagic shock can be classified in children based on their vitals, blood volume, mental status and capillary refill **(Table 7)**.

**TABLE 7:** Classification of haemorrhagic shock in children.

| *Parameter* | *Class I* | *Class II* | *Class III* | *Class IV* |
|---|---|---|---|---|
| Blood volume loss* | Up to 15% | 15–30% | 30–40% | ≥40% |
| Pulse rate | Normal | Mild tachycardia | Moderate tachycardia | Severe tachycardia |
| Blood pressure | Normal/ increased | Normal/ decreased | Decreased | Decreased |
| Capillary blanch test | Normal | Positive | Positive | Positive |
| Respiratory rate | Normal | Mild tachypnoea | Moderate tachypnoea | Severe tachypnoea |
| Urine output | 1–2 ml/ kg/h | 0.5–1.0 ml/ kg/h | 0.25–0.5 ml/ kg/h | Negligible |
| Mental status | Slightly anxious | Mildly anxious | Anxious/ confused | Confused/ lethargic |
| Fluid replacement (3:1 rule) | Crystalloid | Crystalloid | Crystalloid% blood | Crystalloid% blood |

- Adequate blood pressure can be misleading. Assessing capillary refill helps estimate vasoconstriction and compensation levels. Delayed capillary refill (>2 seconds) in the absence of hypothermia suggests that blood pressure is maintained by increased vascular resistance, indicating significant hypovolaemia.
- The SIPA score helps identify severely injured children. This tool accounts for age-dependent changes in vital signs due to blunt trauma.

### *Control External Bleeding*

A rapid assessment should be made for any external signs of bleeding that can be controlled by direct pressure or a tourniquet. The efficacy of tourniquets to control blood loss in military and civilian adults is well-documented; however, less is known regarding their efficacy in children. Combat studies have found that tourniquet or haemostatic dressing application for extremity vascular injury or amputation can be an effective and safe intervention. Based on military experience in both adults and children, a tourniquet should be applied in cases of major haemorrhage from an extremity or amputation.

### *Look for the Internal Bleeding Source*

- The common sites of internal blood loss include the thorax, abdomen, retroperitoneum, long bones and pelvis.

- The pelvis should be examined for stability. If a pelvic fracture is suspected alongside signs of shock, the pelvis should be wrapped in a sheet to provide compression and reduce ongoing bleeding.

### *Decompensated Shock*

- Signs of decompensated shock in children include altered mental status, mottled or cyanotic skin, cool pale extremities, weak peripheral pulses, and delayed capillary refill. Mortality is known to increase in children with traumatic injury and hypotension.
- Age-based normative values for HR and blood pressure show changes from infancy to adolescence. Generally, younger children have higher respiratory and HRs and lower blood pressure, approaching adult values by the age of 12 years.

### *Management*

Haemorrhagic shock in paediatric trauma patients remains a challenging yet preventable cause of death. High-quality evidence to guide specific aspects of haemorrhage control and resuscitation practices in this population is limited. The resuscitation of a child showing evidence of haemorrhagic shock begins with an initial bolus of normal saline or Ringer's lactate (20 ml/kg). Children with life-threatening haemorrhage or decompensated shock require the immediate administration of uncrossmatched red blood cells. If signs of haemorrhagic shock or poor perfusion persist after the initial fluid bolus, blood products should be administered.

According to the Pediatric Traumatic Hemorrhagic Shock Consensus Conference (PTHSCC) guidelines, the use of blood products should be prioritised over crystalloids when resuscitating children in haemorrhagic shock. The guidelines recommend targeting high plasma and high platelet-to-red blood cell ratios (1:1) to minimise plasma and platelet deficits. At present, no one protocol exists for paediatric Massive Transfusion Protocols (MTPs), and the decision to activate the MTP is at the clinician's discretion. Some paediatric centres opt to trigger the release of the first packet of blood products for every high-acuity trauma activation, while others require patients to demonstrate an inadequate response to initial crystalloid resuscitation before activating the MTP. Due to the limited data on which children may require massive transfusion, straightforward and clear criteria are essential for ensuring timely access to blood products. Further research is needed to develop paediatric-specific prediction algorithms or to validate existing adult criteria for use in children. Recent retrospective and prospective observational studies suggest that transfusion strategies—such as limiting crystalloids, maintaining appropriate transfusion ratios, and using whole blood—and IV haemostatic adjunct therapies, can reduce morbidity and mortality in children with traumatic haemorrhagic shock.

## Disability[11-13]

Rapid neurologic assessment should be done using the GCS or the P-GCS, a validated scale for children ≤2 years **(Table 2)**. It is important to assess additional neurological findings, such as pupillary responsiveness and brainstem reflexes (e.g. gag reflex). Unequal or fixed, dilated pupils may suggest cerebral herniation, necessitating urgent interventions to address increased intracranial pressure.

### *Disability Management*

Appropriate management is essential to prevent secondary insult.

- Give supplemental oxygen to keep saturation >95%.
- GCS ≤8, compromised airway indicate a need for early endotracheal intubation and controlled ventilation.
- Hyperventilation [partial pressure of carbon dioxide ($PaCO_2$) <35 mmHg] can lead to cerebral ischaemia due to reduced cerebral blood flow. Therefore, it is essential to keep $PaCO_2$ levels between 35 and 38 mmHg, unless there are indications of impending herniation.
- Rapid fluid resuscitation to maintain cerebral perfusion in patients with hypotension.
- Patients showing signs of cerebral herniation should be treated with IV mannitol at a dosage of 0.5–1 g/kg, or IV hypertonic saline at 2–6 ml/kg of 3% sodium chloride (NaCl) (1-3 mEq/kg) to help reduce intracranial pressure. Whilst there is limited evidence on the optimal osmolar therapy regimen for children with increased intracranial pressure, both mannitol and hypertonic saline are typically effective initial treatments for most paediatric patients.

## Exposure and Environment[1]

Completely undressing the patient during the primary survey allows for quick identification and treatment of multiple injuries. Once advanced procedures are finished, medical providers can log roll the patient while ensuring cervical spine immobilisation to thoroughly assess the back for any injuries to the flank or spine.

## Maintain Normothermia[1,2]

The World Health Organization defines hypothermia in neonates, infants and children as mild 36.0–36.5°C, moderate 32.0–36°C and severe <32.0°C. Due to their larger body surface area relative to weight and higher metabolic rate, children are more susceptible to hypothermia and insensible fluid losses. Hypothermia can exacerbate a critical condition by worsening metabolic acidosis, prolonging coagulation time and negatively impacting heart function. Thus, active efforts should be made to always maintain normothermia. Utilising increased ambient room temperature, radiant warmers, warmed IV fluids and blood, warm and humidified inspired oxygen, and covering the patient with warm blankets after a complete assessment helps to maintain body temperature.

## Initial Radiographic/Ancillary Studies[1,11-15]

Initial trauma labs should be drawn as soon as possible once the child arrives. The following studies are recommended for all children meeting the criteria for trauma activation:

- Complete blood count
- Basic metabolic panel
- *Arterial blood gas (ABG):* The radial artery at the wrist is the most preferred site for ABG sampling as it has adequate collaterals where inadvertent puncture of veins is unlikely. When this is not feasible, popliteal, brachial or femoral arteries can be chosen. Collecting ABG samples in children can be challenging as finding a suitable artery due to small vessel size poses difficulty; children may be more likely to move during the procedure, making it challenging to maintain a stable puncture site. Other problems include increased risk of bleeding or bruising at the puncture site, pain and discomfort for the child, potential for nerve damage, and the need for careful technique to avoid complications, especially in infants and young children who may be more sensitive to the procedure.
- *Urinalysis:* It can serve as an initial screening tool to detect potential urinary tract injuries, particularly kidney damage, by identifying the presence of blood in the urine (haematuria), thus prompting further investigations, such as computed tomography (CT) scans.
- Prothrombin time/international normalised ratio.
- Liver enzymes (aspartate aminotransferase/alanine aminotransferase).
- Amylase
- Type and screen

Initial imaging in paediatric trauma differs significantly from adults, and a selective approach should be utilised to minimise radiation exposure.

*Extended focused assessment with sonography in trauma (e-FAST) examination:* The e-FAST is a quick ultrasound assessment of four abdominal areas: The right upper quadrant, left upper quadrant, subxiphoid region, and pelvis, as well as the lungs and heart. e-FAST may allow for the timely detection of pneumothorax, haemothorax, or cardiac tamponade, with greater sensitivity but lower specificity compared to supine chest radiographs. e-FAST examination can be performed for haemodynamically unstable paediatric trauma patients as a quick bedside tool to identify underlying causes and guide further management. For stable patients, it may also be performed if it will not cause any delays in treatment.

*Intra-abdominal injury detection:* The utility of e-FAST for detecting intra-abdominal injuries in haemodynamically stable children with blunt abdominal trauma is less certain. Due to a significant risk of false negatives, e-FAST should not be used alone to replace abdominal CT in these cases.

*Combination with physical examination:* Preliminary evidence suggests that e-FAST combined with physical examination findings may provide valuable information for clinical decision-making.

*Outcomes in adult versus paediatric trauma:* While FAST has been linked to improved outcomes in adult trauma patients, its routine use in children is limited due to the common presence of solid organ lacerations, which can make FAST less sensitive for detecting critical intra-abdominal injuries.

## SECONDARY SURVEY[1,2]

A secondary survey is a systematic head-to-toe evaluation performed after completing the primary survey and initiating resuscitation as needed to stabilise vital functions. This evaluation includes obtaining the patient's history, conducting a comprehensive physical examination, and performing additional studies and procedures.

While the goal of the secondary survey is thoroughness, the need for rapid treatment may necessitate compromises in certain situations. If the physical examination is abbreviated due to the poor condition of the patient, the medical team must ensure that the full examination is completed after necessary interventions or diagnostic studies. If the patient is transferred to another service or facility, any incomplete examination components should be clearly communicated.

### History

The AMPLE mnemonic can be used to gather a quick, focused history from prehospital personnel, patients, or family members:

- *A:* Allergies
- *M:* Medications
- *P:* Past medical history/pregnancy
- *L:* Last meal
- *E:* Events/environment leading to the injury

*Components of physical examination that deserve special mention include:*

- *Head*: Inspect and palpate the face and scalp.
  - *Eye examination:* Check for haemorrhage, pupillary sign, periorbital ecchymosis (Raccoon eyes).
  - *Ear:* Any blood or fluid, retro-auricular ecchymosis (Battle's sign).
  - Mid face examination: nasal swelling, deformity, bleeding, or clear rhinorrhoea; Palpate maxilla for evidence of LeFort fracture.

- *Cervical spine and neck:* Distended neck veins, C-spine tenderness, subcutaneous emphysema, crepitus over larynx (concerning for laryngeal fracture).
- *Chest:* Inspect and palpate chest, including the clavicle, ribs, and sternum for tenderness, bony deformity, crepitus, open pneumothorax/large flail segment.
- *Abdomen:* Seat belt sign/bruises (Cullen's sign), distension and focal tenderness.
- Perineum/rectum/vagina: Contusion/laceration/haematoma, urethral or vaginal bleeding.
- *Musculoskeletal:* Identify fractures/dislocations, pain on palpation of the pelvic ring, mobility of pelvis with anterior-to-posterior pressure with heels of hands on both anterior iliac spine.

## DAMAGE CONTROL RESUSCITATION[1-3]

Damage control resuscitation (DCR) consists of rapid haemorrhage control, prevention of hypothermia, acidosis, coagulopathy and hypocalcaemia, restriction of crystalloids and balanced administration of blood and blood products. The DCR principles used in children are similar to those in adults. It is important to keep the different physiology of the paediatric population in mind **(Table 8)**.

## SPECIAL SITUATIONS IN PAEDIATRIC TRAUMA

### Traumatic Brain Injury[16-19]

Paediatric traumatic brain injury (TBI) has a bimodal distribution pattern, with very young (0–2 years) and adolescents (15–18 years) more commonly being injured. A disproportionately large head size, weaker neck muscles, decreased agility, lesser fat and connective tissue make children susceptible to severe TBI. Children may present to the trauma bay with altered mental

**TABLE 8:** Physiological differences in children relevant to damage control resuscitation application.

| *Features* | *Description* |
|---|---|
| Mechanism of Injury | Mostly fall from height |
| Cause of death | Commonly, traumatic brain injury rather than haemorrhagic |
| Blood volume | Larger blood volume/unit weight in infants |
| Signs and symptoms of shock | Due to their robust catecholamine-induced compensation, children can maintain blood pressure even after losing 30–45% of their total blood volume |
| Coagulation profile | Until 6 months of life, infants have lower concentrations of coagulation factors and lower functional platelets |

status, loss of consciousness, scalp haematoma, vomiting, seizures and skull fractures. The PECARN (Pediatric Emergency Care Applied Research Network) criteria are utilised for deciding non-contrast computed tomography (NCCT) of the head in a stable child with a GCS of 14 or more. The NCCT head is the investigation of choice for evaluating children with a GCS lower than 14 and with suspected base skull fracture. Brain Trauma Foundation (BTF) guidelines do not recommend repeating CT scans unless there is evidence of neurological deterioration. The type of injury patterns observed in children is similar to adults and includes diffuse axonal injury and intracranial haemorrhage, including epidural haematoma, subdural haematoma, subarachnoid haemorrhage and cerebral contusions. If intracranial hypertension is suspected, osmotherapy should be started with either 3% hypertonic saline or mannitol. 3% hypertonic saline @2–5 ml/kg can be used to target intracranial pressures <20 mmHg and cerebral perfusion pressure of a minimum of 40 mmHg (target serum sodium levels <160 mEq/L). Advanced neuromonitoring with brain tissue oxygen ($PbrO_2$) monitoring ($PbrO_2$ target >10 mmHg) is advocated. Raised intracranial pressures should be managed by increasing sedation/ventilation using midazolam, fentanyl, and propofol along with osmotherapy. Barbiturate coma or decompressive craniectomy may be required for refractory intracranial hypertension **(Table 9)**.

## Spine Trauma[1,7,8]

Spine trauma is relatively uncommon in the paediatric population. Anatomical differences exist between adults and paediatric age groups, with children having weaker neck muscles, less fat and connective tissue, relatively small subarachnoid space, flexible interspinous ligaments and joint capsule, cartilaginous and anteriorly wedged vertebral bodies and flat facet joints. Angular momentum is greater, and the fulcrum exists higher in the cervical spine, accounting for more spinal injuries between the occiput and C3, with upper cervical spine injuries such as atlanto-occipital dislocation and atlantoaxial rotatory subluxation being common in children under 8 years of age. Lower cervical spine injuries are common in older children. Further, up to 50% of spinal cord injuries may exist without radiological abnormalities (SCIWORA) in children <10 years of age. National Emergency X-Radiography Utilization Study (NEXUS) criteria can be used for cervical spine clearance in children with normal development and age above 8 years. It helps determine if a child needs imaging of their spine or not **(Box 1)**. Magnetic resonance imaging (MRI) may also be required in children with spinal cord injury without radiological abnormalities, given the increased risk of ligamentous injuries in the paediatric population.

*If any of the features mentioned in the NEXUS criteria* ***(Box 1)*** *exist, imaging of the cervical spine is indicated.*

**TABLE 9:** Management of intracranial hypertension.

| | |
|---|---|
| Hyperosmolar therapy | Bolus 3% hypertonic saline (2–5 ml/kg over 10–20 minutes) is recommended in patients with intracranial hypertension. Continuous infusion (0.1–1.0 ml/kg/h) to maintain ICP <20 mmHg |
| CSF drainage | CSF drainage through an external ventricular drain is considered to manage raised ICP |
| Seizure prophylaxis | Early seizure prophylaxis (within 7 days), using levetiracetam (20–30 mg/kg every 12 hours) to reduce the occurrence of post-traumatic seizures |
| Hyperventilation | Prophylactic hyperventilation to a $PaCO_2$ <30 mmHg in the initial 48 hours after injury is not recommended. If hyperventilation is used in the management of refractory intracranial hypertension, advanced neuromonitoring for evaluation of cerebral ischaemia is suggested |
| Analgesia and sedation | Appropriate analgesia and sedation, as is the routine during ICU management, should be used. Bolus administration of midazolam and/or fentanyl during ICP crisis should be avoided due to the risks of cerebral hypoperfusion |
| Barbiturate Therapy | High-dose barbiturate therapy, using IV thiopental infusion at a dose of 5–10 mg/kg/h in haemodynamically stable patients with refractory intracranial hypertension despite maximal medical and surgical management |
| Hypothermia | Moderate (32–33°C) hypothermia for ICP control. Prophylactic moderate hypothermia is not recommended over normothermia to improve overall outcomes |
| Decompressive Craniectomy | Decompressive craniectomy to treat neurologic deterioration, herniation, or intracranial hypertension refractory to medical management |

(ICP: intracranial pressure; CSF: cerebrospinal fluid; IV: intravenous; $PaCO_2$: partial pressure of carbon dioxide; ICU: intensive care unit)

**BOX 1:** Emergency X-Radiography Utilization Study (NEXUS) criteria.

*Criteria:*
- Midline cervical tenderness
- Altered level of alertness
- Evidence of intoxication
- Neurological abnormality
- Presence of a painful, distracting injury

## Thoracic Trauma[1-3]

The chest wall in children is more compliant, hence, pulmonary contusion without bony disruption may be seen. Rib fractures are uncommon in children due to increased flexibility. But mobile mediastinal structures

TABLE 10: Chest tube sizes based on age and weight.

| *Age range* | *Weight* | *Chest tube size (Fr: French)* |
|---|---|---|
| Small infant | 6–7 kg | 10–12 Fr |
| Infant (up to 1 year) | 8–9 kg | 10–12 Fr |
| Toddler | 10–11 kg | 16–20 Fr |
| Small child | 12–14 kg | 20–24 Fr |
| Child | 15–18 kg | 20–24 Fr |
| Child | 19–23 kg | 24–32 Fr |
| Large child | 24–29 kg | 28–32 Fr |
| Adult | 30–36 kg | 32–38 Fr |

are associated with tension pneumothorax and haemothorax, which may lead to more circulatory collapse than in adults. Emergent management of tension pneumothorax involves doing a needle decompression in the second intercostal space in the midclavicular line. This is followed by chest tube insertion. The appropriate size of the chest tube for a paediatric patient depends on the child's age and size **(Table 10)**. The size may vary based on the patient's specific medical condition and the clinician's judgment.

## Abdominal Trauma[1,2,14]

Children have relatively larger abdominal organs in proportion to adults, which are less protected by the relatively smaller rib cage. Hence, they are at increased risk of injury. The presence of abdominal tenderness, pain, distention and bruising should alert clinicians to abdominal trauma. e-FAST is incapable of identifying isolated intraparenchymal injuries, which account for up to one-third of solid organ injuries in children. Contrast-enhanced CT abdomen is the investigation of choice if the child is haemodynamically stable. If the child's haemodynamic condition cannot be normalised, they should be mobilised for prompt damage control laparotomy to control haemorrhage. A multidisciplinary team approach is required for managing these children, especially if they are haemodynamically unstable. In addition to the paediatric surgeon, the anaesthesiologist, intensivist, operation theatre staff and transfusion medicine physician should be alerted. Advance notice facilitates collaborative and timely care, rapidly providing properly typed and cross-matched blood products, allowing for immediate transfusion in case of significant blood loss.

## Extremity Trauma[20,21]

Extremity trauma is prevalent in the paediatric population. A clinical suspicion should be raised based on history and bony tenderness. Early fracture stabilisation should be done, especially for fractures involving the growth plates. In contrast to adults, blood loss associated with long bone fractures is less in children. Hence, haemodynamic instability in the presence of an isolated femur fracture should prompt looking for other sources of bleeding, commonly in the abdomen. Peripheral vascular injury, though uncommon, may be seen in this population.

### Burns[22-24]

Accidental scald and contact burns are the most important causes of paediatric burns, with total body surface area involvement less than 10%. Lund and Browder's chart provides a reliable estimation of burn size in the paediatric population. Patients presenting with respiratory distress should raise suspicion of airway burns. Early intubation is recommended, and 100% oxygen should be supplemented, considering the anticipated difficult airway due to airway oedema. Two large-bore IV cannulas should be placed to start fluid resuscitation. The important end points of resuscitation in paediatric patients include urine output of 1–0.5 ml/kg/h, age-appropriate blood pressures, and central venous pressures between 3 and 8 mmHg. Trends of lactates and base deficits should be used for further fluid administration.

## PAIN MANAGEMENT IN PAEDIATRIC TRAUMA[25-29]

Pain in paediatric trauma victims is poorly understood, often under-recognised, and inadequately treated. The pain experienced after trauma in children is a complex interplay of somatic, visceral, and neuropathic pain, compounded by psychological, social, and cultural factors, making pain evaluation particularly challenging. Inadequate pain assessment skills, lack of understanding about pain and analgesics, and excessive concern regarding haemodynamic fluctuations and respiratory depression further contribute to poor pain management. Literature emphasises the necessity of adequate and timely analgesic relief in paediatric patients to avoid complications of chronic pain.

*For moderate to severe trauma:*

- IV opioids are the analgesic method of choice, with the IO route as an alternative.
- IV fentanyl (1–2 μg/kg) is the most common first-line opioid, offering rapid onset, effective pain relief and a favourable safety profile.
- Sub-dissociative (analgesic) doses of ketamine (0.05–15 mg/kg/h IV) are well-suited for analgesia of haemodynamically unstable patients.
- Non-opioid analgesics (IV paracetamol) should be used for their opioid-sparing effects.
- Non-steroidal anti-inflammatory drugs (NSAIDs) are contraindicated in acute moderate-to-severe trauma due to the risk of platelet dysfunction and renal impairment if renal blood flow is compromised.

- Oral ibuprofen (Brufen, Brufen Junior) can be administered if there is no concern for bleeding or potential renal injury. NSAIDs are often used in paediatric trauma to manage pain and inflammation from musculoskeletal injuries, typically as a first-line treatment for mild to moderate pain, due to their analgesic and anti-inflammatory properties. NSAIDs are generally safe and effective, can reduce opioid requirements, do not compromise pain control, and are subsequently associated with similar or reduced frequencies of opioid-related adverse effects. However, while using NSAIDs, careful consideration is needed due to their potential side effects, particularly regarding potential bleeding risks and impact on kidney function, especially in severe trauma cases.
- The use of tramadol and codeine is contraindicated in children under 12 years of age due to the risk of respiratory failure and death.

*For mild-to-moderate trauma:*

- *Distraction techniques*: Utilise guided imagery, music, videos, interactive games, and singing. The presence of parents should be encouraged.
- *Pharmacological therapy*: Typically, it involves a stepwise approach, starting with acetaminophen for mild pain. NSAIDs are also the most commonly used analgesic medications and include Ibugesic (10 mg/kg every sixth hour IV) and ketorolac (0.5 mg/kg every sixth hour IV). Topical anaesthetics can be used as adjuncts or, at times, as an alternative to the oral or IV route. Topical lidocaine derivatives are most commonly used in paediatric emergency settings.
- Analgesia should be administered at regular intervals rather than on an 'as needed' basis. Rescue doses should be available for intermittent and breakthrough pain.

IV opioids are the analgesic method of choice for moderate to severe trauma. Non-opioid analgesics can be used for their opioid-sparing effects, especially in mild to moderate trauma. Single-shot and continuous nerve or plexus blocks are very helpful in limb injuries, where local anaesthetic drugs with or without adjuvants can be infiltrated. Peripheral nerve catheters (PNCs) offer the possibility of extended analgesia beyond the 12–16 hours of analgesia usually obtained from a single-injection block. They have been used extensively in adults, and their use has been increasing in children. PNCs in children have low failure and complication rates that are similar to adult practice. Most importantly, the majority of complications are minor, and there have been no reports of permanent injury.

## CONCLUSION

The initial trauma management of paediatric patients should follow prioritising airway, breathing, and circulation. As paediatric patients have different anatomy and physiology as compared to adults, their response to trauma is different. Evaluation and management of paediatric trauma is unique and should be tailored to a child's weight and age.

## REFERENCES


1. Advanced Trauma Life Support. Student Course Manual by American College of Surgeons Committee on Trauma, 10th edition. United States of America: American College of Surgeons; 2018.
2. Galvagno SM Jr, Nahmias JT, Young DA. Advanced Trauma Life Support® Update 2019: Management and applications for adults and special populations. Anesthesiol Clin. 2019;37(1):13-32.
3. Topjian AA, Raymond TT, Atkins D, Chan M, Duff JP, Joyner BL Jr, et al. Pediatric Basic and Advanced Life Support Collaborators. Part 4: Pediatric Basic and Advanced Life Support: 2020 American Heart Association Guidelines for Cardiopulmonary Resuscitation and Emergency Cardiovascular Care. Circulation. 2020;142(16 Suppl 2):S469-523.
4. Harless J, Ramaiah R, Bhananker SM. Pediatric airway management. Int J Crit Illn Inj Sci. 2014;4(1):65-70.
5. Hansen M, Meckler G, O'Brien K, Engle P, Dickinson C, Dickinson K, et al. Pediatric airway management and prehospital patient safety: Results of a national delphi survey by the children's safety initiative-emergency medical services for children. Pediatr Emerg Care. 2016;32(9):603-7.
6. Kennedy A, Scorpio R, Coppola C. Assessment of the pediatric trauma patient: differences in approach. JECCM. 2018;2.
7. Duhaime AC, Rindler RS. Special considerations in infants and children. Handb Clin Neurol. 2015;127:219-42.
8. Kinjalk M, Jain N, Neogi S, Ratan SK, Panda SS, Sehgal M, et al. Pediatric Age-adjusted Shock Index (SIPA): From injury to outcome in blunt abdominal trauma. J Indian Assoc Pediatr Surg. 2024;29:33-8.
9. Hendrickson JE, Shaz BH, Pereira G, Parker PM, Jessup P, Atwell F, et al. Implementation of a pediatric trauma massive transfusion protocol: one institution's experience. Transfusion. 2012;52(6):1228-36.
10. Guyther J, Wiltjer R. Pediatric trauma. Emergency Medicine Clinics of North America. 2023;41(1):205-22.
11. Burstein B, Upton JEM, Terra HF, Neuman MI. Use of CT for head trauma: 2007-2015. Pediatrics. 2018;142(4):e20180814.
12. Ukwuoma OI, Allareddy V, Allareddy V, Rampa S, Rose JA, Shein SL, et al. Trends in head computed tomography utilization in children presenting to emergency departments after traumatic head injury. Pediatr Emerg Care. 2021;37(7):e384-e90.
13. Ben-Ishay O, Daoud M, Peled Z, Brauner E, Bahouth H, Kluger Y. Focused abdominal sonography for trauma in the clinical evaluation of children with blunt abdominal trauma. World J Emerg Surg. 2015;10:27.
14. Netherton S, Milenkovic V, Taylor M, Davis PJ. Diagnostic accuracy of eFAST in the trauma patient: A systematic review and meta-analysis. CJEM. 2019;21(6):727-38.

15. Stengel D, Leisterer J, Ferrada P, Ekkernkamp A, Mutze S, Hoenning A. Point-of-care ultrasonography for diagnosing thoracoabdominal injuries in patients with blunt trauma. Cochrane Database Syst Rev. 2018;12(12):CD012669.
16. Carney N, Totten AM, O'Reilly C, Ullman JS, Hawryluk GW, Bell MJ, et al. Guidelines for the management of severe traumatic brain injury, fourth edition. Neurosurgery. 2017;80(1):6-15.
17. Gelineau-Morel RN, Zinkus TP, Le Pichon JB. Pediatric head trauma: A review and update. Pediatr Rev. 2019;40(9):468-81.
18. Figaji AA. Anatomical and physiological differences between children and adults relevant to traumatic brain injury and the implications for clinical assessment and care. Front Neurol. 2017;8:685.
19. Kochanek P, Tasker R, Carney N, Totten A, Adelson PD, Selden N, et al. Guidelines for the management of pediatric severe traumatic brain injury, Third Edition: Update of the Brain Trauma Foundation Guidelines. Pediatr Crit Care Med. 2019;20(3S Suppl 1):S1-S82.
20. Kim HHR, Menashe SJ, Ngo AV, Otjen JP, Maloney E, Iyer RS, et al. Uniquely pediatric upper extremity injuries. Clin Imaging. 2021;80:249-61.
21. Centers for Disease Control and Prevention, National center for injury prevention and control. (2020). Web-based Injury Statistics Query and Reporting System (WISQARS) fatal injury data. [Online] Available from https://wisqars. cdc.gov/ [Last accessed June, 2025].
22. Romanowski KS, Palmieri TL. Pediatric burn resuscitation: past, present, and future. Burns Trauma. 2017;5:26.
23. The American Burn Association. Advanced Burn Life Support is designed to provide first responders, nurses, nurse practitioners, physician assistants, and physicians with the ability to assess and stabilize patients with burn injuries during the first critical hours post injury. ABLS programs support emergency preparedness needs for disaster management. [Online] Available from https://ameriburn.org/education/advanced-burn-life-support-abls/abls-handbook/ [Last accessed June, 2025].
24. Wigginton JG, Roppolo LP, Pepe PE. Advances in resuscitative trauma care. Minerva Anestesiol. 2011;77(10):993-1002.
25. Tobias JD, Green TP, Coté CJ, Agarwal R, Anderson CTM, Hardy CA, et al. Codeine: Time to Say "No". Pediatrics. 2016;138(4):e20162396.
26. Frey TM, Florin TA, Caruso M, Zhang N, Zhang Y, Mittiga MR. Effect of intranasal ketamine vs fentanyl on pain reduction for extremity injuries in children: The PRIME randomized clinical trial. JAMA Pediatr. 2019;173(2):140-6.
27. Frenkel O, Liebmann O, Fischer JW. Ultrasound-guided forearm nerve blocks in kids: a novel method for pain control in the treatment of hand-injured pediatric patients in the emergency department. Pediatr Emerg Care. 2015;31(4):255-9.
28. Walker BJ, Long JB, De Oliveira GS, Szmuk P, Setiawan C, Polaner DM, et al. Peripheral nerve catheters in children: an analysis of safety and practice patterns from the pediatric regional anesthesia network (PRAN). Br J Anaesth. 2015;115(3):457-62.
29. Cooney MF. Pain management in children: NSAID use in the perioperative and emergency department settings. Paediatr Drugs. 2021;23(4):361-72.

CHAPTER 17

# Anaesthesia for Airway Procedures in Children

*R Jayanthi, S Ramesh, Narendra Tajne*

## ABSTRACT

Paediatric airway management is uniquely challenging, especially in cases involving stridor or noisy breathing, which may be indicative of a compromised airway. Effective management requires a robust understanding of respiratory physiology, collaborative communication between anaesthesiologists and surgeons, and adaptable anaesthetic plans. Recent advancements in endoscopic techniques have enabled the effective treatment of both congenital and acquired airway problems. High-frequency nasal oxygenation has thus become a valuable technique for tubeless anaesthesia with improved oxygenation and ventilation during these procedures. This still remains uncommon and requires well-selected and strategically prepared patients.

Preoperative assessment for potential complications from previous interventions, such as prolonged intubation or intensive care unit stays, that may lead to subglottic stenosis is considered. Paediatric patients with cardiac disease pose a significant challenge to anaesthetic management and require individualised care to ensure patient safety. Procedures may also be highly variable, necessitating techniques such as tubeless anaesthesia and total intravenous anaesthesia to maintain spontaneous ventilation and adequate oxygenation. Major airway procedures, such as laryngotracheal reconstructions, involve teams that have sufficient experience in facing the challenges that come with them. Good postoperative care and paediatric intensive care unit facilities are mandatory to do such procedures. These patients also need continued follow-up care.

The risks involved with laser airway surgery, including fire hazards and airway access challenges, call for additional safety measures and careful planning. Constant monitoring of physiological parameters is also essential throughout the procedure to ensure patient stability. In general, a multidisciplinary approach that involves thorough preoperative assessment, active collaboration among healthcare teams, and vigilant monitoring can significantly improve outcomes in paediatric patients facing airway surgeries. Adapting anaesthetic strategies to individual patient needs, while ensuring safety protocols, remains essential for addressing the complexities of paediatric airway management effectively.

***Keywords:*** Airway surgery, Dexmedetomidine, Laryngomalacia, Laser surgery, Paediatric anaesthesia, Subglottic stenosis, Tubeless.

## INTRODUCTION

Children having airway issues often present with stridor or noisy breathing, indicating an already compromised airway. The management of these paediatric patients during airway interventions requires a good understanding of respiratory physiology, effective communication with surgical teams, and a lot of experience. The recent development of endoscopic techniques has made it possible to effectively treat both congenital and acquired airway problems. Advanced optical systems and fine instrumentation allow even the smallest airways to be visualised and intervened in. Other key areas of improvement that have improved patient outcomes for complex cases include the availability of improved facilities in neonatal and paediatric intensive care unit (PICUs), combined with advances in paediatric anaesthesia techniques. The anaesthetic plans need to be tailored throughout the procedure to meet the requirements of the surgeon involved. The initial airway evaluations are often dynamic, relying on spontaneous ventilation while ensuring that airway reflexes are bound enough to allow instrumentation and dynamic assessment to be performed. Sometimes the surgical plan is formulated only at this stage. Subsequent anaesthetic management follows the surgical approach being employed.

This chapter aims to address various paediatric airway problems in detail, examine pertinent surgical techniques, and discuss anaesthesia strategies that ensure safe management during airway crises.

## AIRWAY PROCEDURES COMMONLY PERFORMED IN CHILDREN

Airway procedures are done for airway diseases in children that are associated with typical symptoms and a particular age of presentation **(Table 1)**. Airway problems in infants and children may be congenital or acquired.[1,2] Among the fairly widespread congenital problems, the most frequent are laryngomalacia followed by unilateral or bilateral paralysis of the vocal cords, subglottic stenosis (SGS), webs and atresia, subglottic haemangiomas and saccular cysts with a prevalence of 60%, 15–20%, 10–20%, 5%, 1.5–3% and 2%, respectively.[2] Sometimes laryngeal clefts may also be seen, but this is less often a feature. Acquired causes are mainly SGS, which occurs due to intubation and a long-term stay in the intensive care unit.

## CONCERNS AND CHALLENGES WITH AIRWAY PROCEDURES IN CHILDREN

Anaesthetic challenges encountered during airway procedures in children are multifaceted and require careful consideration. One primary concern is the necessity for the anaesthesiologist to share the airway with the surgeon, ensuring the safe provision of anaesthesia while facilitating optimal surgical access. This scenario demands a comprehensive understanding of each professional's responsibilities and requires constant and effective communication. Airway management can become particularly complicated

**TABLE 1:** Airway diseases, their clinical findings and airway procedures in children.

| *Symptom* | *Possible diagnosis* | *Age at presentation* | *Procedure* |
|---|---|---|---|
| Stridor, failure to thrive | Laryngomalacia | Birth to a few months of age | Self-limiting/ supraglottoplasty |
| Stridor, difficult to wean | Subglottic stenosis | Congenital—early infancy, post-intubation—any age | Endoscopic dilatation/ laryngotracheal reconstruction |
| Recurrent aspiration | Laryngeal cleft | Infancy | Repair of laryngeal cleft |
| Breathing difficulty, failure to wean from a ventilator | Cysts in the larynx | Newborn, infancy | Excision of cyst/ aspiration |
| Recurrent breathing difficulty | Papillomatosis | Older child | Laser excision of papilloma larynx, recurrent papilloma excision |
| Stridor, voice change | Unknown aetiology | Any age | Transnasal flexible laryngoscopy |

due to laryngeal pathologies, with restricted or absent access to the airway presented by lesions. For instance, subglottic narrowing, especially in young children, creates unique challenges where traditional endotracheal intubation may not be feasible. Consequently, alternate strategies for airway access, viz. surgical airway, must be readily prepared and available. Furthermore, coordination is essential, as the anaesthesiologist must continuously collaborate with the surgeon and other healthcare professionals throughout the procedure to ensure patient safety and procedural efficacy. Alternate anaesthesia techniques, like tubeless anaesthesia, may have to be employed to facilitate surgical access. Another significant risk factor in these procedures is the potential for fire hazards, particularly with the use of lasers during laryngeal surgeries. The selection of appropriate endotracheal tubes and adherence to preventive techniques are crucial to mitigate this risk. These challenges collectively highlight the complexities of administering anaesthesia in paediatric airway procedures, underscoring the importance of teamwork, proactive planning, and attention to safety protocols in enhancing patient outcomes.

## General Concerns

### *Preoperative Assessment—Previous Treatment History*

Previous interventions, including intubation and extended mechanical ventilation in the PICU, may contribute to the development of SGS. A thorough medical history is essential in determining the underlying cause of stridor, whether it is congenital, infectious or iatrogenic. For children undergoing endoscopic dilation or those who have previously undergone laryngotracheal surgery, it is crucial that airway manipulations are executed with exceptional dexterity and caution to avoid damaging any repaired structures. Understanding the nuances of each patient's past treatment is the key to fostering a safer surgical outcome.

### *Patient Comorbidities*

Comorbidities such as concurrent cardiac conditions can complicate the anaesthetic management of children. These patients often exhibit diminished oxygen reserves and may necessitate a higher fraction of inspired oxygen ($FiO_2$). Therefore, performing a basic haemoglobin estimation and assessing oxygen saturation while the patient is on room air, along with an echocardiogram before the procedure is imperative. Some paediatric patients may already be receiving oxygen supplementation via nasal prongs or a Hudson mask. Endotracheal intubation is required during airway procedures, making these children poor candidates for tubeless techniques.

### *Anaesthetic Plan*[1]

The anaesthetic plan must be carefully crafted to address the challenges of managing the airway before, during, and after surgical intervention. During the initial phases of the procedure, surgeons often require spontaneous ventilation to assess vocal cord movement and upper airway dynamics. As the surgery progresses, the need for complete muscle paralysis may arise. For instance, when operating on the vocal cords, surgeons prefer a non-moving target to optimise surgical conditions.

Additionally, space constraints in paediatric patients are significant, often prompting the use of tubeless techniques that enhance the surgeon's working area. However, these techniques can present challenges for the anaesthesiologist, necessitating careful consideration.

### *Oxygenation and Ventilation*[3]

An essential role of the anaesthesiologist during airway procedures is to balance the need to minimise obstruction of the surgical field with the need to maintain adequate oxygenation and ventilation in the patient. This balance becomes particularly critical in children who already possess limited oxygen reserves. Various ventilation techniques may be employed to achieve this objective, including spontaneous breathing, apnoeic ventilation, jet ventilation and intermittent intubation. The main aim remains the same: to ensure sufficient oxygenation throughout the procedure. Hyperoxygenation is the term used where continuous oxygen is provided either by mask, nasal prongs or nasopharyngeal airway during airway manipulations. This simple manoeuvre can go a long way in preventing desaturation in these critical procedures. It extends the safe apnoea time (the time a child can tolerate without breathing) before oxygen saturation drops to dangerous levels.

### *Hypercapnia*[3]

In addition to oxygenation, the removal of carbon dioxide ($CO_2$) is equally important. Situations may arise where the airway is either intermittently ventilated or completely obstructed by the surgeons, their instruments, or the lesion itself. With the utilisation of tubeless techniques, higher gas flows can help maintain $CO_2$ levels within more tolerable ranges, alleviating some of the potential complications that arise from $CO_2$ retention. Apnoeic oxygenation techniques, such as high-flow nasal oxygenation, can help to slow the rate of partial pressure of $CO_2$ ($PaCO_2$) rise. The end-tidal $CO_2$ ($ETCO_2$) level was reported to increase 1.1 mmHg/min in patients on spontaneous ventilation, with the partial pressure of $CO_2$ increase being 1.8 mmHg/min in apnoeic patients.[3] At the conclusion of lengthy procedures, it is common practice to intubate the patient, assess the $ETCO_2$ values, and ventilate the child for a period to facilitate $CO_2$ washout. In most instances, intubation may be feasible at the end of the procedure, following improvement in airway diameter and pathology.

## Preparation for Anaesthesia

Good planning and understanding the patients' airway and its limitations are the key to a successful outcome. Due to the potential for loss of airway control at any point, it is ideal to commence anaesthesia induction in the main operating room where all equipment, facilities and personnel are available. This is particularly true when a surgical airway is part of the rescue plan. Most procedures start with airway evaluation by the surgeon using transnasal flexible endoscopy. The anaesthetist in this way is also able to see the pathology involved and make a plan in consultation with the surgeon.

He/she can assess at this point the behaviour of the child under anaesthesia. Questions that can be answered at the beginning of the procedure include the following: (1) Will the child tolerate apnoea? (2) What rescue plan can I keep as backup? (3) Is endotracheal intubation possible? (4) Can the child tolerate a tubeless technique, or is endotracheal intubation mandatory? Nevertheless, planning the appropriate theatre environment and keeping ready various options for rescue airway management are important.

Airway procedures can be either diagnostic or therapeutic in nature. Frequently, what begins as a diagnostic evaluation for a symptomatic infant may evolve into a therapeutic procedure, such as dilatation. Having personnel and staff who are familiar with airway procedures is crucial for the smooth execution of airway management tasks.

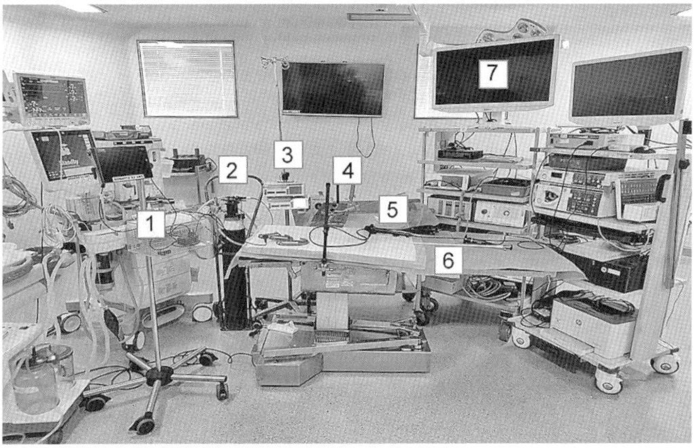


**Fig. 1:** Operation theatre setup for airway procedure. All airway equipment is kept ready in the operating theatre. 1. Videolaryngoscope, 2. Jet ventilation apparatus, 3. Total intravenous anaesthesia, target controlled infusion pumps, 4. Laryngostat, 5. Fibreoptic bronchoscope, 6. Rigid bronchoscope/telescope. 7. Monitors with recording facility. *(For color version, see Plate 9)*

In the operating theatre **(Fig. 1)**, various essential tools and equipment should be readily available. This includes a difficult airway cart equipped with a flexible fibreoptic bronchoscope (FOB), supraglottic airways, small-size endotracheal tubes ranging from sizes 2 to 2.5 mm and tracheostomy tubes of sizes appropriate for the age of the patient **(Table 2)**. Infusion pumps for total intravenous anaesthesia (TIVA) with various drugs diluted as per weight are also prepared in advance. Additionally, a reliable suction source is provided for both the surgeon and the anaesthetist. Local anaesthetic spray, jelly and nasal decongestant drops are kept ready, along with specialised oxygenation equipment such as a jet ventilator and transnasal humidified rapid insufflation ventilatory exchange (THRIVE) if available. It is often necessary to have multiple endotracheal tubes of the same size on standby in case one is needed as a nasopharyngeal airway while reserving the other for future intubation. Surgical instruments typically include rigid bronchoscopes of varying sizes and fine endoscopic equipment. Recording the details of various procedures is vital for monitoring the extent of airway narrowing or recurrence, as well as for documentation purposes **(Fig. 1)**. Today, video laryngoscopes are sometimes the first instruments used to visualise laryngeal anatomy and provide an initial glimpse of the airway.

## Individual Airway Problems[1,2]

This section briefly describes the management of individual airway conditions—congenital and acquired that one may face in the operating room and gives a brief outline of the management of the most frequent of these.

**TABLE 2:** Recommended sizes of bronchoscopes, tracheostomy and endotracheal tubes for different ages.

| *Patient age* | *Bronchoscope (size in mm)* | *Bronchoscope [outer diameter (OD) in mm]* | *Tracheostomy (tube size in mm)* | *Endotracheal tube size (mm)* |
|---|---|---|---|---|
| Premature | 2.5 | 4.2 | 2/2.5 | 2.5 |
| Term newborn | 3.0 | 5.0 | 3/3.5 | 3/3.5 |
| 6–12 months | 3.5 | 5.7 | 3.5/4 | 3.5/4 |
| 1–2 years | 3.7 | 6.4 | 4 | 4/4.5 |
| 2–3 years | 4.0 | 6.7 | 4/4.5 | (Age + 16)/4 |
| 3–4 years | 4.5 | 7.3 | 5 | (Age + 16)/4 |
| 4–5 years | 5.0 | 7.8 | 5/5.5 | (Age + 16/4) |

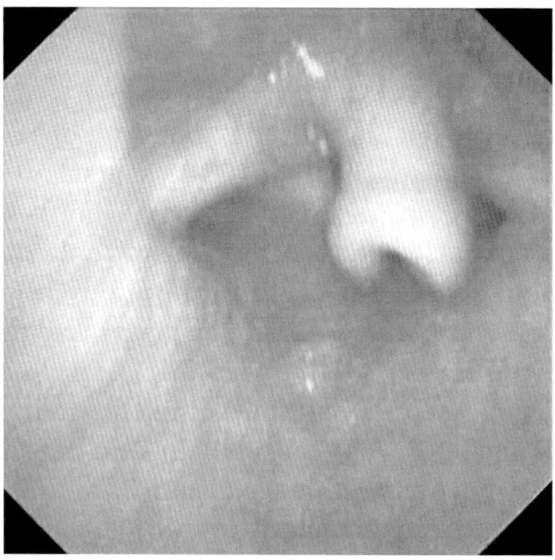

**Fig. 2:** Laryngomalacia. *(For color version, see Plate 10)*

## *Laryngomalacia*[1,2]

Laryngomalacia is one of the most common causes of stridor in newborns, typically occurring in babies 1–2 weeks old. It results from the inward collapse of supraglottic structures during inhalation, leading to a high-pitched inspiratory stridor that worsens with feeding, agitation and crying. This condition often causes significant anxiety for parents. Diagnosis is usually made by performing flexible laryngoscopy in the operating room under light general anaesthesia or while the baby is awake **(Fig. 2)**. The epiglottis is omega-shaped or leafy and closes over the laryngeal inlet with each inspiration. In infants where the problem is significant enough to cause poor feeding and failure to thrive, supraglottoplasty is offered as an option to alleviate the problem. Here, the aryepiglottic folds are refashioned, and an epiglottopexy is done.

### *Unilateral Vocal Cord Palsy*

This accounts for 10–15% of upper airway pathology. Unilateral vocal cord palsy **(Fig. 3)** can occur post-cardiothoracic or oesophageal surgery and presents with hoarseness of voice and aspiration. Unilateral vocal cord palsy following cardiac, oesophageal or mediastinal surgery is due to trauma to the recurrent laryngeal nerve. Nevertheless, the right recurrent laryngeal nerve is seen in the neck and can be damaged during thyroid and parathyroid surgery, while the left recurrent laryngeal nerve loops around the arch of the aorta and is more likely to be injured during patent ductus arteriosus ligation or any procedures around the arch of the aorta. These patients present with mild stridor, hoarseness and feeding difficulty with features of recurrent aspiration. Treatment involves watchful expectancy and enteral feeding till recovery. Rarely, the patients may require tracheostomy.

### *Bilateral Vocal Cord Paralysis*[1,2]

Bilateral vocal cord paralysis (BVCP) **(Fig. 4)** comprises almost half of all cases of vocal cord palsy. These patients present with high-pitched stridor, dyspnoea, apnoeic spells and cyanosis; however, they have a normal voice. The aetiology may be congenital neurological causes in infancy, idiopathic and traumatic. Among the neurological causes, Arnold-Chiari Type 2 malformation, wherein there is cerebellar herniation through the foramen magnum, accounts for about one-third of cases. Associated hydrocephalus

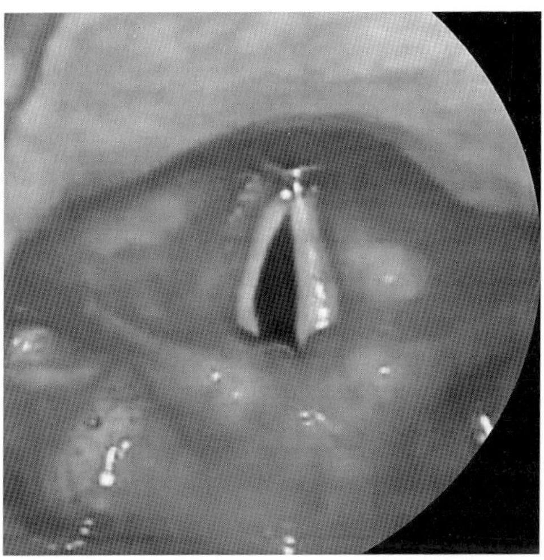

**Fig. 3:** Unilateral (right) vocal cord palsy. *(For color version, see Plate 10)*

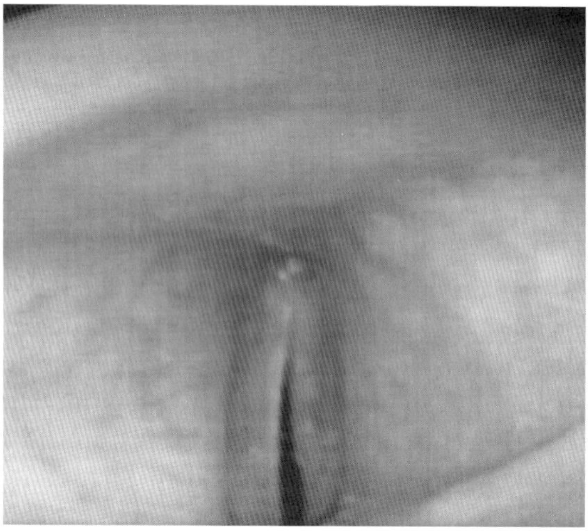

**Fig. 4:** Bilateral vocal cord paralysis. *(For color version, see Plate 11)*

and myelomeningocele can stretch or damage the vagal nuclei, resulting in vocal cord palsy. About 50–65% of patients require tracheostomy. Among the patients with congenital BVCP, 46–64% recover spontaneously in 6–12 months. Hence, no active surgical interventions are recommended up to 2 years of age. Beyond this age, multiple surgical options, both endoscopic and open, have been tried with varying success. Nasal continuous positive airway pressure with enteral feeding in a PICU setting is ideal while recovery is awaited. However, this wait can last up to several weeks and can be very inconvenient for the child and the parents. Some other patients may wait for recovery on tracheostomy before surgical options are suggested.

## *Subglottic Stenosis*[1,2,4]

SGS is defined as a restriction of the subglottic diameter to <4 mm in full-term neonates and <3 mm in preterm infants **(Fig. 5)**. In cases of congenital SGS, infants may present with biphasic stridor at birth, with symptoms appearing when the airway narrows by >50% **(Table 3)**. Lesser narrowing can result in recurrent croup-like episodes. It is better to refer the patient to an experienced paediatric otorhinolaryngologist early, as soon as the condition is suspected, instead of repeated attempts to intubate. Multiple intubation attempts can cause trauma and lead to a 'cannot intubate, cannot ventilate' scenario, which presents life-threatening risks.

In skilled hands, second-generation supraglottic devices, such as the ProSeal laryngeal mask airway and i-gel size 1, can temporarily stabilise the airway and facilitate ventilation while the otorhinolaryngology team is contacted. Congenital SGS often has additional acquired elements due to trauma from prior intubation attempts. The congenital type primarily involves

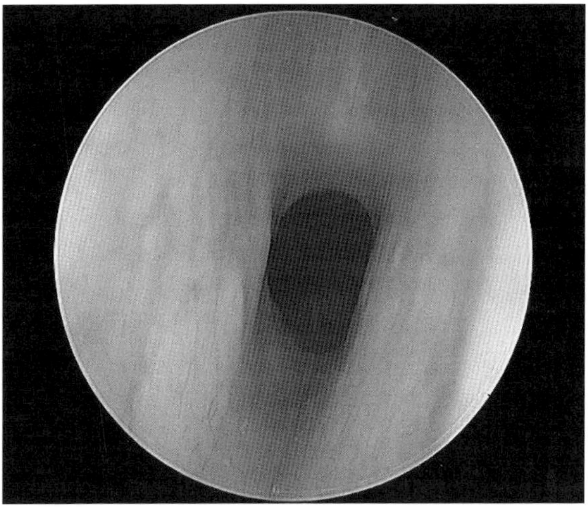

**Fig. 5:** Subglottic stenosis. *(For color version, see Plate 11)*

**TABLE 3:** Cotton-Myer grading of subglottic stenosis.

| *Grade* | *Description* |
|---|---|
| Grade 1 | Lumen obstruction 0–50% |
| Grade 2 | Lumen obstruction between 51 and 70% |
| Grade 3 | Lumen obstruction between 71 and 99% |
| Grade 4 | Complete lumen obstruction |

cartilaginous structures, making dilation with scopes or bougies challenging, while acquired SGS typically involves soft tissue, allowing easier dilation.

Suspicion of SGS requires assessment with flexible laryngoscopy/rigid endoscopy for evaluation of the severity of the stenosis and the diameter of the lumen **(Table 3)**. In older children, careful repeated bougienage with serial dilators can be tried before definitive reconstructive procedures are undertaken. Soft stenosis [as assessed visually or through magnetic resonance imaging (MRI)] is dilated with a balloon dilator [Metic airway balloon catheter (Meril Life Sciences Pvt. Ltd)]. Should these interventions be impossible, one may have to resort to performing a tracheostomy.

Evaluating a newborn with SGS presents high risks and must be carefully managed, preferably under local anaesthesia with supplemental oxygen. The high-pressure, low-volume cuffs of the endotracheal tube are responsible for tracheal mucosal ischaemia, contributing to acquired SGS in intubated patients. Current microcuffed endotracheal tubes are made of polyurethane (a less harmful material) with low-pressure, high-volume cuffs. Also, it is recommended to keep cuff pressures below 20 cm of water using a cuff pressure monitor, especially when prolonged intubation and ventilation are involved, like in the PICU setting.

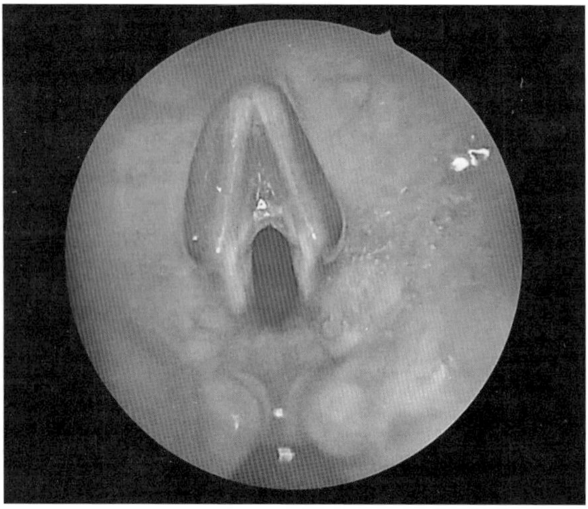

**Fig. 6:** Laryngeal web. *(For color version, see Plate 12)*

### *Laryngeal Web*

Laryngeal web is a relatively rare condition. Most children present at birth, though it may manifest as noisy breathing later. Sometimes laryngeal web can be acquired due to intubation injuries. It may be a small membranous tissue at the cord level or can be thicker, extending down to the subglottic level **(Fig. 6)**. Depending upon the thickness and the extent of the web, the management varies from simple dilatation or laser division to a major reconstructive procedure.

## PREOPERATIVE ASSESSMENT AND PLANNING[5]

A good history is the first step in the preoperative evaluation for airway procedures. The key questions would include the birth history, neonatal intensive care unit stay, previous intubation experiences, and previous airway procedures or anaesthetics. Signs include the nature of the infant's cry, noisy breathing, feeding difficulties and failure to thrive, which might indicate underlying airway problems. In infants, stridor or noisy respiration indicates that the airway diameter may have already decreased by 50%.

More severe symptoms that present in older children include dyspnoea, feeding difficulties, snoring, hoarseness, voice change, poor exercise tolerance and recurrent pneumonia. These children may be on treatment for these symptoms. Sometimes, the breathing difficulty is mistaken for asthma, leading to beta-agonist medication such as salbutamol. The history of intensive care unit admissions and duration of intubation, if any, is essential for the diagnosis of SGS. Red flags that indicate worsening of airway narrowing in children already known to have SGS/airway obstruction include increased oxygen requirement and restlessness.

The narrowing may be exaggerated due to oedema following a viral respiratory illness.

Radiological imaging plays a crucial role in the preoperative assessment, specifically in confirming suspected airway narrowing. Several modalities are employed, each with its own advantages and limitations:

- *X-rays:* Can reveal narrowing of the larynx or indicate recurrent aspiration pneumonia. However, they provide limited detail compared to other imaging techniques.
- *High-definition ultrasound:* This non-invasive method is valuable for assessing tracheal size in newborns and the foetus. However, it requires specialised equipment and expertise, which may not always be readily available.
- *Magnetic resonance imaging (MRI):* Offers detailed information about the airway status. However, it can be challenging to perform in young children due to the need for cooperation and the potential risks associated with anaesthesia, especially in cases of preexisting or unknown airway obstruction. Foetal MRI gives valuable information about soft tissue obstruction in the airway of the unborn child and can be used to assess airway diameter.
- *Computed tomography (CT) scan:* It is generally the preferred imaging modality for evaluating obstructed airways. It is a fast procedure, typically completed in under 5 minutes, and provides detailed images. This speed is particularly advantageous when assessing patients where anaesthesia concerns are present. The recent availability of three-dimensional reconstructions from CT images enhances understanding of the airway anatomy.

In summary, while X-rays and ultrasound have specific applications, *CT scans are often the first-line choice for evaluating airway obstruction* due to their speed and comprehensive assessment capabilities. MRI, although it provides valuable information, is often hampered by practical limitations in paediatric patients. The choice of imaging technique ultimately depends on the specific clinical situation, and often, airway evaluation with a *transnasal flexible laryngoscopy (TNFL)* done in the operating room is the *first and only diagnostic tool.*

For uncooperative children undergoing a CT/MRI—a sevoflurane-based anaesthetic can maintain spontaneous respiration under the supervision of an experienced anaesthetist, ideally in a hospital set up—an environment equipped for emergencies. For more stable patients, MRI can be conducted under sedation, yielding crucial information regarding airway diameter and narrowing. This demarcation of the narrowing allows for the identification of appropriate surgical strategies; larger gaps may require rib grafts with laryngotracheal reconstruction, whereas smaller gaps can be repaired by slide tracheoplasty. A soft membrane causing narrowing will be amenable to cold knife cut and dilatation.

In a child with a stridor, a TNFL done in the operating room is often the first investigation and gives a good deal of information (often before imaging studies such as CT or MRI). During TNFL, a flexible fibreoptic scope is introduced nasally under light general anaesthesia or TIVA to evaluate the upper airway. This assessment includes observing dynamic movements of the vocal cords and identifying any supraglottic pathology. The procedure can assess upper airway collapse, glottic lumen diameter, vocal cord motion, and the extent of subglottic narrowing. Many patients would have associated tracheal conditions, such as tracheomalacia, which is also typically found in tracheoesophageal fistula (TEF).

*Anaesthesia for TNFL:* Patients are to be fasted according to age, and the patient may take clear liquids up to 2 hours before surgery. For infants, haemoglobin levels and echocardiograms may be all that are needed. Anaemia or any background cardiac condition will complicate anaesthetic outcome and increase the danger of hypoxia. In emergency situations, sometimes a full stomach situation might present itself. In such cases, inserting a naso-/orogastric tube after induction and adequate preoxygenation will help. A drying agent, such as atropine or glycopyrrolate, is given on establishing an intravenous line at induction, but sedative premedication is usually avoided. Inhalational induction with sevoflurane in 100% oxygen can be followed by intravenous access, deepening the anaesthetic with a small dose of propofol 1 mg/kg and then spraying the cords with a local anaesthetic spray of lignocaine (3–5 mg/kg). Case 1 (later in this text) illustrates this case. Nasal drops of xylometazoline and lignocaine jelly are used to ensure easy passage of the scope, and a local anaesthetic spray on the vocal cords is added when the scope is passed.

In patients with stridor following TEF repair procedures, a multidisciplinary approach by an otorhinolaryngologist, anaesthetist and gastroenterologist is usually required. A coloured dye is injected via the visible pit or fistula (TEF) within the oesophagus under direct vision with an upper gastrointestinal endoscope (by the gastroenterologist). Simultaneously, the otorhinolaryngologist looks in the trachea via a flexible bronchoscope for evidence of dye leak (at probable TEF site), indicative of recurrent fistula or missed connections. Children who experience recurrences of aspiration and failure to thrive weeks or months after TEF repair typically have a TEF in the trachea's posterior wall just above the carina (that has been repaired) and also have accompanying gastro-oesophageal reflux disease or tracheomalacia and thus require careful assessment.

## OXYGENATION DURING AIRWAY PROCEDURES

Upper airway surgeries pose a great challenge in airway management because the anaesthesiologist and surgeon must share the patient's airway. Advanced techniques, precision equipment such as optical instruments for smaller babies and newer anaesthesia techniques in children allow surgeons to manipulate the upper airway successfully.

Traditionally, general anaesthesia with intubation with a narrow endotracheal tube has been used; this may seem safe and a comfortable choice for the anaesthetist, but is challenging for the surgeon to share the limited space, considering the small area in a child. This is especially true in upper airway procedures. It has the following disadvantages:[3]

- Challenging for the surgeon to share space with the anaesthetist.
- Increased airway resistance due to a narrow endotracheal tube.
- Surgeons can cause damage to the endotracheal tube during surgery.
- The surgical field is cramped, and there is less space to work.
- Inability to reach some areas—posterior part of the larynx, supraglottic area.
- May have to extubate and intubate many times in order to access these areas. This can lead to loss of airway and desaturation (especially in patients who are already compromised).
- All this leads to a prolonged duration of the procedure.

*Methods of oxygenation[1] for airway procedures include:*

- Spontaneous breathing.
- Positive pressure ventilation via an endotracheal tube [often a microlaryngeal tube (MLT) that is smaller and longer] inserted in the proximal trachea. This has its issues as described earlier. But it is still favoured in many infants who cannot tolerate other tubeless techniques **(Fig. 7A)**.
- Jet ventilation—may be supraglottic or subglottic/transtracheal.
- Apnoeic oxygenation using humidified, high-flow nasal oxygen delivery systems or intermittent ventilation.
- Cross-field ventilation with an endotracheal or endobronchial tube within the distal airway (used for open laryngotracheal reconstruction)
- Extracorporeal membrane oxygenation (ECMO) used in intrathoracic open-airway procedures.

## Spontaneous Breathing: Tubeless Anaesthesia Technique[3,5,6]

Deep sedation with spontaneous respiration without endotracheal intubation (tubeless anaesthesia) has definite advantages over conventional general anaesthesia with an endotracheal tube, as the oral aperture, larynx, face, neck, and all other areas apart from the nose remain free to be operated upon. Anaesthesia is maintained by TIVA, and oxygenation is maintained by high-frequency nasal oxygen (HFNO)/THRIVE **(Fig. 7B)**. HFNO[5,6] has emerged as a critical technique for facilitating tubeless anaesthesia. HFNO delivers humidified and heated oxygen at flow rates of up to 70 L/min **(Table 4)**, which enhances oxygenation and ventilation while allowing for prolonged apnoeic oxygenation.

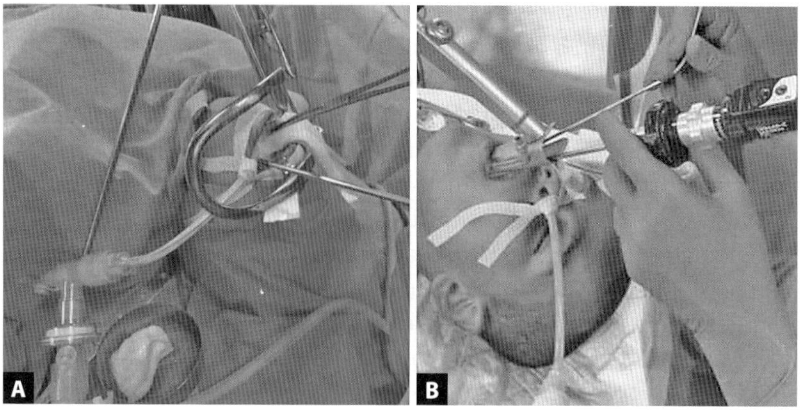

**Figs. 7A and B:** (A) Conventional technique: oral intubation with a small endotracheal tube; and (B) Tubeless technique with nasopharyngeal airway and high-flow oxygen. *(For color version, see Plate 12)*

**TABLE 4:** Oxygen flow rates for high-flow nasal oxygen (HFNO).

| *Patient weight* | *High-flow oxygen rates* |
|---|---|
| 0–12 kg | 2 L/kg/min |
| 13–15 kg | 30 L/min |
| 16–30 kg | 35 L/min |
| 31–50 kg | 40 L/min |
| >50 kg | 50 L/min |

*Physiological effects of HFNO:*[3]

- The continuous high flow of 100% oxygen causes denitrogenation and washout of the anatomical dead space.
- During apnoea, alveolar oxygen absorption exceeds $CO_2$ production because of relative differences in blood solubility, generating a negative pressure gradient that favours the bulk flow of gas from the anatomical dead space into the alveoli, a phenomenon called aventilatory mass flow.
- Increased alveolar ventilation flushes out expired $CO_2$, thereby reducing the rate of $CO_2$ accumulation and dead space rebreathing.
- HFNO generates a low level of continuous positive airway pressure of 2.7–7.4 $cmH_2O$, which helps in alveolar recruitment, prevents atelectasis, reduces shunting and hence improves oxygenation.[3]
- Heated and humidified gases, when supplied, reduce the work of breathing and thereby the energy requirements. They also prevent drying of the nasopharyngeal and tracheobronchial mucosa, improve mucociliary clearance and improve patient comfort. The child is able to tolerate the high flows.

Physiological and clinical studies have shown that HFNO is able to safely support tubeless anaesthesia, maintaining an unobstructed surgical field during laryngeal procedures.

*The advantages of the tubeless technique are as follows:*

- It provides the much-needed space and comfort for surgeons.
- It provides an uninterrupted surgical field for laryngeal surgeries.
- It is a good alternative to conventional anaesthesia if the surgeon/anaesthetist are familiar and choose the correct patients.

Nonetheless, good back-up plans are always the key to safe anaesthesia.

## *STRIVE Hi (Spontaneous Respiration Using Intravenous Anaesthesia and High-flow Nasal Oxygen)*[7,8]

Use of HFNO in spontaneously breathing patients under intravenous general anaesthesia has been shown to benefit oxygenation, ventilation and upper airway patency in a wide range of upper airway procedures. Intravenous induction with propofol, maintaining spontaneous breathing, is a difficult technique to perfect, with a narrow margin for error. In airway procedures, the need for obtunded airway reflexes while maintaining spontaneous respiration makes it challenging. Achieving good operating conditions during endoscopic airway surgery without the use of neuromuscular blockade requires an adequate depth of anaesthesia, application of local/topical anaesthesia, and sometimes the use of a low-dose intravenous remifentanil infusion. The conduct of the STRIVE Hi technique may use propofol target-controlled infusion (TCI) or TIVA when the drug is carefully titrated (manual regime). Remifentanil can be used with propofol as part of the TIVA regime.

The STRIVE Hi technique in adults, as per a study, can maintain adequate oxygenation with a minimal increase in $CO_2$ levels (average 0.2 mmHg/min) during an average procedure time of 44 minutes.[7] Our experience in children shows that oxygenation is well maintained and $CO_2$ levels are acceptable. It is not possible to measure $CO_2$ as the procedures have an open airway; however, the $ETCO_2$ levels while ventilating post-procedure show good clearance of $CO_2$ as shown in adult studies.

Balancing an adequate depth of anaesthesia for spontaneous ventilation techniques is often very difficult and comes with experience. HFNO generates positive airway pressure that ultimately increases the end-expiratory lung capacity and functional residual capacity. Traditionally, fresh gas for oxygenation has been delivered either using a nasopharyngeal tube or an insufflation catheter attached to the anaesthetic breathing circuit. A smaller size uncuffed endotracheal tube is often used as a nasopharyngeal airway for the tubeless technique.

Tubeless anaesthesia with HFNO thus presents promising advantages in upper airway surgery; however, successful implementation will depend on careful patient selection and proactive strategic planning by both anaesthesiologists and surgeons. This collaborative approach will promote more effective and safe management of the airway and ultimately lead to improved patient outcomes in upper airway surgical procedures.

### *Transnasal Humidified Rapid Insufflation Ventilatory Exchange*[9-12]

THRIVE is another technique that is based on HFNO. It is a potentially novel way to achieve oxygenation and ventilation without an invasive device or tidal respiratory movements **(Figs. 8A and B)**. Thrive technique uses a dedicated apparatus that delivers high flows connected to a humidifier. The use of THRIVE is feasible in prolonging the apnoea times in children undergoing anaesthesia and surgery. It is generally well known that children are more likely to develop hypoxaemia during apnoea as a result of higher rates of oxygen consumption, smaller functional residual capacities and higher closing capacities. THRIVE was earlier used to prolong the apnoea time for a premature infant undergoing laryngeal surgery. Time to oxygen desaturation was prolonged even when a 30% air/oxygen mixture was insufflated into the lungs. The possible mechanism proposed is that significant ventilation and gas exchange occur as a result of gaseous mixing and flushing of dead space secondary to the high insufflation flows achievable with HFNO.

We use a modification of the THRIVE principle in our institute, using the standard anaesthesia workstation and all our cases are done with this technique. All children undergo a preoperative evaluation, which includes a detailed history and thorough examination, which forms the cornerstone in formulating an induction plan and estimating the risk of adverse events. We exclude children with anomalies of the nasopharynx, such as choanal atresia and compromised cardiopulmonary function, as they are predisposed to hypoxia due to a narrow apnoeic window. An uncuffed endotracheal tube is placed as a nasal airway, and the standard anaesthesia workstation is used to deliver high flow of oxygen (up to 15 L) through it. A heat and moisture exchange filter serves to provide some humidification. We are thus able to obviate the need for expensive THRIVE equipment. Placement of the tube in

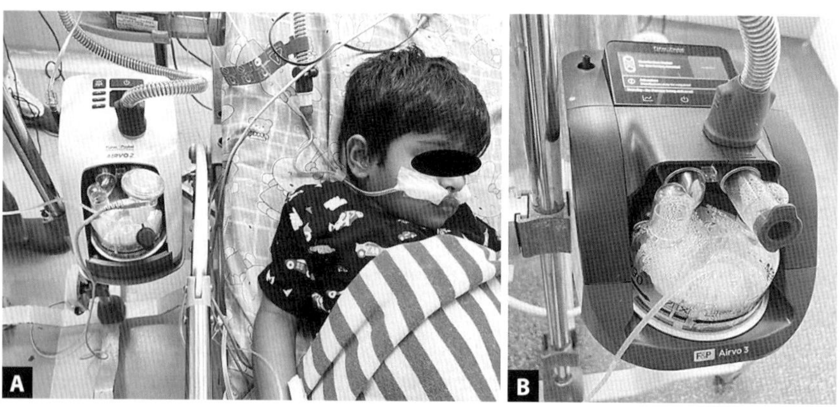

**Figs. 8A and B:** (A) Patient connected to the THRIVE apparatus via nasal cannula and (B) AIRVO 3 (Fisher and Paykel) delivering up to 70 L/min flow with a humidifier (THRIVE device). (THRIVE: transnasal humidified rapid insufflation ventilatory exchange) *(For color version, see Plate 13)*

the nasopharynx (as nasopharyngeal airway) just above the vocal cords not only helps in better visualisation of the operative field for the surgeon, but it also prevents complications related to endotracheal intubation, especially in patients who may already have an endotracheal tube-related injury. Administration of sevoflurane as a supplement to a titrated dose of propofol helps to maintain the depth of anaesthesia, which is possible through the use of the standard anaesthesia workstation. This is a particular advantage as inhalational agents cannot be delivered using the THRIVE device. Though environmental pollution is a concern with this technique, the THRIVE principle used with the anaesthesia machine is a game changer in preventing desaturation and maintaining anaesthesia in this group of patients.

### *Success and Safety of Tubeless Anaesthesia*

Although tubeless anaesthesia has its advantages, it is still not very common in practice. However, it is a viable alternative to conventional anaesthesia if the anaesthesiologist and surgeon collaborate to select suitable patients based on their individual profiles and medical histories after ensuring that they have enough experience to manage this approach. A safe strategy for tubeless anaesthesia requires careful planning and preparation. Nevertheless, appropriate comprehensive backup plans are essential. This includes high-frequency jet ventilation (HFJV) and endotracheal intubation as critical alternatives for maintaining oxygenation and ventilation in case of complications/hypoxia during the procedure. Protocols set by healthcare providers (while using this technique) can improve patient safety and optimise conditions during surgery while performing upper airway interventions.

## Rescue Oxygenation

In a very narrow airway, either initially or during a surgical procedure, if one is unable to ventilate and oxygenate in an emergency, there are only two options: (1) HFJV and (2) the surgical airway. The rigid bronchoscope may sometimes be an option to ventilate in a crisis.

HFJV[13,14] is a technique that involves the delivery of an air-oxygen mixture at high pressure through small-bore catheters. This is achieved by rendering small tidal volumes at very high frequency with either a manual jet ventilating device or a dedicated jet ventilator. Jet ventilation relies on passive expiration and unobstructed airway flow for gas exchange. Given its unique mode of action, it carries specific risks that one should be aware of for safe use. It is also vital to understand that this is an open breathing system where $ETCO_2$ measurements are inaccurate. Alternate methods for measuring $PaCO_2$ with invasive monitoring or continuous transcutaneous $CO_2$ monitoring should be considered. The Manujet is a device that enables jet ventilation through a needle inserted in the side-arm of a rigid bronchoscope **(Fig. 9)**.

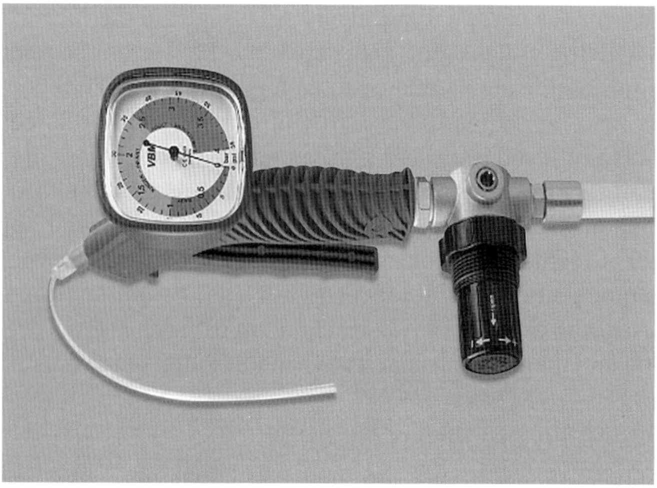

**Fig. 9:** VBM Manujet (VBM Medizintechnik GmbH, Germany). Jet ventilator device showing the pressure gauge, toggle switch and catheter. *(For color version, see Plate 13)*

The HFJV technique is associated with several advantages. The jet ventilation catheter can be placed directly in the airway, through an endotracheal tube or through a supraglottic device. When placed directly in the airway, HFJV can provide optimal conditions for performing tubeless airway surgeries. The use of low tidal volumes with this technique allows limited vocal cord mobility that would be desirable for some laryngeal procedures as well.

There are some risks associated with HFJV. These include barotrauma, airway injury and inadequate gas exchange.

- *Barotrauma:* Any obstruction to the path of egress can cause air-trapping and barotrauma. This may manifest in the form of pneumothorax, pneumomediastinum, subcutaneous emphysema and right ventricular failure.
- *Airway injury:* There are reports of airway injury from prolonged exposure to dry gases at high pressure from jet ventilation. The more recent jet ventilators are able to provide humidification of inspired gases.
- *Inadequate gas exchange (hypoxaemia and hypercapnia):* This is seen especially in patients with severe lung pathology.

## Oxygenation for Open Airway Surgery; Laryngotracheal Reconstruction[15-17]

Open airway procedures include staged laryngotracheal reconstructions (LTR), partial cricotracheal resection (PCTR) or intrathoracic repairs. Most of these patients have a tracheostomy in place, which makes delivering anaesthesia simpler.

### *Single Stage Laryngotracheal Reconstruction*

In single-stage LTR, the tracheostomy tube is removed, and the tracheostoma is closed as part of the reconstruction. Single-stage LTR involves the placement of cartilage grafts into anterior or posterior incisions to dilate the narrowed tracheal lumen. An endotracheal tube is placed into the trachea via the nose. This is later used to calibrate tracheal size during reconstruction and remains as a stent for the airway in the postoperative period. In single-stage PCTR, ventilation takes place through a tracheal stump via a separate sterile endotracheal tube.

### *Double-stage Laryngotracheal Reconstruction*[15]

Double-stage procedures are more straightforward as the tracheostomy is utilised for ventilation during the procedure and retained postoperatively. The patient is eventually decannulated in a staged fashion. A tracheostomy is inserted (if not already in situ) to safeguard the airway postoperatively and the grafted area is stented for approximately 6 weeks. This is followed by the removal of the stent and the tracheostomy tube and a check bronchoscopy is done to confirm airway patency. The tracheostomy is decannulated or surgical closure is done for the tracheostoma subsequently.

### Intrathoracic Procedures (Using Extracorporeal Membrane Oxygenation)[15]

Intrathoracic procedures, including type 4 laryngo-oesophageal clefts, tracheal resections, or slide tracheoplasty, require ECMO support as this can be the only way to oxygenate the patient when the trachea is open for a prolonged time. An endotracheal tube is placed into the airway to provide structure and airway size calibration during reconstruction.

Now that the primary problems with airway procedures and their surgical options have been dealt with, a brief outline of the techniques of maintenance of anaesthesia are outlined below.

## ANAESTHETIC TECHNIQUES: MAINTENANCE OF ANAESTHESIA[18,19]

### Total Intravenous Anaesthesia[18,19]

The technique of TIVA is a popular technique with many advantages in airway procedures with or without an endotracheal tube. The use of propofol for TIVA along with other agents like remifentanil, dexmedetomidine and ketamine is well-known. A correct balance and combination of these drugs for safe anaesthetic management needs a good understanding of the pharmacokinetics and pharmacodynamics of the respective agents. The main advantage of propofol as the base agent for TIVA is that it blunts the laryngeal and airway reflexes, especially in small babies, better than sevoflurane. In a child with a compromised airway, it is important to be able to achieve a plane of sedation with obtunded laryngeal reflexes during the procedure (which may be short), followed by a rapid return of reflexes and wakefulness soon after. Propofol obtunds reflexes very effectively; however, in small babies may cause a significant delay in wake-up and needs to be used with caution, making sure that there are good recovery monitoring facilities. Avoidance of sevoflurane prevents operating room and atmospheric pollution and reduces the cost.[8,9] The intravenous drugs can be administered either by manual TIVA or target-controlled infusion. Propofol can be used alone or in combination with ketamine (with atropine) for short procedures. All children coming for airway procedures benefit from the administration of anti-sialagogue. In longer procedures with open airway or tubeless technique, the addition of 'a touch of' intravenous dexmedetomidine (0.2–0.3 μg/kg) is useful.

## Dexmedetomidine[20]

Dexmedetomidine is a highly specific and selective alpha-2-adrenergic agonist. It has analgesic, amnesic, sedative, and anxiolytic properties.

### *Role of Dexmedetomidine in Paediatric Airway Surgery*

- *Maintaining airway patency:* A key advantage of dexmedetomidine is that it provides sedation while generally preserving respiratory drive and airway patency. This is crucial in airway surgeries where maintaining spontaneous ventilation is often desired.
- *Reducing emergence agitation:* Children often experience emergence agitation after general anaesthesia (especially airway procedures). Dexmedetomidine has been shown to be effective in reducing this, which is particularly important after airway procedures.
- *Opioid-sparing effects:* The analgesic properties of dexmedetomidine allow for a reduction in the use of opioids, which can cause respiratory depression. This is very beneficial in airway procedures.
- *Providing a calm sedation:* It helps to provide a calm and cooperative patient, which is very helpful when dealing with children.

Dexmedetomidine is usually given as an infusion. It is administered as an intravenous bolus of 0.5–1 μg/kg (over 10 minutes) or an infusion of 0.3–1 μg/kg/h. For procedures lasting 30–45 minutes, a single dose initially of 0.3 μg/kg given slowly will suffice for a smooth anaesthetic. It can cause bradycardia and prolonged sedation and is not preferred in infants (with compromised airways) in whom early wake-up is preferred.

## Remifentanil[21]

Remifentanil is an ultra-short-acting potent opioid recently launched in India. As remifentanil is cleared rapidly by non-plasma metabolism, it has a short elimination half-life of 3–6 minutes, which does not change with age. Since it has a very good synergistic effect with propofol, the dose of propofol is reduced (propofol-sparing effect) when used along with remifentanil. Its property of dose-dependent antitussive effect is very useful for short endoscopic procedures of the airway. The dose of remifentanil in the spontaneously breathing patient is 0.05–0.3 μg/kg/min. Spontaneous respiration is preserved well with the propofol/remifentanil combination, especially in children <3 years of age. Remifentanil is ideally started as an infusion at the start of the procedure. It can cause significant bradycardia. In the TCI pump, the remifentanil effect-site concentration (Ce) set is usually 2–4 ng/ml.

Monitoring the depth of anaesthesia during TIVA is by a multimodal approach. Besides factors like movement in response to surgical stimulus, haemodynamic parameters, respiratory pattern, pupil size and lacrimation, the newer modalities like bispectral index (BIS), entropy, auditory evoked potentials, processed electroencephalography and Noxious Stimulus Response Index (NSRI) are all under investigation. The BIS monitor that is commonly available monitors brain electrical activity and provides a numerical value that correlates with the level of sedation and hypnosis. It can be a useful adjunct to clinical signs. BIS values are less reliable in very young infants.

## Inhalational Agents[15,18]

Sevoflurane, which has useful bronchodilator effects, is the preferred agent for inhalational induction and maintenance for airway surgery in children. Its simplicity in usage makes it a popular induction agent in children. The main advantage of using sevoflurane is rapid titrability and a ready-to-use vaporiser, which most of anaesthesiologists are familiar with, as against the more complex TCI and TIVA pumps, which have a learning curve. In children with airway compromise, the induction with sevoflurane may be slightly prolonged. This can be overcome with slight continuous positive airway pressure and assisted breathing. Once the child is deep enough, the cords and trachea can be sprayed with 2% lignocaine. The biggest disadvantage of sevoflurane is atmospheric pollution (in an open airway setting). Finally, the use of TIVA or inhalational agents for maintenance in airway procedures depends on the experience of the user. As the common saying goes—'the type of engine in the car has much less impact on the safety of the journey than the choice of driver.' The key to a smooth, safe anaesthetic in airway procedures is the anaesthetist at the head end, his understanding of the procedure, the needs of the surgeon at various points and his communication with the surgeon.

There are few drugs, but there is much skill and art involved in balancing the combination to provide good operating conditions and a live child.

## LASER SURGERY OF AIRWAY: CHALLENGES[22]

Lasers are used to treat non-vascular lesions in the endotracheal and endobronchial areas as well as division of strictures **(Fig. 10)**. Laser removal of polyps in children with juvenile papillomatosis of the larynx is associated with fewer recurrences. Initial bronchoscopy is essential in determining the type and exact location of the lesion in the airway. Ventilation is maintained through the side arm of a rigid bronchoscope during this phase. Ventilation is adjusted so as not to interfere with the surgeon and is intermittent. While lasers can be very precise in their application, they also pose specific risks that do not relate to airway management. Chief among these concerns is the potential for a fire hazard when lasers are used, especially in the presence of oxygen. Maintaining a $FiO_2$ of <0.3%, using non-combustible material in the airway, such as metal instruments and non-flammable inhaled anaesthetics, are some of the measures taken to prevent airway fires. The endotracheal tubes are wrapped in fire-resistant foil, and the cuff is filled with saline. A smaller-sized endotracheal tube may be used. The micro-laryngeal tubes are longer than conventional ones and are specifically designed to facilitate airway work. Laser-safe tubes are made of rubber, silicone or reinforced with stainless steel. Their cuffs are filled with saline, which may be dyed blue for easy identification in the event of a puncture. The presence of congenital anomalies or prior interventions in the airways may compromise airway access and management in some children who are scheduled for laser airway surgery, such as in vocal cord palsy. The anaesthetic technique needs to be individualised in these patients, in whom many procedures will utilise delicate instruments or require minimal manipulation of the airway. Local anaesthetic spray helps in maintaining the right plane of anaesthesia in such cases.

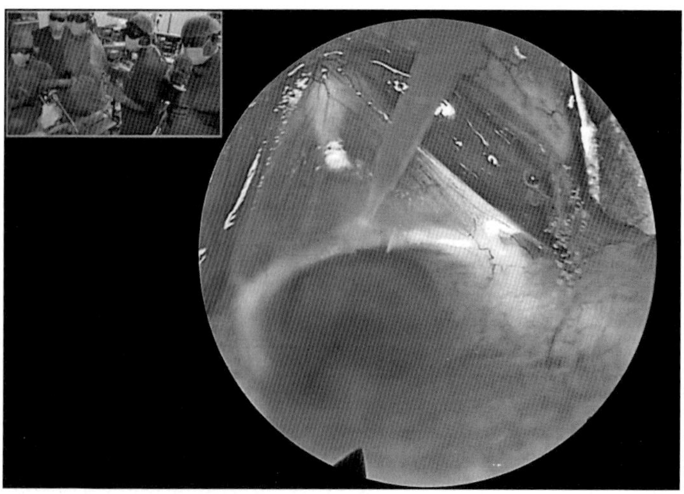

**Fig. 10:** Use of laser for division of laryngeal web. *(For color version, see Plate 14)*

The choice of anaesthetic is another important factor. TIVA or an inhalational agent can be chosen, but it is the job of the anaesthetist to ensure that the patient remains sufficiently oxygenated and maintains normocapnia throughout the operation. In lengthy operations, therefore, strategies against $CO_2$ retention should be undertaken, as an elevated level can contribute to respiratory acidosis.

Protective eyewear for the surgical and anaesthesia teams and awareness about safety principles and fire management algorithms are mandatory while using lasers.

## CASE SERIES TO ILLUSTRATE ANAESTHESIA TECHNIQUES FOR AIRWAY PROCEDURES IN CHILDREN

### Case 1: Diagnostic Procedure (Spontaneous Technique for the Initial Evaluation of Airway Anomalies in a Child)

A 4-month-old child (3.5 kg) with severe inspiratory stridor since birth came for evaluation for TNFL. The preoperative evaluation, including an echocardiography, was done to rule out any associated cardiac condition. The baby was fasted for 4 hours (for breast milk). Once inside the operating room, pulse oximetry and electrocardiography monitors were attached. Induction was with sevoflurane in 100% oxygen. Oxymetazoline nasal drops were applied to both nostrils.

An intravenous line was secured, intravenous glycopyrrolate 30 µg and propofol 2–3 mg/kg were administered. With gentle laryngoscopy, the vocal cords were sprayed with 2% lignocaine (The Golden Trick). Through the left nostril, a size 3 uncuffed endotracheal tube was inserted after good lubrication with xylocaine jelly. This tube was meant to help in the delivery of high-flow oxygen. Jackson Rees anaesthesia circuit was connected to give oxygen at flows of about 7 l/min. Sevoflurane in oxygen at 1% was continued via a nasopharyngeal airway while anaesthesia was maintained with TIVA (propofol infusion). Through the right nostril, a fibrescope was inserted to evaluate for vocal cord mobility, laryngo- and tracheomalacia and any other structural abnormalities. Once the fibrescope was inserted and oxygenation was established, anaesthesia was discontinued to wake-up the infant to facilitate a dynamic evaluation during withdrawal of the scope. This helped to look for laryngomalacia and upper airway collapse. The procedure took about 10 minutes. If the procedure took longer, dextrose containing intravenous fluids (5% dextrose normal saline) could have been started for maintenance.

### Case 2: Supraglottoplasty

An 8-month-old child with noisy breathing since birth, poor feeding and failure to thrive was diagnosed with severe laryngomalacia and posted for epiglottopexy (otherwise called supraglottoplasty). After inhalational induction, an intravenous line was secured. Intravenous glycopyrrolate, propofol 2–3 mg/kg and ketamine 0.5 mg/kg were administered, and nasopharyngeal high-flow oxygen was started. The vocal cords were sprayed with 2% lignocaine. Parson's laryngoscope was assembled and positioned. 0.3 mg/kg atracurium was given at this stage, and the child was intubated (intermittently) with a 3-mm size endotracheal tube, and the procedure was performed. This means that the endotracheal tube was removed by the surgeon briefly for a short part of the procedure, when it was crucial and hindering his work. He then reinserted the endotracheal tube. Nevertheless, an anaesthetist unfamiliar with this technique could request keeping the endotracheal tube in place throughout the procedure. The dictum is 'communication with the surgeon.' Small babies do not tolerate the removal and repositioning of the endotracheal tube and might require a conventional anaesthetic with endotracheal intubation throughout the procedure.

A continuous view of the larynx, the endotracheal tube, good suctioning by the assistant to keep blood and secretions away, and positioning the child suitably (tonsil position) are all key to the success of this technique. All patients require decompression of the stomach with a nasogastric tube (post-procedure) as high oxygen flows can inflate the stomach inadvertently and compromise respiration.

The endotracheal tube is kept postoperatively in such cases for a day or two, or extubation is done on the table, and oxygen support is continued. The babies can receive a dose of intravenous dexamethasone 0.15 mg/kg along with adrenaline nebulisation in the postoperative period, after extubation. Intravenous dexamethasone may be given (up to three doses) to tackle any oedema from airway manipulations.

## Case 3: Open Airway Surgery/Single Stage Laryngotracheal Reconstruction[16,17]

An 11-year-old girl with a history of prolonged ventilation after organophosphorus poisoning developed grade 4 SGS and had a tracheostomy. The child was scheduled for a single-stage LTR. After induction with propofol, fentanyl and paralysis with atracurium, 2% xylocaine was sprayed through the tracheostomy. The tracheostomy tube was removed (following good suctioning). Through the tracheostomy, a 5.5-mm cuffed reinforced endotracheal tube was inserted and fixed to the chest with a transparent dressing **(Fig. 11A)**. Anaesthesia was continued through this tube. A nasogastric tube was inserted in one nostril, and through the other nostril, a 6-mm microcuffed endotracheal tube was inserted and positioned just above the vocal cords **(Figs. 11A and B)**.

Two good intravenous lines and an arterial line were placed. Once the laryngeal reconstruction was done, the endotracheal tube (placed in the nostril) was guided further into the trachea (as a stent), and the reinforced tube (in the tracheostomy) was removed. Anaesthesia was now continued

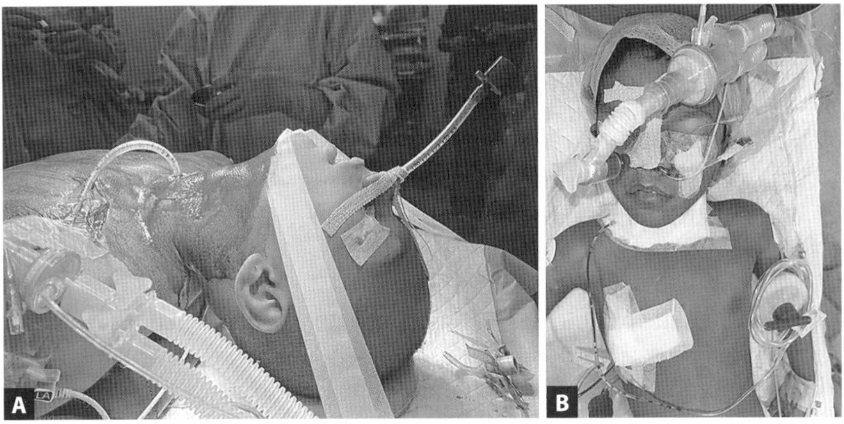


**Figs. 11A and B:** *Laryngotracheal resection:* (A) Preoperatively: A nasotracheal tube is inserted and kept above. Ventilation is maintained via tracheostomy through a flexometallic tube; (B) Postoperatively: Child is ventilated via the nasotracheal tube which also acts as a stent. *(For color version, see Plate 14)*

with the nasal endotracheal tube. Monitoring included direct arterial pressure, electrocardiography, $ETCO_2$, temperature and pulse oximetry. The child was transferred to the PICU for elective ventilation after the procedure. The child was sedated with fentanyl and intermittent atracurium, and the neck was immobilised in the neutral position with the help of sandbags on either side of the head. On the second postoperative day, an opacity was seen in the left lung which was cleared by bronchoscopic suctioning in the PICU itself. After 48 hours, the child was shifted to the operating room; a check bronchoscopy was done, and the child was extubated. Following this, non-invasive ventilation was instituted with $FiO_2$ of 0.3 to keep the tracheal lumen open (pneumatic stenting) in the PICU. After 2 days, the child was comfortable on room air and was discharged on the 10th day from the hospital. The child continued to come for regular follow-up and was doing well. Nevertheless, such patients need to come for follow-up, and TNFL is done initially every 4 weeks to check for airway calibre and tackle any granulation tissue that appears.

## KEY POINTS TO REMEMBER FOR ANAESTHESIA FOR AIRWAY PROCEDURES

- Preoperative evaluation and assessment are the key to understanding the problem.
- Continuous communication with the surgeon and review of all imaging with the surgeon is important.
- Intravenous access is often difficult for patients coming repeatedly.
- Inhalational induction is always better and helps maintain spontaneous ventilation. Intravenous access is mandatory even for minor procedures.

- A good local anaesthetic spray done in the right plane of anaesthesia goes a long way in obtunding the reflexes. It allows instrumentation of the airway and reduces the requirement for anaesthetics.
- TIVA with spontaneous ventilation with HFNO is the technique of choice for all minor interventions.
- Always have backup plans like JET ventilation, rigid bronchoscopy and surgical airway options ready in the operating room.
- Teams with good experience in handling major procedures only need to be involved in major LTR procedures.
- Good PICU teams oriented to these procedures and the requirements for ventilation post-LTR are the keys to success in major reconstruction.
- Good hydration, normoglycaemia and normothermia are essential components for early recovery.
- Postoperatively, steroids and nebulisation with adrenaline can help to reduce oedema following the manipulation of the airway.

## CONCLUSION

Paediatric airway management necessitates a thorough understanding of respiratory physiology, collaborative efforts among healthcare practitioners and patient-specific anaesthetic regimens. Thorough preoperative examination, history-taking and investigations, including imaging, serve as the foundation for the underlying diagnosis. The ability to adapt the method and strategy to the patient's anatomy and history is critical for effective procedure management. These priorities for safety, communication, and continuous monitoring contribute to improving the outcomes of children with airway-related problems by ensuring that interventions are carried out correctly and with minimal complications. This multidisciplinary strategy must be developed to handle all the complications of paediatric airway treatment.

## ACKNOWLEDGEMENT

The authors thank Dr Thirunavukarasu Saravanamuthu, ENT surgeon for sharing his pictures and Dr. S Parthasarathy, anaesthesiologist for helping with the manuscript preparation.

## REFERENCES

1. Oshan V, Walker RW. Anaesthesia for complex airway surgery in children. Cont Educ Anaesth Crit Care Pain. 2013;13(2):47-51.
2. Monnier P (Ed). Pediatric airway surgery: management of laryngotracheal stenosis in infants and children. Part 2, Congenital Anomalies of Larynx and Trachea, 1st edition. Germany: Springer Science & Business Media; 2010. pp.99-147.
3. Min SH, Seo JH. Tube or tubeless: an anesthetic strategy for upper airway surgery. Anesth Pain Med (Seoul). 2023;18(2):123-31.
4. Jagpal N, Sommerfeldt J, Shabbir N. Subglottic Stenosis. In: StatPearls [Internet]. Treasure Island (FL): StatPearls Publishing; 2025.

5. Humphreys S, Schibler A. Nasal high-flow oxygen in pediatric anesthesia and airway management. Paediatr Anaesth. 2020;30(3):339-46.
6. Pearson KL, McGuire BE. Anaesthesia for laryngo-tracheal surgery, including tubeless field techniques. BJA Educ. 2017;17(7):242-8.
7. Booth AW, Vidhani K, Lee PK, Thomsett CM. SponTaneous Respiration using IntraVEnous anaesthesia and Hi-flow nasal oxygen (STRIVE Hi) maintains oxygenation and airway patency during management of the obstructed airway: an observational study. Br J Anaesth. 2017;118(3):444-51.
8. Ji JY, Kim EH, Lee JH, Jang YE, Kim HS, Kwon SK. Pediatric airway surgery under spontaneous respiration using high-flow nasal oxygen. Int J Pediatr Otorhinolaryngol. 2020;134:110042.
9. Patel A, Nouraei SR. Transnasal Humidified Rapid-Insufflation Ventilatory Exchange (THRIVE): a physiological method of increasing apnoea time in patients with difficult airways. Anaesthesia. 2015;70(3):323-9.
10. Humphreys S, Lee-Archer P, Reyne G, Long D, Williams T, Schibler A. Transnasal humidified rapid-insufflation ventilatory exchange (THRIVE) in children: a randomized controlled trial. Br J Anaesth. 2017;118(2):232-8.
11. Jagannathan N, Burjek N. Transnasal humidified rapid-insufflation ventilatory exchange (THRIVE) in children: a step forward in apnoeic oxygenation, paradigm-shift in ventilation, or both? Br J Anaesth. 2017;118(2):150-2.
12. Jagannathan N. Use of THRIVE in children for head and neck procedures: why is it a useful technique? J Head Neck Anesth. 2020;4(1):e23.
13. Chitilian HV, Bao X, Mathisen DJ, Alfille PH. Anesthesia for airway surgery. Thorac Surg Clin. 2018;28(3):249-55.
14. Conlon CE. (2012). High frequency jet ventilation anaesthesia tutorial of the week. [Online] Available from https://resources.wfsahq.org/atotw/high-frequency-jet-ventilation-anaesthesia-tutorial-of-the-week-271 [Last accessed June, 2025].
15. Bradley J, Lee GS, Peyton J. Anesthesia for shared airway surgery in children. Paediatr Anaesth. 2020;30(3):288-95.
16. Mausser G, Friedrich G, Schwarz G. Airway management and anesthesia in neonates, infants and children during endolaryngotracheal surgery. Paediatr Anaesth. 2007;17(10):942-7.
17. Lee AJ, Prager JD, Mandler TN, Chatterjee D, Wine TM, Janosy NR. Anesthesia for laryngotracheal reconstruction in children: A narrative review. Paediatr Anaesth. 2023;33(11):883-93.
18. Lauder GR, Thomas M, von Ungern-Sternberg BS, Engelhardt T. Volatiles or TIVA: Which is the standard of care for pediatric airway procedures? A pro-con discussion. Paediatr Anaesth. 2020;30(3):209-20.
19. Malherbe S, Whyte S, Singh P, Amari E, King A, Ansermino JM. Total intravenous anesthesia and spontaneous respiration for airway endoscopy in children--a prospective evaluation. Paediatr Anaesth. 2010;20(5):434-8.
20. Shukry M, Kennedy K. Dexmedetomidine as a total intravenous anesthetic in infants. Paediatr Anaesth. 2007;17(6):581-3.
21. Lynn AM. Remifentanil: The paediatric anaesthetist's opiate? Paediatr Anaesth. 1996;6(6):433-35.
22. Sjogren PP, Sidman JD. Use of the carbon dioxide laser for tracheobronchial lesions in children. JAMA Otolaryngol Head Neck Surg. 2013;139(3):231-35.

CHAPTER 18

# Frontiers in Paediatric Anaesthesia: Advances in Anaesthetic Care for Foetal and Intrapartum Surgery

*Gita Nath, Sunidhara P Reddy, Shilpa Kedarishetty, Subrahmanyam Maddirala*

## ABSTRACT

With early diagnosis of foetal anomalies and rapid advances in foetal surgery, the responsibilities of the paediatric anaesthesiologist have extended from the neonatal period to include the pre-natal and intrapartum periods. Foetal surgeries include minimally invasive procedures, open mid-gestation procedures and ex utero intrapartum treatment. The main anaesthetic goals are (1) maternal and foetal well-being, (2) managing foetal pain and stress, (3) prevention of premature labour and (4) prevention of maternal haemorrhage. Anaesthetic management for these procedures requires a clear understanding of foetal physiology as well as requirements during the various interventions at different periods of gestation, so that we can ensure favourable maternal and foetal outcomes. It is also necessary to keep abreast with the continuing evolution of surgical, anaesthetic techniques and monitoring technology. Communication and collaboration amongst the various teams managing the patient are crucial in achieving the best possible outcomes in these complex cases.

***Keywords:*** Airway, Anomalies, Foetal, Intrapartum, Mid-gestation, Surgery, Tocolysis.

## INTRODUCTION

Rapid advances in imaging technology have led to early detection of foetal congenital anomalies, presenting a chance to correct those defects which would otherwise prevent successful transition to extrauterine life. Thus, our anaesthetic responsibilities have extended from the neonatal period into the foetal and intrapartum phases. In this chapter, the current knowledge on foetal and intrapartum surgery will be summarised, and more recent developments in this field will be described.

## CONDITIONS IN WHICH FOETAL/INTRAPARTUM SURGERY IMPROVES OUTCOMES

Foetal/intrapartum surgery can improve outcomes in the following conditions:

- Foetal anaemia
- Spina bifida/meningomyelocoele (MMC)
- Congenital diaphragmatic hernia (CDH)
- Lower urinary tract obstruction (LUTO)

- Twin-to-twin transfusion syndrome (TTTS), twin reversed arterial perfusion
- Cardiac defects—critical aortic or pulmonary valve stenosis, hypoplastic left heart syndrome
- Congenital pulmonary airway malformation (CPAM)
- Airway obstruction
- Miscellaneous—amniotic bands

## TYPES OF FOETAL SURGERIES

Foetal surgical interventions can be performed in early pregnancy, during mid-gestation or towards the end of pregnancy.

### Minimally Invasive Interventions

Minimally invasive interventions are performed in the early or mid-gestation period of pregnancy and can be done under local or regional anaesthesia, with or without sedation. Needle-based procedures done under ultrasound control include foetal blood sampling, radiofrequency ablation for selective foetal reduction, balloon valvuloplasty for aortic stenosis and placement of shunts for urinary obstruction or hydrothorax.

Foetoscopy or FETENDO involves percutaneous insertion of tiny scopes under ultrasound guidance to perform procedures such as tracheal occlusion for CDH, laser photocoagulation for TTTS and amniotic band release, foetal cystoscopy for LUTO and foetoscopic MMC repair **(Figs. 1A and B)**.[1]

For these procedures, the position of the placenta and baby is confirmed by ultrasonography, and a needle/foetoscope is introduced through the anterior abdominal wall into the uterus. The baby is immobilised with a combination of fentanyl and muscle relaxant injected into the thigh, after which the foetal intervention is performed.

### Open Mid-gestational Foetal Surgeries

Open mid-gestational foetal surgeries are usually done in the second trimester through a hysterotomy to access the foetus. This approach has

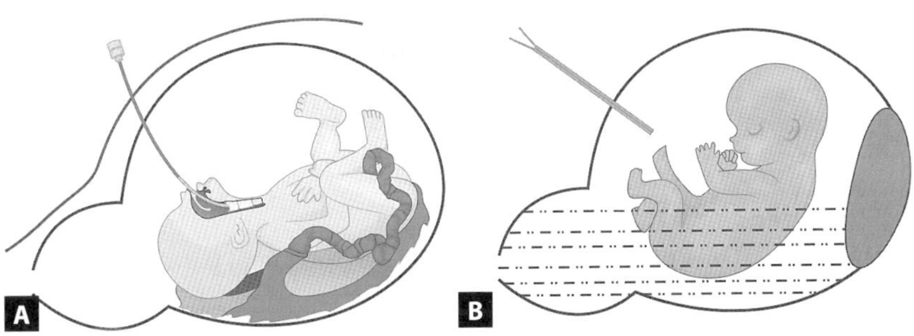


**Figs. 1A and B:** (A) Insertion of tracheal balloon for congenital diaphragmatic hernia; (B) Partial amniotic carbon dioxide insufflation.

been used for MMC repair, vesicostomy for LUTO, excision of CPAM and temporary tracheal occlusion for CDH. These are increasingly being replaced by minimally invasive operations.[1]

### Ex utero Intrapartum Treatment

Ex utero intrapartum treatment (EXIT) is also called operation on placental support (OOPS) and is the performance of lifesaving interventions, whilst the foetus is still oxygenated via the placental circulation. These interventions may be classified based on the indications given as follows:[2]

- EXIT to airway—cervical teratoma, CDH with tracheal occlusion, laryngeal atresia, stenosis, large neck mass and congenital high airway obstruction syndrome (CHAOS)
- EXIT to resection—CPAM, bronchogenic cyst and mediastinal tumours
- EXIT to extracorporeal membrane oxygenation (ECMO)—complex congenital heart diseases, hypoplastic left heart syndrome with intact atrial septum
- EXIT to separation—conjoined twins

For EXIT procedure, under maternal anaesthesia, the uterus is opened as for caesarean section. The foetus is partially delivered out and the required treatment is given, for instance, securing the airway for an obstructive airway lesion. During this time, the uterus is kept relaxed, and intrauterine pressure is kept up so that the placenta does not separate. Thus, foetal oxygenation is maintained till the treatment is complete.

## ANAESTHETIC CONSIDERATIONS FOR FOETAL SURGERIES

### Maternal Concerns

The various anatomical and physiological changes in pregnancy are well known. The important points to be kept in mind include (1) need to avoid aortocaval compression, (2) airway management—prevention of aspiration, possible difficult intubation, (3) rapid desaturation due to diaphragmatic elevation and (4) balancing haemodynamic effects of tocolytic agents with maintenance of uteroplacental blood flow. Ensuring maternal safety is paramount, since foetal surgery to improve outcome confers no direct benefit to the mother.

### Foetal Physiology

The combined (biventricular) cardiac output in the foetal parallel circulation is normally 425-550 ml/kg/min. The blood volume of 110-160 ml/kg is distributed between the foetus and placenta.[3] Cardiac output is rate-dependent, and any stressor such as hypoxia, hypothermia and noxious stimuli leads to bradycardia (heart rate < 100 beats/min). Despite a partial pressure of oxygen ($PO_2$) of 30 mmHg in the umbilical vein, adequate oxygen delivery is ensured by the increased oxygen affinity and higher concentration of foetal haemoglobin. Since maternal coagulation factors do not cross the placenta, prothrombin and activated partial thromboplastin times are prolonged.

Though thalamocortical pathways for pain perception only develop by 23-30 weeks of gestation, development of the cortical subplate and subcortical structures enables foetal pain perception even in the first trimester. Irrespective of conscious pain perception, lack of descending modulatory or inhibitory pathways makes the foetus extremely sensitive to pain, which is poorly localised and perceived over a large area, possibly resulting in long-term sequelae such as altered pain sensitivity and impaired neurocognitive development.[4]

Noxious stimuli increase levels of foetal stress hormones, including cortisol, β-endorphins and catecholamines. Truncal needling decreases the middle cerebral artery pulsatility index, indicating redistribution of blood flow to the brain, as part of the stress response. These changes also cause placental vasoconstriction, decreased foetal blood flow, bradycardia and increased uterine irritability.[4,5]

## Foetal Anaesthesia

Extraction index [foetal/maternal (F/M) ratio of drug concentration] of individual drugs depends on their molecular weight, lipid solubility and ionisation. Volatile anaesthetic concentrations exceeding 2 minimum alveolar concentration (MAC) are effective at anaesthetising the foetus, since the extraction ratio of sevoflurane is 0.38. With morphine and fentanyl having F/M ratios of 0.6 and 0.5, respectively, maternal analgesic drugs do not suffice to produce adequate foetal analgesia and muscle relaxants cross the placenta in negligible amounts. A combination of opioid (fentanyl 20 μg/kg), muscle relaxant (rocuronium 2 mg/kg) and anticholinergic (atropine 20 μg/kg) as an intramuscular injection directly to the foetus provides adequate foetal analgesia and immobility. Remifentanil infusion at 0.1 μg/kg/min in the mother has been found to be useful for foetal immobilisation and maternal sedation **(Table 1)**. For non-innervated tissue, such as placenta or umbilical vessels, specific foetal analgesia is not required.[5]

## Neurodevelopmental Effects of Foetal Exposure to Anaesthesia

Animal studies have shown that both inhalational and intravenous anaesthetic agents cause apoptosis in the developing brain, but these findings cannot be directly applied to humans. The vulnerable period in human foetuses

**TABLE 1:** Drugs used for foetal anaesthesia.

| *Drug* | *Foetal/maternal ratio* | *Route of administration* | *Dose* |
|---|---|---|---|
| Sevoflurane | 0.38 | Maternal inhalation | 2 MAC in mother will produce 0.76 MAC in foetus |
| Propofol | 0.5–0.8 | IV infusion to mother | Unreliable, not recommended |
| Morphine | 0.6 | IV to mother | Unreliable, not recommended |
| Fentanyl | 0.5 | IV to mother | Unreliable, not recommended |
| Remifentanil | 0.88 | IV infusion to mother | Effective when mother is under regional anaesthesia |
| Administered directly to foetus | | | |
| Fentanyl 20 µg/kg<br>Rocuronium 2 mg/kg or Vecuronium 0.2 mg/kg<br>Atropine 20 µg/kg | | Combine in 0.2–0.5 ml volume and give intramuscularly to foetus | Effective at attenuating foetal stress response and producing immobility |

(IV: intravenous; MAC: minimum alveolar concentration)

and infants extends from the middle of second trimester till 2–3 years of age. Clinical studies have shown that a single, short exposure to anaesthesia has no detrimental effect in young children, but the same cannot be said of repeated or prolonged anaesthesia. It is also difficult to separate the possible effects of anaesthesia from those of the primary surgical condition which necessitates anaesthesia.

Anaesthetic exposure during minimally invasive foetal surgery is much less compared to open surgery or EXIT procedure, where high concentrations of volatile agents are used to maintain uterine relaxation. There is still no direct evidence showing foetal neurotoxic effects because of anaesthetic exposure, but it may be preferable to use alternative agents to relax the uterus such as nitroglycerin, terbutaline, atosiban or magnesium.[6]

## Foetal Oxygen Delivery

Foetal oxygen delivery depends on the uterine blood flow, which in turn depends on maintaining an adequate blood pressure. Uterine blood flow is compromised by foetal procedures, hypotension, maternal pain and stress, uterine contractions and aortocaval compression. Hypotension caused by tocolytic agents and volatile anaesthetics should be countered by vasopressors such as phenylephrine. Umbilical cord compression or kinking due to amniotic fluid loss or foetal manipulation is detrimental to the foetus.

### Foetal Monitoring

During minimally invasive and open surgery, the foetal heart rate is monitored every 3–5 minutes with Doppler ultrasonography. Foetal cardiac interventions are done with continuous echocardiography monitoring. During EXIT procedure, pulse oximetry can be used after delivery of an arm. Though it reads the heart rate, the actual arterial oxygen saturation ($SaO_2$) values are difficult to interpret.

### Foetal Resuscitation

Foetal bradycardia may be precipitated by maternal causes, including hypoxia or hypotension, increased uterine tone, umbilical cord compression and placental abruption. Other causes are foetal cardiac dysfunction, vagal response and hypothermia.

Pre-placental measures to increase foetal oxygen delivery are optimising maternal oxygenation and ventilation, maintaining maternal haemodynamics with left uterine displacement, vasopressors and fluids. Other measures are improving uterine relaxation and checking for placental abruption.

Post-placental measures include relief of any cord compression, repositioning the foetus and increasing the uterine volume by fluid infusion. Additionally, adrenaline or atropine can be injected into the foetal heart (cardiocentesis) or umbilical cord (cordocentesis). Foetal blood transfusion and foetal chest compressions (directly or through the uterine wall with ultrasound transducer) can be done. If all these measures fail, the foetus should be delivered emergently and neonatal resuscitation should be carried out.[1]

## ANAESTHESIA FOR FOETAL SURGERY

Key goals of anaesthetic management include the following:

- Maternal safety and comfort
- Foetal well-being
- Foetal pain and stress management
- Prevention of premature labour
- Prevention of maternal haemorrhage

### Pre-operative Evaluation and Planning

Anaesthetic evaluation should include a detailed review of maternal obstetric history, comorbidities, previous anaesthetic exposures, drug allergies and obstetric complications. A thorough physical and systemic examination, including airway assessment, should be performed. The pre-operative investigations required are complete blood picture, blood grouping and typing. Reservation of cross-matched packed red blood cells is to be ordered for open mid-gestation surgeries and EXIT procedures.

Evaluation includes anatomical and physiological assessment by reviewing foetal imaging and echocardiography. This includes a meticulous ultrasound examination and preferably magnetic resonance imaging to delineate the lesion to help in planning the management. The baseline heart rate, weight for drug dosing and position of placenta and foetus should be documented. Irradiated, leucodepleted O-negative packed red cells cross-matched to the mother's blood group should be reserved for the foetus.

A multidisciplinary team meeting comprising obstetricians, foetal medicine experts, anaesthesiologists (separate teams for obstetric and paediatric management), foetal or paediatric surgeons, otorhinolaryngologists and neonatologists should be held well in advance to discuss, plan and simulate the conduct of the procedure. The team should collectively counsel the family about the planned procedure, surgical and anaesthetic risks and possible need for emergent delivery, and informed anaesthetic and surgical consent should be taken. Communication between team members is very important for the smooth algorithmic flow of interventions, especially with changing contingencies. These procedures should be conducted in a tertiary or a quaternary care centre where specialists from different disciplines work together.[7]

## Anaesthesia for Minimally Invasive Interventions

Ultrasound-guided needle-based procedures are usually performed under local or neuraxial anaesthesia, with or without sedation, with standard monitoring and antibiotic cover. Foetoscopic surgeries were earlier performed via laparotomy but are now done percutaneously in many centres. If complex or prolonged, they will require general anaesthesia.

Tocolysis is mandatory in the perioperative period to prevent premature labour. Fluid restriction (<750 ml) will prevent pulmonary oedema due to tocolytics and intraoperative amnioinfusion. Foetal analgesia and immobility are achieved by intramuscular injection into the deltoid or the gluteal muscles, if required for the procedure.[8]

## Anaesthesia for Open Mid-gestation Procedure[7-9]

These are done at late mid-trimester gestation (26–28 weeks), under general anaesthesia with or without epidural analgesia. Invasive monitoring and adequate intravenous access are necessary in addition to standard American Society of Anesthesiologists monitoring.

### *Goals of Anaesthesia*

- *Preserve uteroplacental perfusion:*

- Maintain 15° left uterine displacement.
- Maintain haemodynamics within 15% of baseline values.

- *Maintenance of anaesthesia:*
  - Volatile agents at 2–3 MAC for uterine relaxation
  - Alternatively, supplemental intravenous anaesthesia (SIVA) with propofol and remifentanil infusions (0.1–0.2 mg/kg/h) and 1–1.5 MAC of volatile agents only during hysterotomy. This technique reduces foetal cardiac dysfunction and need for resuscitative interventions when compared to inhalation agents alone.[10]
- *Surgical procedure:*
  - After laparotomy and uterine exposure, position of the placenta is confirmed with intraoperative ultrasound under sterile conditions.
  - Haemostasis is ensured by avoiding the placental margins and using a specialised absorbable uterine stapler.
  - The operative site of the foetus is then brought into position or delivered partially for surgical access.
- *Uterine relaxation:*
  - Volatile agents or SIVA technique as discussed above
  - Additional tocolysis with nitroglycerin infusion (0.5–1 μg/kg/min), indomethacin (50–100 mg oral or per rectum), magnesium sulphate (4 g loading dose followed by 2 g/h) or beta-adrenergic agonists such as terbutaline
  - Prevent hypotension caused by tocolytics with vasopressor infusions (noradrenaline or phenylephrine).
- *Prevent placental separation:*
  - Supplement lost amniotic fluid with warm saline infused by a large-bore catheter into the uterine cavity.
- *Monitor foetal well-being:*
  - Foetal echocardiography to monitor heart rate and ventricular function
  - Watch for foetal blood loss.
  - Ultrasonographic assessment of umbilical and middle cerebral artery blood flow
  - Foetal heart rate, cardiotocography and visual monitoring of umbilical cord pulsations
  - Resuscitative doses of adrenaline (1 μg/kg) and atropine (20 μg/kg) should always be kept ready.
  - Proactive planning for emergent delivery and neonatal resuscitation in a situation of foetal distress, placental separation, or onset of uterine contraction
- *Foetal anaesthesia and analgesia:*
  - Intramuscular injection of opioids, neuromuscular agents and anticholinergics as mentioned earlier

- *Emergence:*
  - Ensure continued tocolysis when withdrawing inhalational anaesthetic agents.
  - Adequate reversal of neuromuscular blockade, especially when using magnesium sulphate
  - Smooth emergence and extubation to prevent any stimulus which may precipitate uterine dehiscence, placental separation, pre-term labour or foetal distress
  - Multimodal analgesia with or without epidural infusion
  - Post-operative tocolysis to prevent pre-term labour; usually continued with calcium channel blockers throughout pregnancy.

## Anaesthesia for EXIT[7-9]

This is usually performed electively at 36–37 weeks of gestation, commonly done under general anaesthesia with or without post-operative epidural analgesia. Neuraxial anaesthesia for EXIT carries the risk of maternal haemodynamic compromise due to autonomic blockade compounding the effects of tocolysis and atonic post-partum haemorrhage (PPH).

The goals of anaesthesia and anaesthetic protocols are very similar to those of open mid-gestation procedures, with the following differences:

- *Use of uterotonic drugs* for the prevention of atonic PPH
- *Avoidance of magnesium sulphate* due to prolonged tocolytic action. Nitroglycerin infusion is preferred for tocolysis.

### *Partial Delivery of Foetus*

After hysterotomy, the foetal head, upper torso and arm are delivered to secure the airway. Placental separation is prevented by infusing warm crystalloid solution into the uterine cavity. Foetal oxygen saturation can be monitored by pulse oximetry placed on the foetal hand, and the foetal anaesthetic cocktail is injected into the deltoid muscle.

### *Securing the Airway*

A pre-planned and algorithmic approach to secure the airway should be followed, with a pre-fixed time allocated for each manoeuvre (e.g. 5–10 minutes each for direct laryngoscopy, bronchoscopy and tracheostomy) **(Flowchart 1)**. Equipment required for all these approaches should be cleaned, sterilised and kept ready **(Fig. 2)**. Confirmation of tracheal tube placement is done by capnography, lung sliding on ultrasound, visible chest rise and auscultation **(Figs. 3 and 4)**. Failure to secure the airway by multiple manoeuvres should lead to ECMO cannulation. A high index of suspicion should be maintained for barotrauma and inadvertent pneumothorax.

**Flowchart 1:** Airway management in EXIT procedure.

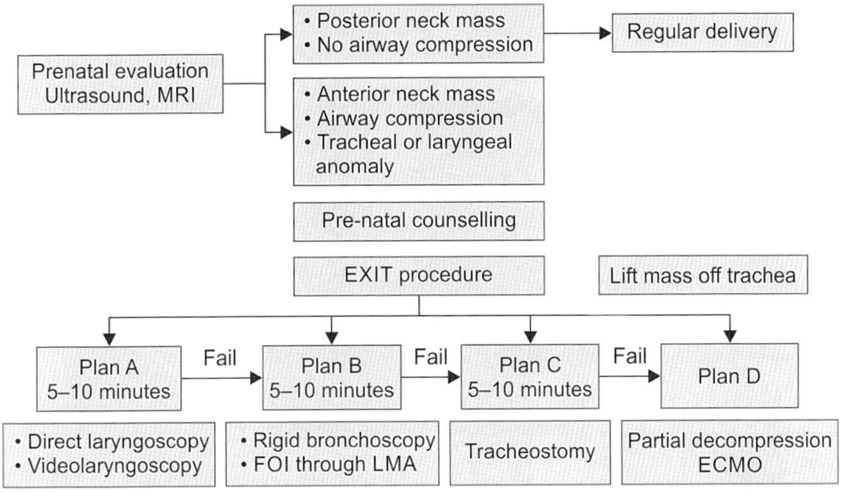


(ECMO: extracorporeal membrane oxygenation; EXIT: ex utero intrapartum treatment; FOI: fibreoptic intubation; LMA: laryngeal mask airway; MRI: magnetic resonance imaging)

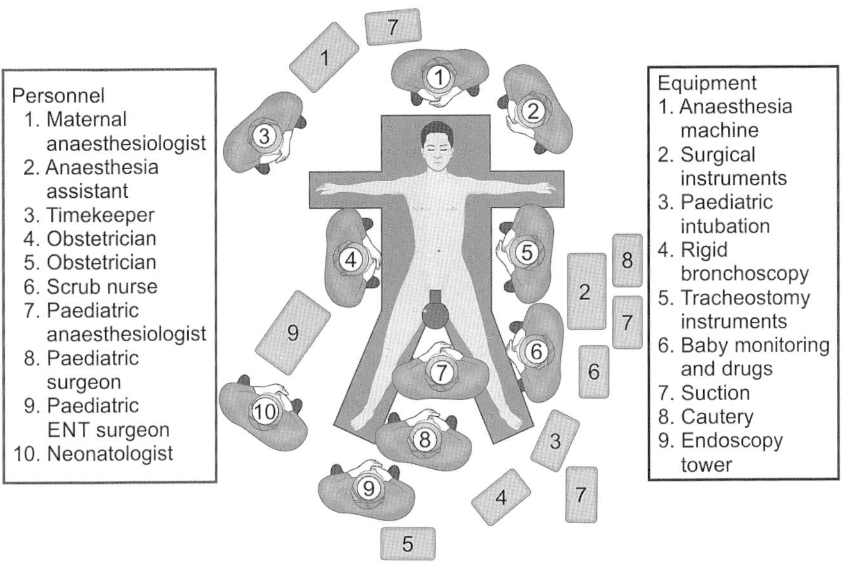


**Fig. 2:** Arrangement of personnel and equipment for EXIT procedure. (ENT: ear, nose and throat; EXIT: ex utero intrapartum treatment) *(For color version, see Plate 15)*

After the airway is secured, the foetus is delivered and handed over to the neonatology team for further resuscitation and care. Uterine tone is now increased by reducing MAC of the inhalational agent and administration of uterotonic drugs (oxytocin or carbetocin, methergine, carboprost and

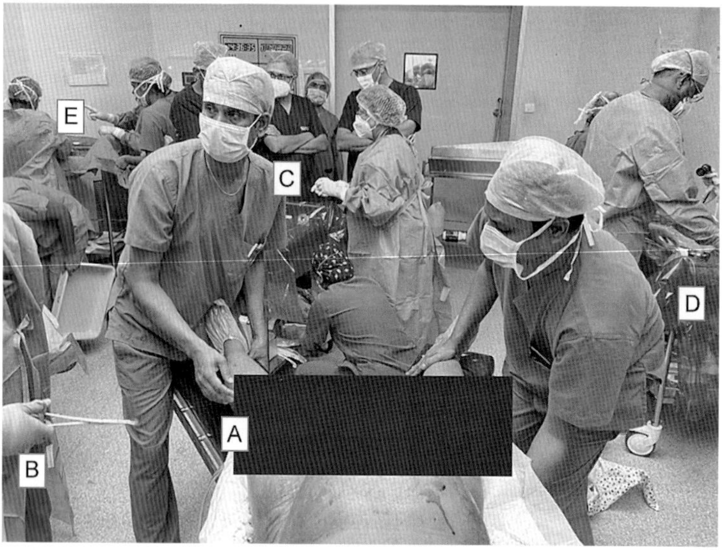


**Fig. 3:** Preparation for EXIT procedure. (A) Patient is positioned in lithotomy; (B) Surgeon is ready to operate; (C) Airway trolley; (D) Bronchoscopy trolley; (E) Tracheostomy trolley. (EXIT: ex utero intrapartum treatment) *(For color version, see Plate 15)*

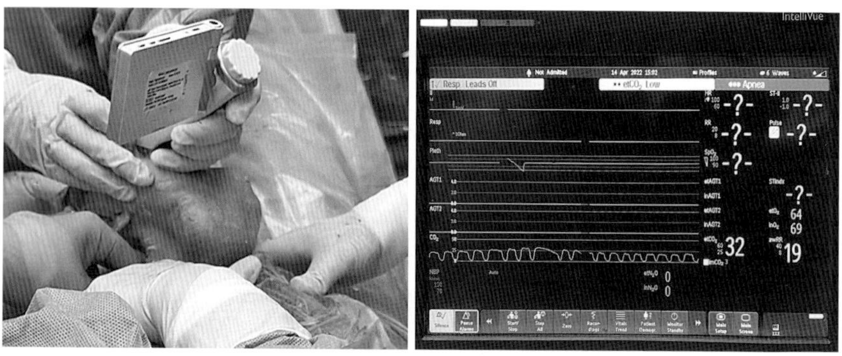


**Fig. 4:** Securing airway during EXIT. (EXIT: ex utero intrapartum treatment) *(For color version, see Plate 16)*

misoprostol), and the uterus is closed. Tranexamic acid can be administered to reduce PPH.

For non-airway-related EXIT such as for CPAM or conjoint twins, the airway should be secured before the foetal procedure in case urgent delivery is required. For all EXIT procedures, a second team of paediatric surgeons, paediatric anaesthesiologists and nursing staff should be on standby to complete the surgery on the newborn, if the EXIT procedure is terminated earlier than planned. Emergence and post-operative considerations are the same as discussed in open mid-gestation procedures, except that uterotonics are given rather than tocolytics.

## RECENT DEVELOPMENTS IN FOETAL SURGERY

### Partial Amniotic Carbon Dioxide Insufflation (Fig. 1B)

This was introduced by Kohl after several years of study in sheep to perfect the technique. It greatly improves the visibility of the foetus and intrauterine structures and enables the performance of precise and complex operations.[11]

General anaesthesia with muscle relaxation is used to keep the intrauterine pressure low. The patient is ventilated to normocapnia, and hypotension is avoided to maintain uteroplacental perfusion. An 18-G needle is inserted into the uterine cavity under ultrasonographic guidance, followed by infusion of 500 ml of warm Ringer's lactate (RL) solution. Under ultrasonographic guidance, three to four percutaneous ports are inserted into the uterus, and 1 L of amniotic fluid is removed. After ensuring the presence of a normal uteroplacental Doppler flow signal, carbon dioxide ($CO_2$) insufflation is started. Uterine 'opening pressure'—the pressure at which $CO_2$ starts flowing—is measured, and the insufflation pressure maintained at 4 mmHg above it.

Sustained $CO_2$ insufflation pressures cause a decrease in umbilical venous flow, foetal pre-load and blood pressure. This results in increased umbilical artery resistance which diverts flow to lungs through the ductus arteriosus, thereby increasing deoxygenated blood mixture. Maternal pressor response to intrauterine $CO_2$ insufflation can be alleviated by additional intravenous morphine. Over-insufflation may result in placental abruption and chorioamniotic separation. Conversely, the workspace may become smaller because of increased uterine or abdominal muscle tone or leakage of $CO_2$ into the mother's peritoneal cavity.[11]

Partial amniotic carbon dioxide insufflation (PACI) has been used for improved visibility and precision in several foetoscopic procedures, including laser ablation for TTTS, umbilical cord transection or ligation, amniotic band removal and the newer foetoscopic repair of MMC.

### Evolution of Spina Bifida/Meningomyelocoele Repair

Meningomyelocoele repair has been the commonest mid-gestational operation done, since the publication of the landmark Management of Myelomeningocele Study (MOMS), which showed the dramatic reduction in ventricular shunting and improved motor outcome when surgery was done prenatally. However, the risks of pre-term delivery and uterine thinning or dehiscence increased (89 and 35%, respectively), since an open technique with hysterotomy was used.[12] The surgical technique was similar to what is done postnatally, namely dissection of the neural tissue followed by a three-layer repair.

Concurrently with the introduction of minimally invasive foetal surgery, the surgical technique was modified. A less invasive technique was devised,

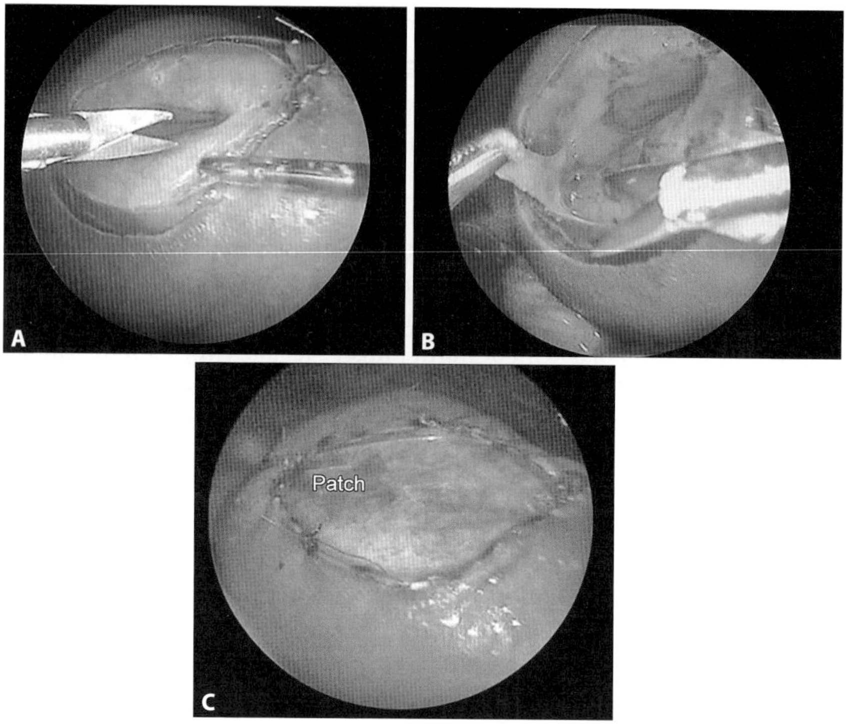


**Figs. 5A to C:** Foetoscopic repair of meningomyelocoele. (A) Lesion circumcised; (B) Meticulous dissection of neural tissue; (C) Closed with water-tight patch. *(For color version, see Plate 16)*

where the neural tissues are carefully dissected and then a water-tight closure is done with a biocellulose patch. This allows cerebrospinal fluid to accumulate over the patch, preventing adhesions and neural compression **(Figs. 5A to C)**. Several authors have observed better neurological outcomes with minimally invasive MMC repair.[13-15] Foetoscopic repair has the advantage of avoiding a uterine scar.

## Congenital Diaphragmatic Hernia

This is a developmental defect in the diaphragm which allows abdominal organs to herniate into the chest and leads to pulmonary hypoplasia and pulmonary arterial hypertension. Larger defects are diagnosed earlier in pregnancy and result in lower survival. Open anatomical repair via maternal laparotomy and hysterotomy was introduced in the 1990s but did not improve survival (in liver-down CDH) compared to post-natal repair. Liver-up CDH had a very high risk of foetal death due to umbilical vein kinking when the liver was placed in the abdomen.[16] Observing that CHAOS was associated with hyperplastic lungs, the procedure of tracheal occlusion was developed for improving lung volume and function. Initially, this was done via hysterotomy,

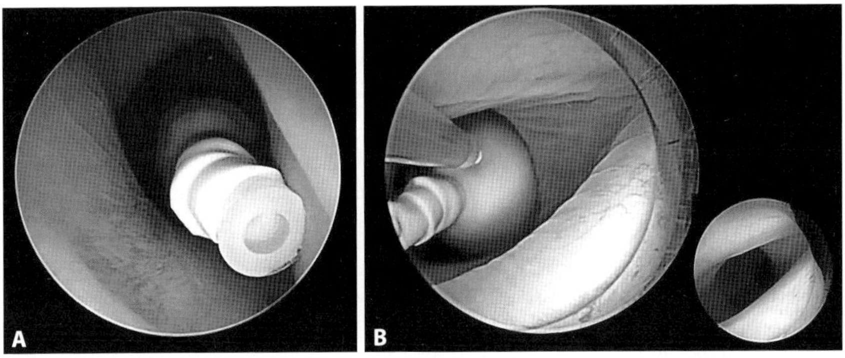


**Figs. 6A and B:** (A) Insertion of tracheal balloon; (B) Balloon puncture and removal.
*(For color version, see Plate 17)*

with an external tracheal clip or internal foam plug, necessitating an EXIT procedure for removal of the obstruction.[11]

The current technique of *foetoscopic endoluminal tracheal occlusion* (FETO), done at 26–29 weeks' gestation, consists of inserting a rigid foetoscope percutaneously and inserting a balloon into the foetal trachea. This is inflated with 0.6 ml of saline and left in situ, occluding the airway, and helps in accumulation of pulmonary fluid. It is done under local anaesthesia with conscious sedation with midazolam (1–2 mg) and remifentanil target-controlled infusion (2–3 ng/ml), which also helps to reduce foetal movement. At 34 weeks of gestation, the balloon is ruptured foetoscopically or percutaneously under ultrasonographic guidance **(Figs. 6A and B)**. An EXIT procedure is performed to remove the balloon if the patient goes into labour before balloon removal.[11]

Due to varying results, the FETO procedure is considered investigational and not standard of care. Further advances include development of a 'Smart-TO' balloon which will not need a second procedure,[17] and the use of transplacental sildenafil[18,19] which may work synergistically with tracheal occlusion to improve the development of pulmonary vasculature.

## Congenital Pulmonary Airway Malformation

This consists of a mass of polycystic, hypertrophic bronchioles in communication with the bronchial tree. It needs to be differentiated from bronchopulmonary sequestration, congenital lobar emphysema and even CDH because of the bowel loops. The size of the mass rather than the type of lesion determines its effect. Lesion size is measured by the CPAM volume ratio (CVR), calculated as 'CPAM volume/head circumference.' Maximum CVR <1 predicts that the disease will be asymptomatic at birth. CVR >1, especially with mass effect, can lead to lung compression, mediastinal compression, oesophageal obstruction and polyhydramnios. Massive lung masses lead to foetal hydrops and congestive heart failure.[20,21]

Open mid-gestational lung resection was introduced in the 1990s[22] and was the mainstay in the management of CPAM with hydrops till steroid therapy was introduced. This involves maternal laparotomy and hysterotomy, and the anaesthetic management has been described earlier. Currently, open resection is done for a pre-viable foetus with hydrops and solid lesions, if there is no response to steroids. For a viable foetus with delayed diagnosis and a likelihood of difficulty in neonatal resuscitation, the EXIT procedure may be done.

Maternal steroid (two doses of intramuscular betamethasone 12.5 mg) is the first-line therapy for large microcystic CPAM with impending hydrops.[20] Large cystic lesions may be drained by placing an ultrasonography-guided thoracoamniotic shunt (pig-tailed catheter through a trocar). Other options are embolisation, radiofrequency or laser ablation of feeding vessels. After ensuring maternal and foetal immobility, alcohol ablation of large macrocystic (5–10 ml 95% alcohol, withdrawn after 5 minutes) and microcystic (0.1–0.2 ml at multiple locations) CPAM has been shown to shrink the lesion and improve cardiac function. FETO has been used as a last resort to achieve lung growth.[11]

## CONCLUSION

With the advances in foetal surgery, the responsibilities of the paediatric anaesthesiologist have extended from the neonatal period to include the pre-natal period as well. It has become imperative for us to have a clear understanding of foetal physiology and requirements during the various interventions at different periods of gestation, so that we can ensure favourable maternal and foetal outcomes.

## KEY POINTS

- Foetal surgeries include minimally invasive procedures, open mid-gestation procedures and Ex-utero intrapartum treatment.
- Main anaesthetic goal is maintenance of maternal and foetal wellbeing.
- Foetal concerns include maintenance of foetal physiology, and minimising foetal pain and stress.
- Maternal concerns include prevention of premature labour and maternal haemorrhage.
- Multidisciplinary collaboration and communication are the keys to achieving the best possible outcomes.

## REFERENCES

1. Hoagland M, Chatterjee D. Anesthesia for fetal interventions—an update. Adv Anesth. 2021;39:269-90.
2. Hoagland MA, Chatterjee D. Anesthesia for fetal surgery. Paediatr Anaesth. 2017;27:346-57.

3. Rychik J. Fetal cardiovascular physiology. Pediatr Cardiol. 2004;25:201-9.
4. Thill B. The fetal pain paradox. Front Pain Res (Lausanne). 2023;4:1128530.
5. Bellieni CV. Analgesia for fetal pain during prenatal surgery: 10 years of progress. Pediatr Res. 2021;89:1612-8.
6. Cinquegrana D, Boppana SH, Berman D, Nguyen TT, Baschat AA, Murphy J, et al. Anesthetic neurotoxicity in the developing brain: an update on the insights and implications for fetal surgery. Anesth Pain Med (Seoul). 2024;19(Suppl 1): S96-104.
7. Nath G, Subrahmanyam M, Jayanthi R, Singh R, Ramesh S, Ahuja V. Recent advances in anaesthesia for intrauterine and foetal surgery. Indian J Anaesth. 2023;67:11-8.
8. Kodali BS, Bharadwaj S. Foetal surgery: anaesthetic implications and strategic management. Indian J Anaesth. 2018;62:717-23.
9. Chatterjee D, Arendt KW, Moldenhauer JS, Olutoye OA, Parikh JM, Tran KM, et al. Anesthesia for maternal-fetal interventions: a consensus statement from the American Society of Anesthesiologists committees on obstetric and pediatric anesthesiology and the North American Fetal Therapy Network. Anesth Analg. 2021;132:1164-73.
10. Marsh BJ, Sinskey J, Whitlock EL, Ferschl MB, Rollins MD. Use of remifentanil for open in utero fetal myelomeningocele repair maintains uterine relaxation with reduced volatile anesthetic concentration. Fetal Diagn Ther. 2020; 47:810-6.
11. Kohl T. Lifesaving treatments for the tiniest patients—a narrative description of old and new minimally invasive approaches in the arena of fetal surgery. Children (Basel). 2022;10:67.
12. Adzick NS, Thom EA, Spong CY, Brock JW 3rd, Burrows PK, Johnson MP, et al. A randomized trial of prenatal versus postnatal repair of myelomeningocele. N Engl J Med. 2011;364:993-1004.
13. Kohl T. Percutaneous minimally invasive fetoscopic surgery for spina bifida aperta. Part I: surgical technique and perioperative outcome. Ultrasound Obstet Gynecol. 2014;44:515-24.
14. Verbeek RJ, Heep A, Maurits N, Cremer R, Hoving EW, Brouwer OF, et al. Fetal endoscopic myelomeningocele closure preserves segmental neurological function. Dev Med Child Neurol. 2012;54:15-22.
15. Herrera SRF, Leme RJDA, Valente PR, Caldini EG, Saldiva PH, Pedreira DA, et al. Comparison between two surgical techniques for prenatal correction of meningomyelocele in sheep. Einstein (Sao Paulo). 2012;10:455-61.
16. Harrison MR, Adzick NS, Longaker MT, Goldberg JD, Rosen MA, Filly RA, et al. Successful repair in utero of a fetal diaphragmatic hernia after removal of herniated viscera from the left thorax. N Engl J Med. 1990;322: 1582-4.
17. Sananès N, Basurto D, Cordier AG, Elie C, Russo FM, Benachi A, et al. Fetoscopic endoluminal tracheal occlusion with Smart-TO balloon: study protocol to evaluate effectiveness and safety of non-invasive removal. PLoS One. 2023;18:e0273878.
18. Russo FM, Toelen J, Eastwood MP, Jimenez J, Miyague AH, Vande Velde G, et al. Transplacental sildenafil rescues lung abnormalities in the rabbit model of diaphragmatic hernia. Thorax. 2016;71:517-25.

19. Russo FM, De Bie F, Hodges R, Flake A, Deprest J. Sildenafil for antenatal treatment of congenital diaphragmatic hernia: from bench to bedside. Curr Pharm Des. 2019;25:601-8.
20. Kunisaki SM. Narrative review of congenital lung lesions. Transl Pediatr. 2021;10:1418-31.
21. Gupta B, Chaudhary K, Hayaran N, Neogi S. Anesthetic considerations in patients with cystic pulmonary adenomatoid malformations. J Anaesthesiol Clin Pharmacol. 2021;37:146-52.
22. Harrison MR, Adzick NS, Jennings RW, Duncan BW, deLorimier AA, Goldberg JD, et al. Antenatal intervention for congenital cystic adenomatoid malformation. Lancet. 1990;336:965-7.

CHAPTER 19

# Common Adverse Events and Their Mitigation Strategies in Paediatric Anaesthesia: Learn how to Minimise Risks and Ensure the Best Outcomes!

*Indrani Hemantkumar, (Brig) Rahul Yadav, Aavula Muralidhar, Pooja Bihani*

## ABSTRACT

Paediatric anaesthesia involves a precious population with a very low margin of safety and demands taking the utmost care to ensure patient safety. The perioperative period is a vulnerable period wherein the perioperative interventions of anaesthesia can lead to undesirable or harmful outcomes or complications, namely adverse events. Common events include respiratory, cardiovascular, allergic and medication related, among others.

Multiple patient factors such as age, gender of the baby, American Society of Anesthesiologists (ASA) physical status and nutritional status of the child and pre-existing medical conditions such as congenital heart disease and upper respiratory tract infection can affect the occurrence of adverse events. The complexity, type, nature and duration of surgery; use of narcotics; location and completeness of pre-operative checkup; location of administration of anaesthesia/sedation; intraoperative anaesthesia technique; ventilatory strategy; anaesthesia provider experience and attentiveness and neurotoxicity of anaesthetics are some other factors that can influence the perioperative adverse events.

Appropriate mitigation strategies for the adverse events include continuous perioperative monitoring and vigilance including pharmacovigilance, minimising human factors, use of trigger tools in the identification and measurement of adverse events, simulation and drills for training the perioperative team to deal with critical events and the availability of dedicated paediatric anaesthesia equipment and personnel.

***Keywords:*** Adverse event, Identification, Mitigation, Paediatric, Perioperative, Risk, Strategies.

## INTRODUCTION

Paediatric anaesthesia is a critical field, where the stakes are particularly high due to the vulnerable nature of the patient population. Administering anaesthesia to children poses unique challenges and risks that differ significantly from those in adults. Adverse events in paediatric anaesthesia, although relatively rare, can have serious and long-lasting consequences. Many adverse events can result in permanent harm, and the majority are classified as preventable. Therefore, understanding these potential risks and implementing effective mitigation strategies is crucial for anaesthesiologists to ensure the best outcomes. Targeted safety interventions can help to prevent adverse events. The causes and implications of adverse events encountered in paediatric anaesthesia are explained in this chapter. Furthermore, the chapter explores a range of mitigation strategies that can be employed to minimise these risks. A comprehensive guide for anaesthesiologists, highlighting best practices and innovative approaches to enhance patient safety and improve outcomes in paediatric anaesthesia, is provided by analysing both the challenges and solutions.

## WHAT IS AN ADVERSE EVENT?

An adverse event is an injury, large or small, ranging from mild to severe, caused by the use of a drug, test or medical treatment. An adverse drug event is an injury, large or small, caused by the use/non-use of a drug. Adverse events lead to unintended or undesirable healthcare outcomes. Severe or serious unexpected adverse events that lead to serious negative patient outcomes, potentially involving harm, risk of harm or serious disruption, are considered as 'critical incidents.' A critical incident can be caused by the patient's disease or human error during the administration of anaesthesia or other healthcare interventions, and it threatens the safety and well-being of the patient.[1] All critical incidents are adverse events. A study identified 295 (0.55%) critical incidents from 53,541 cases of paediatric anaesthesia (3,471 cardiothoracic surgeries). Cardiac arrest accounted for 25 (8.5%) cases of the 295 critical events.[2]

Common major adverse events in the perioperative period in children include respiratory adverse events such as laryngospasm, bronchospasm, apnoea, arterial desaturation and delayed detection of oesophageal intubation; cardiovascular events such as cardiac arrest, hypotension, bradycardia and arrhythmias; allergic reactions; medication-related events; nausea; vomiting; agitation and emergence delirium.[3]

## FACTORS THAT INFLUENCE ADVERSE EVENTS IN PAEDIATRIC ANAESTHESIA

Adverse events in paediatric anaesthesia are influenced by multiple factors, including age, gender, type of surgery, emergency or elective nature, and American Society of Anesthesiologists (ASA) physical status. Understanding these factors helps in tailoring anaesthesia management to minimise risks and improve outcomes.[2]

### Age of Child

#### *Neonates (0–28 Days)*

*Common adverse events:* Respiratory distress, bradycardia, hypothermia and hypoglycaemia.

*Challenges:* Immature organ systems, increased sensitivity to anaesthetic agents and difficulty in securing the airway.

Newborn premature babies are a very high-risk group, whose physiology differs from those born full term or older infants. The premature brain has limited autoregulatory function and is more susceptible to hypoperfusion due to immaturity of cerebral blood flow dynamics. Newborns who are exposed to sedative drugs are associated with a higher incidence of apnoea, airway obstruction and haemodynamic complications, which can result in hypoxia, hypercarbia and hypotension.

### *Infants (1 Month to 1 Year)*

*Common adverse events:* Respiratory complications, dehydration and electrolyte imbalances

*Challenges:* Rapid changes in physiology and higher metabolic rates

### *Toddlers and Pre-schoolers (1–5 Years)*

*Common adverse events:* Airway obstruction, emergence delirium and allergic reactions

*Challenges:* Smaller airway diameters and difficulty in communicating symptoms or discomfort

### *School-age Children (6–12 Years)*

*Common adverse events:* Respiratory events, nausea, vomiting and anxiety-related complications

*Challenges:* Varied responses to pre-medication and anaesthesia due to psychological factors

### *Adolescents (13–18 Years)*

*Common adverse events:* Cardiovascular instability, substance abuse-related complications and anxiety

*Challenges:* Variability in physiological responses and potential comorbid conditions

The results of a large prospective multicentre cohort study to determine the incidence and nature of severe critical events in children undergoing anaesthesia showed a large variability across the participating centres in 33 European countries. Respiratory-related severe critical events were the most frequent complications reported in all age groups, whereas cardiovascular incidents were predominantly reported in neonates and infants.[4]

### *Gender of Child*

- *Males:* Generally higher incidence of respiratory complications such as laryngospasm and bronchospasm
- *Females:* Higher incidence of post-operative nausea and vomiting (PONV)

## ASA Physical Status of Child

### *ASA I (Healthy)*

*Common adverse events:* Minor respiratory events and anxiety-related issues

*Challenges:* Typically lower risk, but vigilance is still necessary to prevent unexpected complications

### *ASA II (Mild Systemic Disease)*

*Common adverse events:* Respiratory complications and exacerbation of underlying conditions

*Challenges:* Increased sensitivity to anaesthetics and potential for mild systemic disease to influence anaesthesia management

### *ASA III (Severe Systemic Disease)*

*Common adverse events:* Haemodynamic instability, exacerbation of systemic diseases and respiratory complications

*Challenges:* Need for careful pre-operative assessment and optimisation of medical conditions

### *ASA IV (Severe Systemic Disease that is a Constant Threat to Life)*

*Common adverse events:* Severe cardiovascular and respiratory events, organ failure and perioperative mortality

*Challenges:* High risk of complications requiring meticulous planning and monitoring

### *ASA V (Moribund Patient Not Expected to Survive Without the Operation)*

*Common adverse events:* High perioperative mortality, multi-organ failure and extreme haemodynamic instability

*Challenges:* Often palliative or life-saving surgery with very high risks

## Use of Narcotics

*Common adverse events:*

- *Respiratory depression:* Over-sedation leading to hypoventilation or apnoea
- *Nausea and vomiting:* Increased risk of aspiration and electrolyte imbalance
- *Hypotension:* Especially in combination with other anaesthetics
- *Bradycardia:* Due to vagal stimulation

## Regional Anaesthesia

*Common adverse events:*

- *Local anaesthetic toxicity:* Due to accidental intravascular injection or overdose
- *Nerve injury:* From improper needle placement
- *Haemodynamic instability:* Especially with high spinal or epidural anaesthesia

## Sedation for Non-operating Room Anaesthesia

*Common adverse events:*

- *Airway obstruction:* Due to inadequate airway management
- *Hypoxaemia:* From sedation-induced respiratory depression
- *Aspiration:* Increased risk in non-fasting patients
- *Hypothermia*

## Inhalational Anaesthetics Causing Adverse Events

*Common adverse events:*

- *Cardiovascular instability:* Hypotension or arrhythmias
- *Emergence delirium:* Agitation and confusion during recovery
- *Malignant hyperthermia:* A life-threatening reaction to certain inhalational agents, though rare

A systematic review and meta-analysis revealed that propofol in paediatric anaesthesia significantly mitigated the occurrence of laryngospasm, vomiting and agitation, albeit with an elevated risk of apnoea when compared to sevoflurane anaesthesia. Also, especially in patients receiving laryngeal mask airway, propofol anaesthesia significantly reduced the incidence of laryngospasm and agitation.[5]

## Intraoperative Ventilation Strategies

*Common adverse events:*

- *Barotrauma:* Due to high ventilatory pressures
- *Atelectasis:* From inadequate ventilation
- *Hypercarbia or hypocarbia:* Due to improper ventilator settings

## Deep versus Awake Extubation or Removal of Supraglottic Airway Device

*Common adverse events:*

- *Airway obstruction:* Higher risk during deep extubation
- *Laryngospasm:* Particularly during light anaesthesia or awake extubation
- *Aspiration:* If protective reflexes have not fully recovered

## Pre-operative Location

- *Inadequate pre-operative assessment facilities* for thorough assessment can lead to missed diagnoses such as congenital heart disease or unoptimised medical conditions as in idiopathic hypertrophic pyloric stenosis, etc.
- *Limited access to specialised paediatric care* where paediatric specialists are not available.
- *Lack of child-friendly environments* which are stressful or non-child-friendly environments can increase anxiety and cooperation issues.
- *Insufficient pre-operative testing capabilities* of essential diagnostic tests (e.g. blood tests, imaging studies) can result in incomplete pre-operative evaluations.

*Some of the common pre-operative locations and their contributions to adverse events are as follows:*

- *Non-operating room anaesthesia (NORA) suites:* The location is generally far from the operating room, and the equipment may not be serviced in time. Adequate and expert help is not available when there is an adverse event.
- *Primary care clinics:* There are limited resources for comprehensive pre-operative assessments and a lack of paediatric anaesthesia expertise. Incomplete history taking, missed comorbidities and improper fasting instructions can lead to complications.
- *Outpatient surgery centres* focus on quick turnover, and might lead to rushed or superficial evaluations leading to adverse events.
- *Hospital pre-operative units*, especially those without dedicated paediatric anaesthesiologists and comprehensive pre-operative protocols
- *Emergency departments* with high patient volume and urgency can result in hurried evaluations and prioritisation of acute over chronic conditions. This can result in failure to adequately stabilise chronic conditions before surgery, leading to complications such as respiratory distress or haemodynamic instability.[6]

## Provider Experience and Perioperative Attentiveness

Provider experience and vigilance play a crucial role in paediatric anaesthesia, and inadequate experience or attention can potentially contribute to adverse events in several ways:

- *Dosage calculation errors:* Paediatric patients require precise dosing based on weight and age. Inexperienced providers may miscalculate or misinterpret dosage guidelines, leading to either under- or over-medication.

- *Airway management challenges:* Children have smaller airways and are more prone to airway obstruction or difficulty in intubation. Experienced providers are better equipped to handle these challenges promptly and effectively.
- *Monitoring and response to changes:* Anaesthesia can affect a child's vital signs rapidly. Experienced providers are more adept at monitoring these changes and responding promptly to prevent complications such as hypotension or hypoxia.
- *Decision-making under pressure:* Paediatric cases can be stressful, especially during emergencies. Experienced providers are typically more confident in making critical decisions quickly, such as adjusting anaesthesia levels or transitioning to alternative methods.
- *Communication and team coordination:* Anaesthesia involves coordination with surgical teams and other healthcare professionals. Inexperienced providers may struggle with effective communication or teamwork, which can delay responses to adverse events.
- *Knowledge of paediatric physiology and pharmacology:* Understanding the unique physiology and pharmacology of children is essential. Inexperienced providers may lack the depth of knowledge needed to anticipate and manage physiological responses to anaesthesia.
- *Distractions during critical periods of anaesthesia:* This can be due to social media, overwork and exhaustion leading to mental and physical fatigue of the anaesthesiologist. This can lead to human errors that can compromise patient safety.[3]
- Overall, whilst experience alone does not guarantee safety, it significantly reduces the likelihood of adverse events by enhancing technical skills, decision-making abilities and situational awareness in paediatric anaesthesia.[7]

## Time in the Perioperative Period

Perioperative adverse events can occur before, during and after surgery.[8,9]

### *Pre-operative Period*

Pre-operative anxiety and behavioural stress response are undesirable and can lead to long-term psychologically traumatic consequences. Risk factors associated with this response include young age, especially pre-school, previous surgery, association with a previous unpleasant perioperative encounter, lack of pre-operative visit/orientation, shy and inhibited temperament and anxious parents.[10] Adverse events of drugs given for pre-medication can also occur in this period, e.g. apnoea and respiratory depression. Excessive crying can lead to laryngospasm after induction or extubation.

### *Intraoperative Period*

Respiratory complications include bronchospasm, laryngospasm, airway obstruction caused by anatomical issues, secretions or improper tube positioning, desaturation and aspiration. Cardiovascular complications include bradycardia, tachycardia, hypotension, hypertension and cardiac arrest. Neurological complications may include seizures, which can be triggered by hypoxia, metabolic disturbances or anaesthetic agents. Other adverse events include allergic reactions to anaesthetic agents, local anaesthetic systemic toxicity, malignant hyperthermia, surgical bleeding, medication errors and hypothermia.

### *Post-operative Period*

Respiratory complications such as hypoxia, atelectasis and post-operative apnoea and cardiovascular complications such as hypotension or hypertension and arrhythmias may occur. Other problems include emergence delirium, pain and discomfort, PONV, shivering, delayed recovery, prolonged drowsiness, sleep disturbances and mood swings.

## Surgical Risk Factors

- *Complexity of the surgery:* More complex and longer surgeries such as major cardiac, neurological or thoracic surgeries tend to have higher risks of complications.
- *Type of surgery:* Emergency surgeries have higher risks compared to elective surgeries. Similarly, surgeries involving the airway, chest or abdomen are associated with higher respiratory complications.
  - *Airway/otorhinolaryngological surgery:*
    - *Common adverse events:* Airway obstruction, laryngospasm and bleeding
    - *Challenges:* Proximity to the airway and the potential for swelling or bleeding postoperatively
  - *Cardiac surgery:*
    - *Common adverse events:* Arrhythmias, haemodynamic instability and coagulopathies
    - *Challenges:* Complex and prolonged procedures with significant physiological stress
  - *Abdominal surgery:*
    - *Common adverse events:* Fluid and electrolyte imbalances, pain management issues and respiratory complications
    - *Challenges:* Intraoperative fluid management and post-operative pain control
  - *Orthopaedic surgery:*
    - *Common adverse events*: Blood loss, thromboembolic events and fat embolism

  - *Challenges*: Long surgical times and the need for immobilisation postoperatively

*Emergency versus elective surgery:*

- *Emergency surgery:*
  - *Common adverse events*: Haemodynamic instability, inadequate pre-operative assessment and higher risk of anaesthesia-related complications
  - *Challenges:* Limited time for preparation, existing medical conditions and often more critical physiological states
- *Elective surgery:*
  - *Common adverse events:* PONV, pain management issues and anxiety
  - *Challenges:* Pre-operative fasting, psychological preparation and managing expectations

- *Duration of surgery:* Prolonged surgeries increase the risk of hypothermia, blood loss and prolonged exposure to anaesthesia.
- *Invasiveness of the procedure:* Invasive procedures carry higher risks of bleeding, infection and trauma to surrounding tissues.[11]

## Medical and Anatomical Risk Factors

- *Pre-existing medical conditions:* Children with congenital heart disease, respiratory conditions (e.g. asthma), neurological disorders or metabolic conditions are at a higher risk. Conditions such as obesity or malnutrition can also increase the risk of complications. Perioperative respiratory adverse events are often associated with viral upper respiratory tract infections (URIs), especially with the presence of fever within 48 hours of the anaesthetic. Their incidence is as high as 30% in children with symptomatic URI and 40% in children undergoing tonsillectomy.[12] Nevertheless, an audit in a tertiary care centre revealed that respiratory complications were the most frequent (33%). Infants, especially those with congenital heart disease, were identified as at a higher risk for perioperative cardiac arrest. Twenty-eight percent of the patients who suffered events died within 48 hours.[13]
- *Previous anaesthetic history:* There may be a history of complications in prior anaesthetic exposure, especially in children with a family history of malignant hyperthermia or other genetic conditions associated with muscular weakness.
- *Medication use:* Concurrent medications can interact with anaesthetic agents or impact physiological stability. Polypharmacy, especially in children with chronic conditions, increases the risk of drug interactions.
- *Immunocompromised status:* Children with weakened immune systems (e.g. due to cancer, human immunodeficiency virus or immunosuppressive therapy) are at a higher risk of infections and sepsis.

- *Allergies:* Known allergies to medications, latex or other substances used in the surgical environment can lead to adverse reactions.
- *Nutritional status:* Malnourished or obese children have a higher risk of perioperative complications, including respiratory issues.
- *Airway anatomy:* Airway management will be risky in children with anatomical anomalies (e.g. cleft palate, large tonsils).

## Patient Transport/Transfer

Accidental extubation, arterial desaturation, cardiovascular adverse events such as bradycardia, hypotension due to unintentional cessation of intravenous vasopressor infusion, and cardiac arrest can occur.

## Neurotoxicity of Anaesthetics

Long (>3 hours) duration of administration or repeated doses of anaesthetic drugs and sedatives during surgeries or procedures in children <3 years of age may affect the development of the children's brains. General anaesthetics and sedative drugs such as desflurane, etomidate, halothane, isoflurane, ketamine, lorazepam, methohexital, midazolam, pentobarbital, propofol and sevoflurane can cause neurotoxic effects in children <3 years of age.

These neurotoxic effects by neonatal exposure to anaesthesia may result in long-term detrimental functional outcomes in later childhood or adulthood, such as deficits in memory, learning, attention and motor function.

Studies in animals have shown that exposure to sedative/anaesthesia agents can cause neurotoxicity through neuronal apoptosis, impaired neurogenesis, neuroinflammation, modulation of neuronal plasticity, disruption of glial cytoarchitecture in immature astrocytes and disturbances in the ultrastructural properties of developing synapses. Recently, there has been evolving evidence of the role played by the microglia, which are the resident immune cells in the central nervous system, on brain development and maturation. Using immune molecules such as chemokines and complement molecules, microglia can alter synaptic transmissions and plasticity in the brain under normal physiologic conditions. Two recent studies on the impact of anaesthesia on the developing brain including the (1) General Anaesthesia Compared to Spinal Anaesthesia (GAS) study and (2) the Paediatric Anaesthesia Neurodevelopmental Assessment (PANDA) study have given some reassurance that single, short exposure to anaesthetic agents might not result in persistent cognitive impairment in children; however, multiple exposures were found to be associated with modest decrease in processing speed and fine motor coordination.[14-16]

## ADVERSE EVENTS IN NEONATAL INTENSIVE CARE UNIT PATIENTS

The neonatal intensive care unit (NICU) is a perioperative area with a potential for a high risk of adverse events because its population is at a particularly increased risk owing to a rapidly changing physiology and small margin of error.[3] The most common adverse events known to occur are nosocomial infections, endotracheal tube-related events (e.g. tube malposition, post-extubation stridor, unplanned intubation/accidental extubation), catheter-related complications (e.g. peripheral intravenous infiltration as well as central catheter complications, such as catheter malfunction, clot or breakage requiring change or removal), adverse drug events, hypotension, fluid overload (pulmonary oedema), bleeding, skin problems such as burn/blister, hypoglycaemia, prolonged hyperglycaemia, pruritus, cardiac or respiratory arrest, renal dysfunction, readmission to NICU within 48 hours, pneumothorax, return to surgery, electrolyte abnormalities such as hyperkalaemia requiring treatment, oversedation, decubitus ulcers, rash, reintubation within 24 hours of extubation, tube- and drains-related (i.e. Foley catheter, chest tube, external ventricular drain) complication, seizures (new since admission), arrhythmia requiring treatment, cardiac depression/compromise, allergic reaction, respiratory depression/compromise, central nervous system bleed (not on admit), acid-base imbalance, anaemia unspecified, deep vein thrombosis, dehydration, neurological complication, surgical complications and others.[17]

## MITIGATION STRATEGIES FOR PERIOPERATIVE ADVERSE EVENTS

Perioperative adverse events can have negative impacts such as premature case termination, longer hospitalisation stays and costs and medicolegal litigations in case of serious harm caused by the adverse event. Although most perioperative adverse events can be promptly detected and managed and will not lead to any sequelae, the risk of life-threatening progression remains. The adverse events should be evaluated after identification for severity, preventability, ability to mitigate and ability to identify the event earlier. There are few practical methods available to study and identify adverse events.[17,18] More than one half of all identified adverse events are preventable, with 40% of events falling into the more severe harm categories. Understanding and addressing the risk factors and adopting the following strategies can significantly improve the perioperative outcomes:

- *Pre-operative management:* Detailed evaluation of the child's medical history, physical examination and necessary laboratory tests help in identifying high-risk patients and optimising their medical conditions before surgery.

- Vigilance after administration of the pre-medicants can prevent adverse events. Pre-medicants can reduce anxiety and tachycardia, prevent crying and thereby laryngospasm.
- *Tailored anaesthesia plan:* One should individualise the anaesthesia plan based on the child's specific risk factors and should ensure the availability of appropriate anaesthetic agents and equipment for managing potential complications.
- *Multidisciplinary approach:* Involvement of a team of specialists, including paediatric anaesthesiologists, surgeons and intensivists, for comprehensive care is needed for prevention of complications.
- *Parental involvement:* Engaging parents in the perioperative process and decision making provide comfort and reduce the child's as well as parental anxiety.
- *Monitoring and vigilance:* Continuous monitoring of vital signs and readiness to manage complications during the perioperative period are mandatory, and advanced monitoring techniques should be used when necessary. Pharmacovigilance can help in the prevention of drug-related adverse events.
- *Use of risk prediction systems:* These use patient-specific variables and mathematical models calibrated against large data sets to provide a quantitative assessment of risk. Risk stratification should be routinely documented for high-risk patients. Different scoring systems are available, which can be categorised into surgery and patient-specific risk scoring tools. The *Snoring, Trouble Breathing, Un-Refreshed (STBUR) Screening Questionnaire* can be considered as a routine pre-operative screening tool in children undergoing elective procedures.[19] It is an example of a pre-operative assessment and prediction tool for perioperative respiratory adverse events. It has been validated in identifying children with symptoms of obstructive sleep apnoea who are at risk of perioperative respiratory adverse events. A positive screening on the STBUR questionnaire is associated with an increased risk of perioperative respiratory adverse events in paediatric surgical patients.
    - *Components of the STBUR questionnaire:* Whilst sleeping, does your child SNORE more than half the time? SNORE LOUDLY? Have TROUBLE breathing or struggle to breathe? Stop breathing during the night? Wake up feeling unrefreshed in the morning?
- *Intraoperative strategies:*
    - *Airway:* Desaturation is addressed by increasing oxygen delivery, adjusting ventilator settings and resolving the underlying cause. Repositioning of the airway and confirming proper tube placement can be done if needed. Bronchospasm can be managed by administering bronchodilators and adjusting ventilation settings. Laryngospasm is treated with positive-pressure ventilation, muscle

relaxants and sometimes reintubation. Airway obstruction is treated by treating the underlying cause such as suctioning, repositioning the airway and ensuring proper tube placement. Aspiration is managed through suctioning the airway, administering antibiotics and providing supportive respiratory care. Devices for difficult airway management, including high-flow nasal cannula, supraglottic airway device, videolaryngoscope and ultrasonography, can be employed in routine anaesthesia practise. Use of easily titrable anaesthetic agents, use of advanced monitoring and equipment and familiarity with this equipment can contribute in a large way to provide safe anaesthesia.

- *Cardiovascular adverse events:* Bradycardia can be managed by administering atropine and addressing causes such as hypoxia or vagal stimulation. Tachycardia is treated by controlling pain, administering fluids and identifying the underlying cause. Hypotension is managed through fluid boluses, vasopressors and adjusting the depth of anaesthesia. Hypertension is treated by pain control, adjusting anaesthesia depth and administering antihypertensive medications. In the event of cardiac arrest, immediate cardiopulmonary resuscitation and advanced cardiac life support protocols are initiated.
- Seizures can be managed with anticonvulsants and by addressing the underlying cause. Awareness during anaesthesia is managed by ensuring adequate depth of anaesthesia and addressing any patient distress.
- Allergic reactions to anaesthetic agents are managed by discontinuing the offending agent and administering antihistamines, steroids and epinephrine if necessary. Malignant hyperthermia requires discontinuing triggering agents, administering dantrolene and providing supportive care, including cooling and hydration.
- Surgical bleeding can be managed by ensuring surgical haemostasis, administering blood transfusions and replacing fluid volume.
- *Medication-related complications:* Adverse drug reactions are managed by discontinuing the offending medication and providing supportive care. In cases of medication errors, monitoring for adverse effects and administering antidotes if available are necessary. It has to be kept in mind that the pharmacokinetics of premature babies are different from the full term due to immaturity of the hepatic and renal systems, and hence the dose and dosing frequency have to be adjusted.
- Adoption of correct ventilatory and fluid management strategies, use of point-of-care ultrasonography and opioid-sparing strategies with the use of multimodal analgesia can help reduce intraoperative adverse events.

- *Post-operative care:*
  - Respiratory complications can be managed by supplemental oxygen and addressing the underlying cause, encouraging the child for deep breathing exercises and using incentive spirometry, monitoring and supportive care.
  - Cardiovascular complications such as hypotension or hypertension can be managed by fluid therapy, vasopressors or antihypertensive medications. Arrhythmias require appropriate monitoring, antiarrhythmic drugs and addressing the underlying cause.
  - Pain and discomfort can be treated with multimodal analgesia (non-steroidal anti-inflammatory drugs, regional anaesthesia).
  - PONV needs maintenance of appropriate hydration and age-appropriate antiemetic medications.
  - Emergence delirium presenting as confusion and agitation upon waking from anaesthesia needs reassuring the child, providing a calm environment, and sometimes administering sedatives.
  - Delayed recovery and prolonged drowsiness need monitoring with treatment of underlying cause and delayed return to normal function requires rehabilitation and supportive care.
  - Post-operative behavioural changes such as sleep disturbances or mood swings are managed with supportive care and counselling if needed.
- *Availability of dedicated facilities, including specialised personnel trained in paediatric anaesthesia and access to appropriate equipment and resources:* These can contribute to the reduction in perioperative risk for paediatric patients. However, access to all the resources may be limited in resource-constrained settings.
- *Use of trigger tools to identify adverse events:* Trigger tools are used for accurate identification of adverse events and for measurement of their rate over time. Triggers are clues. A trigger is a data element within a health record that identifies the presence of an adverse event that has occurred or is about to occur.[20] A trigger tool is a targeted review of medical record carried out manually or via computers.[21] Trigger tools have been developed by various hospitals and societies. Triggers are derived from clinical, medication or laboratory tests. Triggers can be global (that can be used in various healthcare settings) or specific (for specific healthcare areas); for example, NICU-focused trigger tools are useful to identify adverse events in the NICU and find their incidence.

The triggers most commonly used in the NICU to identify adverse events are nosocomial infection, antibiotic use, unplanned extubations, hypotension, respiratory arrest, death, catheter infiltration/burn, naloxone (Narcan) administration, anticoagulant administration, rising serum creatinine, necrotising enterocolitis, seizures, use of phenobarbital, electrolyte abnormality, abnormal cranial imaging, hyperglycaemia and return to surgery.[18]

Trigger tools specific for the paediatric perioperative period are yet to be developed.

- *Strategies in the intensive care unit:* Avoiding prolonged sedation for young patients in the paediatric intensive care unit and using ventilator-weaning protocols with daily spontaneous breathing trials, promotion of early mobility or the use of non-invasive ventilation, if possible, may decrease the need for prolonged sedation. The inclusion of neuroprotective agents such as dexmedetomidine in the sedative and analgesic regimens can improve long-term outcomes.
- *Effective communication*, teamwork and coordination between anaesthesiologists, surgeons, radiologists, operation theatre staff, intensive care unit personnel, laboratory personnel and other specialists are important.
- *Simulation* and *drills* can assist in evaluating protocols or processes, critical incidents, etc. without involving patients. They are effective tools that can teach non-technical skills. The simulated setting allows participants to make mistakes safely and to learn from these mistakes whilst avoiding patient harms that might otherwise occur.
- *Minimising human factors that can lead to serious adverse events is very important.* Examples of such human factors include negligence in checking the anaesthesia workstation leading to machine-related issues, breathing circuit disconnection, inadvertent gas flow change, syringe swap; gas supply problem, intravenous apparatus disconnection; laryngoscope malfunction, premature extubation, and not conducting a detailed pre-anaesthesia checkup. A study revealed that human factor-related events accounted for 61.0% of all critical incidents associated with paediatric anaesthesia in a tertiary children's hospital.[2] Such critical incidents can be avoided by following certain protocols strictly; for example, before starting any case, a *checklist* is mandatory to prevent technical and non-technical complications. There is evidence that the use of new equipment which adds safety, following protocols and awareness of the relevance of critical incidents can improve safety. Handing over of critical cases between doctors and nurses also play a vital role in the management of cases in critical units.[3] Maintaining standard of care in assessment, anaesthetising the patient and close monitoring can identify adverse events early so that treatment can be given effectively. The anaesthesiologist should not be sleep deprived or exhausted.
- *Regular audit and analyses of perioperative adverse events in children and neonates:* Reporting, regular audit and analysis of perioperative critical incidents allow the identification of the cause of critical incidents, understanding of the current situation and the development of a

prevention strategy. These can help to understand the weaknesses of the perioperative care system that led to the adverse events. This can further facilitate the establishment of standards of care and implementation of patient safety and quality improvement projects aimed at reducing the risk of severe critical events.[4] This can improve and maintain quality and safety in paediatric perioperative care. However, currently, the reporting standards for adverse events are poor.[22]

- *Development of safety resources through organisations:* These include the paediatric perioperative crisis and airway checklists through the Society for Paediatric Anaesthesia (SPA) and patient safety organisations such as Wake Up Safe (WUS). WUS collects data on perioperative anaesthesia-related adverse events from multiple member institutions.[3]

## CONCLUSION

Adverse events and critical incidents in paediatric anaesthesia represent significant challenges that require immediate attention and expert management to safeguard the health and well-being of young patients. The regular implementation of strategies for reducing errors and adverse events can improve children's safety during the perioperative period. High-quality large-scale studies on the influence of surgical procedure type, anaesthesia management strategies, human errors and patient attributes on perioperative adverse events are needed. Evidence-based prevention strategies for adverse events in the paediatric perioperative period need to be developed.

## REFERENCES

1. Currie M. A prospective survey of anesthetic critical events in a teaching hospital. Anaesth Intensive Care. 1989;17(4):403-11.
2. Cho SA, Lee JH, Ji SH, Jang YE, Kim EH, Kim HS, et al. Critical incidents associated with paediatric anaesthesia: changes over 6 years at a tertiary children's hospital. Anesth Pain Med (Seoul). 2022;17(4):386-96.
3. Lorinc AN, Walters CB, Lovejoy HK, Crockett CJ, Reddy SK. Hot topics in safety for pediatric anesthesia. Children. 2020;7(11):242.
4. Habre W, Disma N, Virag K, Becke K, Hansen TG, Johr M, et al. Incidence of severe critical events in paediatric anaesthesia (APRICOT): a prospective multicentre observational study in 261 hospitals in Europe. Lancet Respir Med. 2017;5(5):412-25.
5. Li Caiping, Zhu Y. Impact of sevoflurane and propofol on perioperative respiratory adverse events in pediatrics: a systematic review and meta-analysis. J Perianesth Nurs. 2025;40:158-68.
6. Herman AD, Jaruzel CB, Lawton S, Tobin CD, Reves JG, Catchpole KR, et al. Morbidity, mortality, and systems safety in non-operating room anaesthesia: a narrative review. Br J Anaesth. 2021;127:729-44.
7. Fehr JA, Boulet JR, Waldrop WB, Snider R, Brockel M, Murray DJ, et al. Simulation-based assessment of paediatric anaesthesia skills. Anesthesiology. 2011;115:1308-15.

8. Regli A, von Ungern-Sternberg BS. Diagnosis and management of respiratory adverse events in the operating room. Curr Anesthesiol Rep. 2015;5:156-67.
9. Sury MR, Palmer JH, Cook TM, Pandit JJ. The state of UK anaesthesia: a survey of National Health Service activity in 2013. Br J Anaesth. 2014;113(4):575-84.
10. Moynihan R. Preoperative behavioral stress response in children: Is there a role (What is the role) for oral pre-medication in outpatient surgery? J Oral Maxillofac Surg. 2007;65(9):29.
11. Tait AR, Malviya S, Voepel-Lewis T, Munro HM, Seiwert M, Pandit UA. Risk factors for perioperative adverse respiratory events in children with upper respiratory tract infections. Anesthesiology. 2001;95:299-306.
12. Saynhalath R, Efune PN, Nakonezny PA, Alex G, Sabers JN, Lee M Clintsman Jr, et al. Association between preoperative respiratory symptoms and perioperative respiratory adverse events in paediatric patients with positive viral testing. J Clin Anesth. 2023;90:111241.
13. Khoso N, Ghaffar WB, Abassi S, Khan FA. Pediatric anesthesia severe adverse events leading to anesthetic morbidity and mortality in a tertiary care center in a low- and middle-income country: a 25-year audit. Anesth Analg. 2021;132:217-22.
14. Pinyavat T, Warner DO, Flick RP, McCann ME, Andropoulos DB, Hu D, et al. Summary of the update session on clinical neurotoxicity studies. J Neurosurg Anesthesiol. 2016; 28:356-60.
15. Donat CK, Scott G, Gentleman SM, Sastre M. Microglial activation in traumatic brain injury. Front Aging Neurosci. 2017;9:208.
16. Davidson AJ, Disma N, de Graaff JC, Withington DE, Dorris L, Bell G, et al. Neurodevelopmental outcome at 2 years of age after general anaesthesia and awake-regional anaesthesia in infancy (GAS): an international multicentre, randomised controlled trial. Lancet. 2016; 387:239-50.
17. Sharek PJ, Horbar JD, Mason W, Bisarya H, Thurm CW, Suresh G, et al. Adverse events in the neonatal intensive care unit: development, testing, and findings of an NICU-focused trigger tool to identify harm in North American NICUs. Pediatrics. 2006;118(4):1332-40.
18. Resar RK, Rozich JD, Classen DC. Methodology and rationale for the measurement of harm with trigger tools. Qual Saf Health Care. 2003;12(Suppl2):ii39-45.
19. Tait AR, Voepel-Lewis T, Christensen R, O'Brien LM. The STBUR questionnaire for predicting perioperative respiratory adverse events in children at risk for sleep- disordered breathing. Paediatric Anesth. 2013;25:510-6.
20. Institute for Healthcare Improvement. (2018). Introduction to trigger tools for identifying adverse events. [online] Available from https://www.ihi.org/resources/tools/introduction-trigger-tools-identifying-adverse-events. [Last accessed June, 2025].
21. Griffin FA, Resar RK. IHI global trigger tool for measuring adverse events. In: IHI Innovation Series white paper, 2nd edition. Cambridge, MA: Institute for Healthcare Improvement; 2009.
22. Dillner P, Eggenschwiler LC, Rutjes AWS, Berg L, Musy SN, Simon M, et al. Incidence and characteristics of adverse events in paediatric inpatient care: a systematic review and meta-analysis. BMJ Qual Saf. 2023;32:133-49.

CHAPTER 20

# Paediatric Anaesthesia in a Resource Challenged Set-up: Providing Top-notch Care with Limited Resources!

*Sukhminder Jit Singh Bajwa, Anita Shirley Joselyn, Shilpa Tiwaskar, Swati Jindal*

## ABSTRACT

Absence of age-appropriate anaesthesia equipment and monitoring devices or trained paediatric anaesthesia personnel to provide perioperative care for children can be considered as a resource-limited setting in the context of paediatric anaesthesia. The precautionary measures which anaesthesiologists should take whilst anaesthetising a child in a resource-limited setting include selecting children with normal airway and no haemodynamic compromise, scheduling paediatric patients first in the morning, meticulous pre-operative assessment, careful operating room preparation and well chalked-out perioperative care. Anaesthesiologists can ensure the safety of a paediatric patient by equipping themselves with their own armamentarium and gadgets required for safe paediatric anaesthesia, by upgrading their knowledge regularly by attending academic events and by training other healthcare workers available in the theatre to help with anaesthesia care. These measures can make the resource-limited surroundings at par with multispeciality hospitals whilst ensuring the provision of high-quality, safe perioperative care in children.

***Keywords:*** Paediatric, Paediatric anaesthesia, Resource-challenged.

## INTRODUCTION

Paediatric anaesthesia has undergone a dramatic evolution over the last three decades. Development of newer monitoring gadgets, newer drugs and various innovative techniques has made the life of a paediatric anaesthesiologist comfortable to a large extent. However, in a developing nation like ours, majority of paediatric surgical cases are handled in peripheral and remote set-ups with limited resources. Moreover, availability of modern infrastructure, equipment, gadgets, drugs and other resources is confined primarily to a few larger institutes and hospitals. Hence, the morbidity and mortality in the perioperative period for paediatric patients continue to be high in developing countries.[1,2]

The growth and development of healthcare facilities in a developing country is largely dependent on the availability of trained personnel, funding and resources in terms of equipment and manpower across different parts of the country. In addition to the above, prevalence of local practises and myths can also impede the growth and development of healthcare facilities. India is unique as it faces challenges of great disparity in health care between a rural and urban set-up just similar to the existing gaps and variations in our cultural and geographical diversities. The healthcare set-ups range from being at par or better than those in a developed country to places with a scarcity of basic healthcare resources and infrastructure.

The paediatric population constitutes approximately 40% of the total population of India. The field of paediatric and neonatal surgery has advanced significantly in the recent years. This has been matched by a colossal growth in research and development in the branch of paediatric and neonatal intensive care. The provision of good-quality, safe anaesthesia with limited personnel and resources for these little patients is a huge challenge as they require a very specialised and focused approach. This chapter elaborates on different methodologies which can be adopted to provide quality perioperative care for paediatric patients in a resource-limited setting.

## DEFINING A RESOURCE-LIMITED SETTING: A SUBJECTIVE AND OBJECTIVE CONUNDRUM!

A simple definition of a 'resource-limited setting' is a healthcare set-up with scarce resources. The care provided in such a setting will include only basic or primary care with referral to higher centres for definitive care. Resource in a healthcare setting refers to the supply of medication and equipment, availability of qualified healthcare personnel and the ability of patients to pay the cost of treatment.

When defining a resource-limited setting in the context of paediatric anaesthesia, absence of age-appropriate equipment (such as airway gadgets, monitoring equipment), absence of appropriate infrastructure such as dedicated operation theatres for paediatric population, high-dependency units or intensive care units (ICUs) for recovery and absence of trained paediatric anaesthesia personnel to provide perioperative care for children can be considered as important aspects.[3] Examples of resource-limited settings for paediatric anaesthesia include rural primary- and secondary-level hospitals, mission hospitals, private nursing homes and municipal/government hospitals. Bigger hospitals wherein less importance is given to age-specific surgical population can also be included.

## ESTABLISHING PRE-ANAESTHETIC EVALUATION AND PATIENT PREPARATION PRACTICES

Increased survival rates in children, even with complex medical and surgical diseases, necessitate a comprehensive pre-operative assessment to ensure optimal outcome of these potentially vulnerable patients. Children can present with multiple pathophysiological conditions, including anaemia and malnutrition. A delayed presentation for surgery means that the child has been coping up with the condition for a long time. Invariably, such patients have a decreased immunity and are more prone to respiratory tract infections. In such scenarios, the decision to postpone or proceed with surgery depends on the expertise of the concerned anaesthesiologist and the resources available to provide post-operative respiratory support. In the absence of expertise and post-operative ICU facilities, there should be a lower threshold for cancellation of a child who has an upper respiratory tract infection after consultation with the surgeon and also after informing the parents about the involved risks. Children requiring cardiac and neurosurgeries, complex orthopaedic surgeries, pre-term neonates or syndromic children with difficult airways or those presenting for procedures which require post-operative ICU care should be referred to adequately resourced centres.

Ideally, pre-anaesthetic evaluation should be done at least 1 day prior, mostly 1–2 weeks earlier for elective surgeries and on the day of surgery for emergency procedures. The aim is to thoroughly analyse, optimise and decide if limited resources are sufficient for surgery and anaesthesia to proceed safely. The risk stratification is done as per existing norms and should be documented in the pre-anaesthesia assessment form. Psychological reassurance to both, the child and parents should be provided at the time of the pre-operative visit.

Pre-operative investigations should include basic blood tests such as complete blood count and urine routine/microscopy. Other investigations should be done based on the child's comorbidities and complexity of the planned procedure/surgery. Children with anaemia are usually optimised by blood transfusion. Pre-medication can be administered if required based on the available trained staff and monitoring facility in the pre-operative wards.

Long hours of fasting are generally avoided. A child should be scheduled as the first case in the morning. Clear liquids (water/water with sugar/pulp-free juice) are allowed for up to 2 hours as per the latest guidelines. Feeding breast milk to the infant is allowed for up to 2 hours before anaesthesia induction. The child is fasted for up to 4–6 hours before anaesthesia in case of history of intake of light meals or solid food.

## ANAESTHESIA PLANNING AND PREPARATION FOR THE SURGICAL INTERVENTION

- Operation theatre preparation in a limited-resource setting is crucial to improve patient safety and prevent untoward perioperative events.[4] Based on the surgery planned, a checklist of necessary drugs, equipment and other supplies should be given to trained theatre staff the previous day. Apart from the material resources, the requirement and availability of trained personnel cannot be ignored. In case there is a need for a second anaesthesiologist, they should be called and checked for availability 1 day prior, and the hospital should be informed of any renumeration to be paid.

- *Anaesthesia machine:* Boyle's anaesthesia machine used for adults will be used invariably for paediatric cases in small and peripheral hospitals where paediatric cases are not regularly done. Even though the manufacturing of halothane has been stopped, a few nursing homes still have halothane vaporiser (bottle) on the Boyle's machine, and most have added sevoflurane vaporiser to the back bar **(Figs. 1 and 2)**. Whilst checking the anaesthesia machine, attention should be paid to the active status and availability of soda-lime stock for replacement.
- *Oxygen supplies—the lifeline of operation theatres:* Most of these centres have only oxygen cylinders and no piped supply of medical gases. It is important to check if there is an adequate supply of oxygen cylinders to cover the perioperative period. It will be helpful to calculate the oxygen requirement based on the minute ventilation of the patient and hours of anticipated use. The oxygen key should be handy, and the second oxygen cylinder mounted on the stand with flowmeter and the oxygen tubing should be ready.

  It is recommended to check the reading in the pressure gauge on opening the oxygen cylinder with the key. Oxygen E-type cylinder, which is mostly attached to the Boyle's machine when full, has a capacity of 680 L.

  All oxygen cylinders when full will have oxygen stored at a pressure of 2,200 pounds per square inch (psi) and a force of 150 kg/cm$^2$. So, if the cylinder reading is 1,200 psi, it has 1,200 × 680 L divided by 2,200 = 370 L.

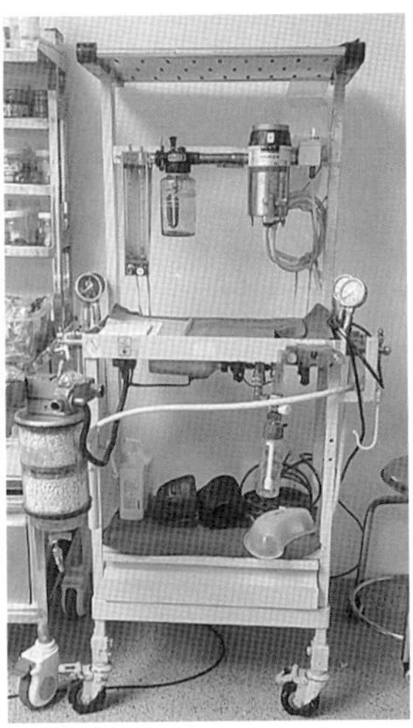

**Fig. 1:** Boyle's machine with sevoflurane vaporiser. *(For color version, see Plate 17)*

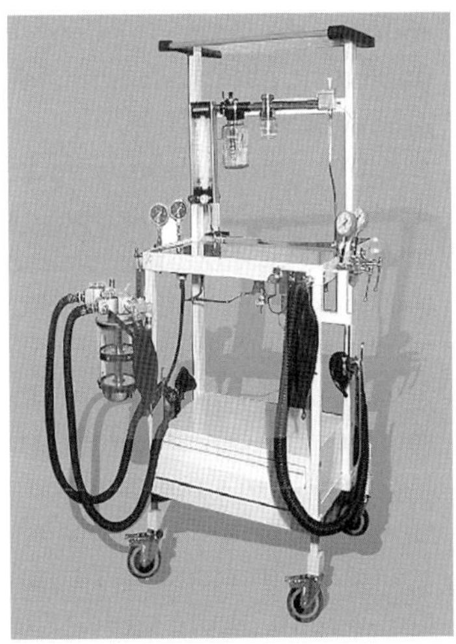

**Fig. 2:** Boyle's machine with halothane vaporiser. *(For color version, see Plate 17)*

Apart from that, one should also ensure that smaller oxygen cylinders are also available with Mox regulator assembly in case the need for transportation of the patient to a higher specialised centre arises.

- *Simple mathematical vigilance and essential checks:* One should always remember that the fresh gas flow required to prevent rebreathing in Jackson–Rees (JR) circuit is usually two to three times the minute ventilation (MV) in patients with spontaneous breathing and equal to the MV in patients with controlled breathing. For example, in a 15 kg patient who is on controlled ventilation, the tidal volume is approximately 120 ml (8 ml/kg) and MV is 120 × 16 = 1,920 ml = approximately 2 l.
  - So, if the flow is 2 l/min, 370 L will last for how long? 2 l/min = 120 l/h; that means approximately 3 hours. This can last for an extra 3 hours if 50% nitrous oxide is used.
  - If the reading is in kg/cm$^2$, then 2,200 psi = 150 kg/cm$^2$. If the reading shows 100 kg/cm$^2$, then 100 × 14.23 = 1,423 psi.
  - If 2,200 psi is 680 ml, then 1,423 psi = 439.8 ml.
  - At 2 l/min, 120 l/h; so it will go on for 3.66 hours.

These simple calculations as mentioned above can be helpful in ensuring patient safety and in providing the comfort zone to the attending anaesthesiologist.

- *Airway equipment*: Endotracheal tubes (ETTs) that can be used for different paediatric age groups start from size 2.5 mm for uncuffed tubes and 3.0 mm for cuffed tubes. The anaesthesiologist can calculate the required size of the tube based on the age of the child and should ideally keep ready one size smaller and one size bigger than expected, especially whilst using an uncuffed ETT. Sometimes, the hospital will request the anaesthesiologist to get the tracheal tubes required for paediatric patients. Supraglottic airway devices can serve as both airway management devices and rescue devices in difficult airway scenarios. A roller gauze should be kept ready for throat packing if required. A paediatric Ambu bag, paediatric laryngoscope with a working bulb and new battery should be available. A small towel can be folded, kept below the neck of the child as a shoulder roll and fixed with micropore during airway management.
- *Monitoring*: The anaesthesiologist should be aware of the make of the monitor and the monitoring modalities available.[4] They should check the availability of smaller blood pressure cuffs, pulse oximeter probes and small electrocardiography leads.
- *Suction catheters*: 6–10 numbers, as needed, appropriate for age and weight of the child. The working suction bottle, with tubing and connector, should be checked. The availability of nasogastric tubes of sizes 8–12 Fr should be checked.

- *Positioning*: Additional small operation theatre towels should be available to cover the baby. A small green plastic drape if available can be used to cover the baby below sterile sheets, to prevent heat loss. A paediatric head ring or doughnut can be prepared by winding bandage to an adult doughnut.
- *Intravenous (IV) access and fluid therapy*: Adequate numbers of paediatric IV cannulas (20, 22, 24 and 26G), three-way connectors, IV securing tapes, burette sets and regular IV sets should be available. A cardboard sheet (from any packing) in the shape of a small rectangle, wound with white bandage can be used as a splint for IV line. An electric kettle or small water steriliser (used for instrument sterilisation) can be kept ready for warming fluids. The nearest blood bank should be notified, and packed red cells should be kept ready if blood loss is expected. It will be ideal to have blood available in smaller units (e.g. 50 or 100 ml bags for children weighing <10 kg) along with a blood transfusion set. The cross-match for blood transfusion should always be sent, and the blood sample can be taken during securing of the IV line.
- *Drugs*: All anaesthetic and emergency medications diluted as per the weight of the child should be available. Paediatric suppositories of diclofenac and paracetamol should be kept ready, as per availability.
- It is important to check the *operation table functioning*, and whether the table has the capacity to provide a head-low or head-up position.
- *Regional blocks*: Local anaesthesia vials, 2% lidocaine with adrenaline and 0.5% bupivacaine, 22G hypodermic needle, 1 inch and 1.5 inches, to give caudal anaesthesia or regional blocks should be available.
- The *pre-operative waiting area* can be made child-friendly with toys and colourful pictures of pet animals and cartoon characters in order to decrease the pre-operative anxiety of the child and family. A white/blue glove can be filled with air, and faces can be drawn over it with a marker pen. Nursery rhymes and cartoons can be played on phone.

In addition to the above theatre preparation, the anaesthesiologist can also carry some of the following basic equipment whilst working in a resource-limited setting:

- *Capnometer* to confirm proper placement of the ETT and proper placement of supraglottic airway device whenever and wherever feasible.
- *Paediatric Ambu bag*, a small blood pressure cuff and portable pulse oximeter. It will be extremely helpful in all situations if the hospital does not have these gadgets.
- Various sizes of *paediatric face mask*, oral or nasal airways.
- Straight blade and curved blade *laryngoscope*, extra bulbs and batteries of laryngoscope, bougie and paediatric Magill's forceps.
- JR circuit, additional ventilating bag for JR circuit, connectors and additional plastic connectors for attaching JR circuit to Boyle's machine

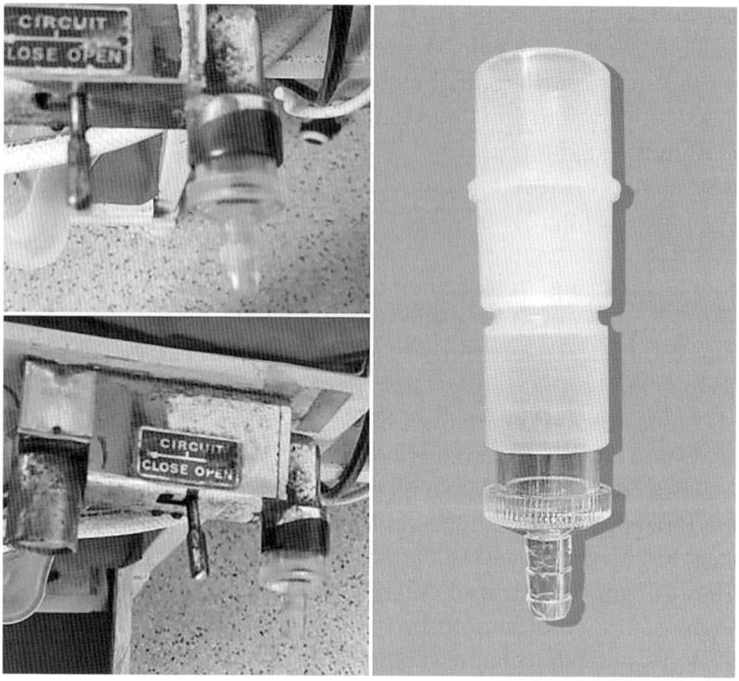


**Fig. 3:** Connectors. *(For color version, see Plate 18)*

[some connectors would go inside the common gas outlet, whilst other white connectors would go over it **(Fig. 3)**, universal connector no. 5 and 5.5]. Universal connectors have multipurpose use and can get attached to the nasal airway, common gas outlet, 16G IV cannula and 3 cc syringe assembly for needle cricothyrotomy or tracheotomy in a 'cannot intubate, cannot ventilate' situation.

- Supraglottic airway device as an airway rescue device whenever and wherever feasible.
- Peripheral nerve stimulator (PNS) for block along with Stimuplex needle.
- An emergency small bag or kit which should contain all the essential drugs such as atropine, phenylephrine, adrenaline and many more should always be carried by the practitioners.

## INTRAOPERATIVE MANAGEMENT

### Airway

Assessment of the airway is crucial in a child, and a clear airway management plan has to be made before inducing the child. In an anticipated difficult airway scenario, the anaesthesiologist should have a plan A and plan B which should also be communicated to the team. Each member of the team (anaesthesia technician, nurse and surgeon) should be allocated clear roles and responsibilities. In situations of limited manpower, nurses, technicians or surgeons can be taught basic skills such as bag and mask ventilation, securing IV access and monitoring to help the anaesthesiologists. Difficult airway algorithm for paediatric patients should be printed and kept handy for reference in the theatre. It is always better to paste it on the side walls. The airway should be secured for prolonged surgeries, prone positioning and surgeries where position change is required intraoperatively, in full stomach conditions and in smaller babies. A good depth of anaesthesia before airway manipulation should be ensured and extubation should be done preferably when the child awakens and is able to protect his/her airway.

## Monitoring

Most of the smaller hospitals have a monitor capable of monitoring vitals as per American Society of Anesthesiologists (ASA) minimum monitoring standards, except for the end-tidal carbon dioxide monitoring. In addition to ASA standard monitoring devices, a pre-cordial stethoscope should be used if available. Blood sugars and temperature should be measured during induction and repeated as required.

## Intraoperative Fluid Management

The appropriate size and number of IV cannula should be established before the child is handed over to the surgical team. Handheld vein finders can help in securing an IV line in children who have difficulty with IV access.

Hypotonic solutions such as 5% dextrose should be avoided, and only isotonic crystalloid solutions such as normal saline or Ringer's lactate should be used intraoperatively. A 1 or 2.5% glucose can be administered if there is documented hypoglycaemia intraoperatively. The administration of fluids can be through a micro drip (burette) or regular IV (macro drip) set (*60 micro drops = 1 ml and 16 macro drops = 1 ml*). The above calculation can be used in the absence of infusion pumps.

The requirement of maintenance intraoperative fluid should be calculated according to the Holliday-Segar formula **(Table 1)**. If fasting orders are followed appropriately, there is no requirement of replacing fasting deficit. Fluid boluses of 5–10 ml/kg are used for hypotension, and subsequent boluses can be administered based on the child's haemodynamic response.

**TABLE 1:** Calculation of maintenance intraoperative fluid.

| *Weight (in kg)* | *Maintenance fluid/hour* |
|---|---|
| 3–10 | 4 ml/kg/h |
| 10–20 | 40 + 2 × (weight – 10) ml/h |
| 20–60 | 60 + 1 × (weight – 20) ml/h |
| >60 | 100 ml/h |

## Temperature Management

A multiparameter monitor with temperature probe for continuous temperature monitoring is not always available in resource-limited settings. Hence, rectal and oral thermometers can be used to measure pre-operative and post-operative temperature wherever necessary. Heating mattresses or forced air warmers are expensive and not easily available. To maintain normothermia, the theatre ambient temperature can be maintained higher prior to induction (22–23°C). One can cover the child's head and peripheries with Gamgee roll or with warmed simple operation theatre towels. The baby can be covered with a small plastic drape to prevent heat loss. Hot water can be poured in a glove and the glove can be placed over the baby's body over a towel. Hot water bags or hot IV fluid bags should not be placed directly on the child as these can cause thermal burns. Post-extubation, smaller babies should be handed over to the mother for making skin contact which can help to warm the baby. These precautions can help in reducing morbidity during prolonged surgeries or where blood loss is extensive.

## Pain Management

Pain relief is an absolute necessity as the myth of lesser pain in children has been refuted, and it has been clearly established that children also feel almost the same level of pain as adults. Multimodal analgesia with local anaesthetics, IV analgesics and rectal suppositories can provide adequate perioperative analgesia.

Monitoring for post-operative pain is a very important step in pain management. Use of age-appropriate pain scales [Face, Legs, Activity, Cry, and Consolability (FLACC) Scale, Wong–Baker Faces Scale, Numerical Rating Scale and Visual Analogue Scale] can be used. These scales are easily available and can be printed and kept in the post-anaesthesia care unit (PACU).

Non-pharmacological pain management techniques such as therapeutic massage, breastfeeding, sucrose and distraction with toys or books can be employed to reduce the need for systemic analgesics.

Non-opioid, systemic analgesics should be the mainstay of pain management for mild-to-moderate surgeries. Paracetamol should be liberally used in children in the perioperative period. The dosing and frequency should be as per recommendation, and the first dose should be administered pre-emptively before surgical incision. Oral and rectal administration have unpredictable onset of action, and the IV route of administration should be used **(Table 2)**.

Inflammation plays a significant role in the development of post-operative pain. Non-steroidal anti-inflammatory agents such as diclofenac (IV, suppositories) and ibuprofen (oral) can be used in the perioperative period to reduce the need for opioids. Anti-inflammatory effects of

**TABLE 2:** Dosage of paracetamol.

| *Age of child* | *Route* | *Dose (mg/kg)* | *Frequency* | *Maximum dose per day (mg/kg/day)* |
|---|---|---|---|---|
| Pre-term neonate | IV | 7.5 | Q8H | 40 |
| Term neonate and infant | IV | 10 | Q6H | 60 |
| >1 year of age | IV | 15 | Q6H | 75–100 |

(IV: intravenous; Q8H: every 8 hours; Q6H: every 6 hours)

corticosteroids involve inhibition of the formation and release of pro-inflammatory cytokines. Corticosteroids stabilise the cell membranes of neurons in the peripheral tissues and exert an antinociceptive effect at the spinal level. Dexamethasone (IV 0.1–0.5 mg/kg) is an adjuvant most frequently used to treat pain in children. It decreases the intensity of pain and opioid requirements in the post-operative period and prevents post-operative nausea and vomiting. Moreover, it is easily available in most of the peripheral set-ups.

Though opioids remain the mainstay of analgesics for intraoperative pain relief in children, the licensing and availability of fentanyl and morphine are a challenge in resource-limited settings. So, based on the availability, tramadol and agonists–antagonists such as pentazocine and nalbuphine can be used. The European Society for Paediatric Anaesthesiology (ESPA) has advocated to avoid ondansetron for nausea and vomiting due to tramadol. The ESPA has also suggested to avoid metoclopramide with tramadol for the risk of seizures.

IV Lidocaine can be used perioperatively in children. It lowers pain intensity in the early post-operative period, reduces the incidence of nausea and vomiting, accelerates the restoration of gastrointestinal function, induces preventive analgesia and has anti-inflammatory and immunomodulatory effects. Its use in the perioperative period as a component of multimodal analgesia enables the reduction of opioid doses. Care should be taken in liver and kidney dysfunction. Dose is 0.5 mg/kg loading (pre-emptive) followed by 1.5 mg/kg/h.

Presently, *alpha-2 adrenergic drugs* are widely used in the perioperative multimodal management of pain in children. They act by stimulating alpha-2 receptors in the posterior horn of the spinal cord and supraspinally at the locus coeruleus. They inhibit glutamate and substance P release. They lower the intensity of pain in the post-operative period, allow opioid doses to be decreased and reduce the incidence of nausea. IV dexmedetomidine, administered at a dose of 0.3–1 μg/kg bolus and 0.3–0.7 μg/kg/h, is preferred over clonidine due to less side effects such as hypotension, bradycardia and excessive sedation.

**TABLE 3:** Drug dosages for various types of regional anaesthesia.

| *Block* | *Dose* |
|---|---|
| Caudal (caudal epidural) | • 0.5 ml/kg to achieve a sacral surgical level<br>• 1.0 ml/kg to achieve a high lumbar surgical level<br>• Maximum dose 1 ml/kg = 2.5 mg/kg<br>• 1.25 ml/kg can be given to achieve a low thoracic surgical level<br>• If child is <20 kg, 0.175–0.125% is preferred |
| Peripheral nerve block such as femoral and supraclavicular | • 0.2–0.5 ml/kg<br>• Maximum dose 1 ml/kg = 2.5 mg/kg |
| Peripheral nerve block such as axillary block | 0.1–0.2 ml/kg |
| Wound (local) infiltration and field block | Maximum dose 1 ml/kg = 2.5 mg/kg |
| Transversus abdominis plane block | 0.2–0.3 ml/kg per side, per block |
| Rectus sheath block | 0.1–0.2 ml/kg per side, per block |
| • Ilioinguinal and iliohypogastric block<br>• Penile block | 0.3–0.5 ml/kg = 0.75–1.25 mg/kg |

*Regional blocks* should be employed whenever applicable to reduce the need for systemic medication and to enhance the quality of perioperative analgesia. One important thing related to regional block is that it should be exercised by the most experienced person who has the requisite knowledge and skills.

Before the start of surgery, landmark-guided blocks can be administered. The anaesthesiologist can use a PNS if available. Commonly employed regional techniques include caudal/ilioinguinal/iliohypogastric/transversus abdominis plane/rectus sheath/femoral/supraclavicular/axillary blocks, local infiltration or field block at the incision site. All precautions for regional techniques such as consent, site and side confirmation, sterile precautions, toxic dose calculation, monitoring of vitals during injection, repeated aspiration to rule out intravascular placement and incremental and slow injection should be followed **(Table 3)**.

## POST-OPERATIVE RECOVERY

A designated PACU with trained staff and monitors should ideally be available for post-operative recovery of the children; however, it might not be available in all healthcare centres. The anaesthesiologist should ensure that a designated area with a monitor is available close to the theatre. Emergency medication, crash cart and defibrillator if available should be checked every day in the PACU. The child should be awake with protective reflexes, haemodynamically stable and normothermic before reaching the PACU. A nurse should be present in the PACU to receive the handover and monitor the child. Placards with common post-operative complications such as laryngospasm or airway obstruction and medication doses, resuscitation algorithm, normal age-appropriate limits of vitals in children and recovery/discharge criteria should be available in the PACU for easy reference.

## 'TRAINING' AS THE WAY FORWARD TO MAINTAIN SAFE PAEDIATRIC ANAESTHESIA IN A LIMITED RESOURCE SET-UP

Trained paediatric anaesthesiologists will not always be available in a peripheral hospital or rural centres. Invariably, a general anaesthesiologist will be required to provide paediatric perioperative care. In this scenario, a practitioner in a resource-limited setting can keep themselves updated with the latest developments in paediatric anaesthesia, by attending online free webinars, locally held continuous medical education (CME) programmes including the academic programmes sponsored and managed by the Indian Society of Anaesthesiologists (ISA) National, debates, forums and discussions. There is a dedicated separate session on paediatric anaesthesia in the National Conference of the ISA (ISACON), held annually. Some keen practitioners use records from surgeries and publish case reports, case series and their own innovations and research if and when time permits. Anaesthesiologists should also train themselves in neonatal and paediatric resuscitation courses regularly. There are training programmes run by international charity foundations or non-government organisations which collaborate with tertiary care centres in India to train occasional paediatric anaesthesiologists regarding safe children's surgery.[5-8]

Paediatric anaesthesia as a speciality was first started at the Christian Medical College in Vellore, Tamil Nadu, India. After this, many new centres started paediatric anaesthesia fellowship programmes, including the one sponsored by the Indian Association of Paediatric Anaesthesiologists (IAPA). Short-term fellowship programmes offered by paediatric speciality centres and tertiary hospitals are a sustainable way to train anaesthesiologists to provide safe and high-quality perioperative care in a peripheral set-up. There are various fellowships as well as higher speciality training programmes [e.g. for the degree of Doctorate of Medicine (DM) in Paediatric Anaesthesia] that are being conducted all across India. College of ISA (CISA) is coming up with various innovative programmes, including paediatric anaesthesia training through simulation across the nation. Nonetheless, simulation is a great way of learning, and practitioners should attend the simulation courses that are being offered in order to update their skills and knowledge.

## FUTURE OF PAEDIATRIC ANAESTHESIA IN A RESOURCE-LIMITED SETTING

With the availability of many trained paediatric surgeons in areas of limited resources, anaesthesiologists are expected to provide safe paediatric anaesthesia. Apart from training, having a good clinical acumen, doing meticulous assessment and preparation, providing goal-oriented intraoperative care, following safety checklists and being well versed in crisis management and resuscitation protocols can help to provide top-quality care with minimal resources.

Anaesthesiologists should be more trained in regional anaesthesia skills to provide good regional analgesia as part of multimodal analgesia since the availability of narcotic analgesics might be limited. Use of ultrasound, especially point-of-care ultrasonography skill, can help in the quick identification of a crisis situation and its management. Enhanced recovery after surgery protocols should be followed for all surgeries in the perioperative period with more emphasis on minimising pre-operative fasting, early post-operative feeds, goal-directed fluid therapy and multimodal analgesia. Nonetheless, the major challenges for the development of healthcare facilities in remote locations include the availability of financial support and the ability to retain trained personnel.

## CONCLUSION

Today's anaesthesiologists have to make themselves more efficient in providing perioperative anaesthesia care for children, by increasing their own armamentarium and gadgets and also training the staff available in the theatre. The precautionary measures which the anaesthesiologists should take whilst anaesthetising a child in a resource-limited setting include selecting ASA grade I and II patients with a normal airway and no haemodynamic compromise, keeping the child as the first case in the morning, meticulous pre-operative assessment and careful operating room preparation. In addition to the above, upgrading their knowledge by attending conferences and workshops and creating awareness about anaesthesia and its risk and necessities amongst surgical colleagues and hospital owners is important. Anaesthesiologists by their own efforts can make the resource-limited surroundings at par with any multispeciality hospital whilst ensuring the provision of high-quality, safe perioperative care for children.

## REFERENCES

1. Barbour R, Deka P. Paediatric anaesthesia for low-resource settings. BJA Educ. 2017;17:351-56.
2. Zoumenou E, Gbenou S, Assouto P, Ouro Bang'na Maman AF, Lokossou T, Hounnou G, et al. Pediatric anesthesia in developing countries: experience in

the two main university hospitals of Benin in West Africa. Paediatr Anaesth. 2010;20(8):741-7.
3. Ndikontar Kwinji R, Evans F, Gray RM. Challenges with pediatric anesthesia and intraoperative ventilation of the child in the resource-constrained setting. Paediatr Anaesth. 2022;32(2):372-79.
4. Tegegne BA, Lema GF, Fentie DY, Bizuneh YB. The preparedness of preoperative anesthesia equipment's and monitors for pediatric patients. Ann Med Surg (Lond). 2023;85(7):3423-27.
5. Powell WF Jr, Echeto-Cerrato MA, Gathuya Z, Gray RM, Hodges S, Nabukenya MT, et al. Delivery of safe pediatric anesthesia care in the first 8000 days: realities, challenges, and solutions in low- and middle-income countries. World J Surg. 2023;47(12):3429-35.
6. Sen I, Dave N, Bhardwaj N, Juwarkar C, Beegum S. Specialised training in paediatric anaesthesia: Need of the hour. Indian J Anaesth. 2021;65(1):17-22.
7. Pulvirenti R, Gortan M, Cumba D, Gamba P, Tognon C. Pediatric surgery and anesthesia in low-middle income countries: current situation and ethical challenges. Front Pediatr. 2022;10:908699.
8. De Graaff JC, Johansen MF, Hensgens M, Engelhardt T. Best practice & research clinical anesthesiology: safety and quality in perioperative anesthesia care. Update on safety in pediatric anesthesia. Best Pract Res Clin Anaesthesiol. 2021;35:27-39.

CHAPTER 21

# Changes and Advancements in the Paediatric Anaesthesia Curriculum: Stay Informed on the Latest Developments and Provide the Best Education

*Madhuri Kurdi, Poonam Motiani, Aruna Parameswari, Milon V Mitragotri, Deepshikha R*

## ABSTRACT

The post-graduate anaesthesia education in our nation underwent a major revamp in 2019 with the introduction of the competency-based medical education curriculum. Paediatric anaesthesia is considered a superspeciality, and the learning objectives have been clearly mentioned in the curriculum. The primary goal is to ensure quality and safety in paediatric anaesthesia. Many anaesthesia post-graduates are now opting for the superspeciality fellowship course in paediatric anaesthesia. The syllabus of this fellowship course is well defined. Considering that there are anatomical and physiological differences, especially in young infants, paediatric anaesthesia has evolved in terms of drugs, equipment, devices, anaesthesia techniques and the clinical application of regional anaesthesia. There is an increase in the number of non-operating room surgical procedures, complex surgeries such as foetal ex-utero intrapartum treatment procedure and minimally invasive paediatric robotic surgeries. Childhood obesity and children with comorbidities are currently on the rise. This has led to the need for parallel changes and advancements in the paediatric anaesthesia teaching curriculum. This chapter provides an overview of the current paediatric anaesthesia curriculum framework in our nation, the contemporary challenges, innovations and future directions in the paediatric anaesthesia curriculum.

***Keywords:*** Anaesthesia, Competency, Curriculum, Education, Learning, Postgraduate, Teaching.

## INTRODUCTION

Anaesthetising a paediatric patient has always been challenging from time immemorial, mainly because of the unique anatomy and physiology of the 'small' patient demanding the 'big' expertise of the anaesthesiologist. Nevertheless, with the increasing complexities of surgeries in the neonates and paediatric patients, the need for quality and safe conduct of anaesthesia and rapid yet smooth recovery with a pleasant post-operative course have been realised. This has led to refinements and marked changes in the art and science of paediatric anaesthesia, from the traditional Miller blade, Rendell-Baker-Soucek face mask, Jackson-Rees circuit, inhalational induction, blind/palpatory method to make veins prominent for cannulation to the low-flow technique, video laryngoscopes, microcuffed endotracheal tubes, supraglottic devices, dual-control modes of ventilation, heat and moisture exchange filters, total intravenous anaesthesia and ultrasound-guided peripheral intravenous and central venous cannulation. Regional anaesthesia is becoming popular even in centres that practised general anaesthesia in neonates and children as a routine.[1] All this has led to the need to redefine current paediatric anaesthesia curriculum and training modules of post-graduate students in paediatric anaesthesia.

## CURRENT TRENDS IN PAEDIATRIC ANAESTHESIA EDUCATION

Nowadays, medical education is undergoing a paradigm shift from time-based training towards competency-based training by supplementing the conventional knowledge-based curriculum.[2]

The competency-based medical education (CBME) curriculum for post-graduates in anaesthesiology was launched in the year 2019 by the National Medical Commission of India. Its main focus is on specific learning objectives, including theoretical knowledge, technical skills and attitude development provided by well-trained educators. This is a well-planned and supervised course of 3-year duration for the delivery of safe and effective anaesthesia.[3] Paediatric anaesthesia has been considered a superspeciality in this curriculum. In the West, there is a 1-year specialisation course for paediatric anaesthesia after post-graduation in general anaesthesia. In India, a 3-year Doctorate of Medicine (DM) degree as well as 1-/2-year fellowship courses in paediatric anaesthesia are offered by accredited government and private hospitals **(Table 1)**. Post-graduate students of anaesthesiology willing to do superspecialisation in paediatric anaesthesia can opt for any of these courses. The details of the various courses are available from individual websites of the National Board of Examinations in Medical Sciences, the institutes, and the Indian Association of Paediatric Anaesthesiologists (IAPA) website (for fellowship accredited by IAPA).[4]

### Current Paediatric Anaesthesia Curriculum Framework: Components, Goals, Syllabus, Teaching and Evaluation

The goal of the ongoing paediatric anaesthesia training programmes in India is to train anaesthesiologists to ensure the safe delivery of anaesthesia to this vulnerable group of patients.

The current post-graduate [Doctor of Medicine (MD) and Diplomate of National Board (DNB)] syllabus in anaesthesiology has specific learning objectives related to paediatric anaesthesia. This includes the ability of the student to practically apply the knowledge of the anatomical changes, physiology and pharmacology in the paediatric patients and neonates. The student has to be well versed with the pre-operative fasting guidelines, anaesthetic equipment, blood volume estimation and fluid

**TABLE 1:** Superspecialisation courses in paediatric anaesthesia (1-, 2- and 3-year courses).

| *Name of course* | *Institution/university* | *Location* |
|---|---|---|
| Accredited by National Board of Examinations in Medical Sciences (NBEMS) (duration 2 years) | Rainbow Children's Hospital | Bengaluru, Karnataka |
| | Apollo Hospital | Chennai, Tamil Nadu |
| | Chacha Nehru Bal Chikitsalaya (CNBC) | Delhi |
| | Post Graduate Institute of Child Health | Noida, Uttar Pradesh |
| | Employees State Insurance Corporation (ESIC) Medical College Hospital and Super Specialty Hospital | Hyderabad, Telangana |
| | Rainbow Children's Hospital | Hyderabad, Telangana |
| | Government Medical College | Srinagar, Jammu and Kashmir |
| | Society for Rehabilitation of Crippled Children (SRCC) Children's Hospital | Mumbai, Maharashtra |
| Accredited by Indian Association of Paediatric Anaesthesiologists (IAPA) http://www.iapaindia.com/accredited-institutions.html Duration: 1 year (Post-MD Anaesthesia) 2 years (Post-Diploma Anaesthesia) | G Kuppuswamy Naidu Memorial Hospital (GKNM) | Coimbatore, Tamil Nadu |
| | Sri Ramachandra Institute of Higher Education and Research | Chennai, Tamil Nadu |
| | Amrita Institute of Medical Sciences (AIMS) | Kochi, Kerala |
| | Kasturba Medical College (KMC) | Manipal, Karnataka |
| | Rainbow Hospitals | Marathahalli, Bengaluru, Karnataka |
| | SRCC Children's Hospital | Mumbai, Maharashtra |
| | Rainbow Hospitals | Hyderabad, Telangana |
| | K G Patel Children Hospital | Vadodara, Gujarat |
| | CNBC | New Delhi |
| | Post Graduate Institute of Child Health | Noida, Uttar Pradesh |
| | Madhukar Rainbow Children's Hospital | Malviya Nagar, Delhi |
| Post-Doctoral PA Fellowship (duration 1 year) | All India Institute of Medical Sciences (AIIMS) | Jodhpur, Rajasthan |

*Contd…*

*Contd...*

| *Name of course* | *Institution/university* | *Location* |
|---|---|---|
| Affiliation: Rajiv Gandhi University of Health Sciences, Karnataka (duration 1 year) | Bangalore Medical College and Research Institute | Bengaluru, Karnataka |
| | Indira Gandhi Institute of Child Health | Bengaluru, Karnataka |
| | Bapuji Medical College | Davanagere, Karnataka |
| Accredited by Dr MGR Medical University Paediatric Anaesthesia Fellowship (duration 1 year) | Kanchi Kamakoti CHILDS Trust Hospital | Chennai, Tamil Nadu |
| | Christian Medical College | Vellore, Tamil Nadu |
| Accredited by Maharashtra University of Health Sciences (MUHS) (duration 1 year) | Grant Medical College and Sir Jamshedji Jeejeebhoy Hospital (JJ Hospital)<br>King Edward Memorial (KEM) Hospital and Seth GS Medical College<br>Lokmanya Tilak Municipal General Hospital (LTMGH) and Medical College,<br>Bai Jerbai Wadia Hospital for children | Mumbai, Maharashtra |
| Accredited by:Indian College of Anaesthesiologists (ICA) Paediatric Cardiovascular Anaesthesia Fellowship (duration 18 months) | Narayana Hrudayalaya, Bangalore | Bengaluru, Karnataka |
| Fellowship in Paediatric Cardiac Anaesthesia (duration 1 year) | Postgraduate Institute of Medical Education and Research | Chandigarh |
| Fellowship in Paediatric Cardiac Anaesthesia (duration 1 year) | All India Institute of Medical Sciences (AIIMS) | New Delhi |
| World Federation of Societies of Anaesthesiologists (WFSA) Paediatric Anaesthesia Fellowship (duration 6 months) | Children Anaesthesia Services www.suryahospitals.com | Mumbai, Maharashtra |
| | Christian Medical College | Vellore, Tamil Nadu |
| Doctorate of Medicine (Paediatric Anaesthesia and Intensive Care) (duration 3 years) | Postgraduate Institute of Medical Education and Research | Chandigarh |
| Doctorate of Medicine (Paediatric and Neonatal Anaesthesia) (duration 3 years) | King Edward Memorial (KEM) Hospital and Seth GS Medical College | Mumbai, Maharashtra |

(PA: Paediatric anaesthesia)

*Source*: Partly compiled with permission from Sen et al.[4] Permission to reproduce this table obtained from the Indian Journal of Anaesthesia.

management, transport of a sick baby, induction and maintenance of anaesthesia by different routes, and the various techniques of regional anaesthesia in children, including caudal, dorsal penile and inguinal block and spinal and epidural block. The student has to demonstrate expertise in the recognition and treatment of apnoea, laryngospasm, acid–base and electrolyte disturbances in children, anaesthetic management of children with congenital syndromes, neonatal and paediatric resuscitation, paediatric pain management and paediatric intensive care, including ventilatory management and central venous cannulation. The recognition and assessment of a child with upper respiratory tract infection, malignant hyperthermia and the anaesthetic management of foreign body in the bronchus/oesophagus, Wilms' tumour, congenital diaphragmatic hernia, tracheo-oesophageal fistula, foetal surgery and diagnostic and therapeutic procedures outside the operating room have been given impetus in the syllabus. The student has to acquire all this experience in paediatric anaesthesia, preferably in the last 12 months of the course.[3]

The 1-year IAPA fellowship programme offered by many accredited government and private institutions facilitates the development of knowledge, attitudes and skills necessary to provide advanced perioperative care to paediatric patients (including critically ill ones) for surgeries or painful procedures under general anaesthesia, regional anaesthesia or sedation **(Table 1)**.

The syllabus includes the following:

- Attaining knowledge regarding anatomical, physiological, psychological and pharmacological differences and variations in the various subsets of paediatric patients, including the neonate, the premature baby and infants; difficult airway management and devices used; high-risk pregnancies: pre-eclampsia, gestational diabetes, jaundice, thyroid deficiency, etc.; high-risk children, including those on ventilators, with heart diseases and severe asthma, etc.; neonatal and paediatric emergencies such as necrotising enterocolitis, diaphragmatic hernia, tracheo-oesophageal fistula, volvulus, torsion testis, appendicitis, etc.; bronchoscopy for foreign body; fluid management in neonates, children and high-risk patients; local anaesthetic pharmacology as applied to children and neonates; neuraxial and systemic opioids, non-steroidal anti-inflammatory drugs and non-opioid adjuncts for analgesia in children and neonates; spinal, epidural, caudal and combined spinal–epidural anaesthesia for paediatric and neonatal usage and the recognition and treatment of complications of anaesthesia and regional blocks in children.
- Conducting under supervision, anaesthesia for paediatric surgery including neonatal surgeries and laparoscopic surgeries in both children

and neonates, plastic surgery including burns and cleft lip/palate, dental surgery, otorhinolaryngological surgery including tracheostomies and bronchoscopy, neurosurgery including ventriculoperitoneal shunts, trauma, etc., and orthopaedic surgery including congenital malformations and trauma.

- *Achievement of skills:* Placement of peripheral intravenous lines, central lines, spinals, epidurals, caudals and peripheral nerve blocks and management of difficult airway.
- Development of interpersonal and communication skills to communicate effectively with children and their families, colleagues and other health professionals, thereby ensuring safe patient care; ability to work effectively as a team member; also in situations of crisis or difficult interpersonal conflicts in the operative team; effectively communicate when handing over patients to another team; maintain comprehensive and clear medical documentation in a timely manner and to attain ability to analyse a medical error or a critical incident.

Clinical teaching includes the review of perioperative management of each patient which is supplemented with lectures on various topics, journal club meetings (review of current paediatric anaesthesiology articles), case discussions of challenging cases, interdepartmental meetings with obstetricians and paediatricians and annual paediatric anaesthesia meetings and continued medical education programmes.

Research is another facet of the fellowship curriculum and includes the publication of at least one study and/or one case report (or submit for publication) related to paediatric anaesthesia by the end of the course.

The evaluation process includes 6-monthly examinations (written and viva voce), maintenance of a log book (documented log of all cases and procedures done) and an exit examination conducted by the IAPA Fellowship Committee yearly/concerned university.

## CONTEMPORARY CHALLENGES IN PAEDIATRIC ANAESTHESIA CONTEMPLATING THE NEED FOR A SYLLABUS AND CURRICULUM CHANGE

There are several contemporary challenges faced by paediatric anaesthesiologists. There are an increasing number of procedures done outside the operating room with their own implications on the quality and safety of care provided to these children. Non-operating room anaesthesia (NORA) is limited by the lack of availability of contemporary anaesthesia machines and monitoring equipment, airway devices, and personnel for help along with lack of familiarity with the new procedures. The incidence of adverse events is more in these locations, and paediatric anaesthesia training should focus on NORA training in addition to operating room training.[5]

There has also been an increase in less invasive and more complex procedures such as paediatric robotic surgery with its own anaesthesia implications. Pre-anaesthetic evaluation whilst assessing suitability for robotic surgeries emphasises on identifying factors that can affect physiologic response to changes from pneumoperitoneum and tolerance to robot-assisted paediatric surgeries. Potential difficulty in accessing the patient after docking requires planning of vascular access (including central line and arterial catheter), securing endotracheal tube, nasogastric tube, monitoring devices and fluid management. The application of lung-protective ventilatory strategies with optimum positive end-expiratory pressure to prevent atelectrauma and the quantification of intraoperative fluid loss are important. Potential risks of cerebral oedema with increasing duration of pneumoperitoneum and Trendelenburg positioning and hypothermia are some of the other concerns in robotic surgeries. Operating room safety is compromised by the distance between the operating team and the patient. Safety can be improved by time-trained simulations to develop proficiency in docking/undocking and other critical procedures.[6] Similarly, with the development of maternal and foetal medicine, it is time to introduce training in foetal ex-utero intrapartum treatment (EXIT) procedures as a part of paediatric anaesthesia training. With the shift to regional anaesthesia and ultrasound-guided blocks, skill development in this aspect of anaesthesia during training, both during post-graduation and during fellowships, still remains limited. This could be due to the lack of universal availability of ultrasound to the anaesthesiologists in the operating rooms, lack of formal training in ultrasound-guided paediatric regional anaesthesia and lack of availability of experienced teaching faculty. Another challenge in contemporary paediatric anaesthesia is the increase in the number of children with obesity, multiple comorbidities and unusual syndromes coming for complex surgeries. Specialised paediatric anaesthesia training becomes mandatory in such high-risk situations. In addition, a paediatric anaesthesiologist working in a low-resource setting will encounter a diverse range of other challenges in ensuring the provision of safe anaesthesia with limited resources. Data collected from low- and middle-income countries show higher perioperative mortality and adverse perioperative respiratory events in children, especially neonates and infants and amongst children with additional risk factors such as complex congenital cardiac diseases, American Society of Anesthesiologists (ASA) class >3 and emergency surgeries. A wide range of equipment sizes such as face masks, oropharyngeal airways, laryngeal mask airways, tracheal tubes, laryngoscopes and intravenous cannulae are required to adequately anaesthetise a diverse paediatric population, and there are often shortages or non-availability in a resource-poor setting. There are scenarios where the available equipment has to be reused multiple times after rudimentary decontamination procedures. The range of anaesthetic drug preparations might be narrow, the available drug preparations may be out of date and those that require refrigeration may have been stored at ambient temperature, hampering their efficacy. Piped oxygen is often unavailable with oxygen usually being provided by cylinders. End-tidal agent and carbon dioxide monitoring is almost universally absent. The availability of other forms of non-invasive monitoring such as non-invasive blood pressure, electrocardiogram and pulse oximetry may vary between centres. Inconsistent supply of homogenous blood components and lack of standard infection control practices are not uncommon.[7,8]

Newer curricula in paediatric anaesthesia education need to be devised keeping all the above challenges in mind and also the need to improve safety and quality in anaesthesia delivery and the ethical and legal issues involved in paediatric anaesthesia care.

## UPDATES ON PAEDIATRIC ANAESTHESIA SAFETY AND QUALITY IMPROVEMENT

Ensuring safety and quality improvement (QI) in paediatric anaesthesia is indispensable and is monitored as a part of the Joint Commission International Accreditation and National Accreditation Board for Hospitals and Healthcare Providers. Some of the international collaboratives towards safety in paediatric anaesthesia include the following:

- The Wake Up Safe (WUS) initiative in the United States of America. Member institutions of WUS submit data on any serious adverse event, and three anaesthesiologists who were not involved in the event have to analyse the event with a root cause analysis to identify the causal factors.[9]
- The National Confidential Enquiry into Perioperative Deaths (NCEPOD) in the United Kingdom. In 2011, NCEPOD published data on paediatric surgical patients.[10]
- The Australian Patient Safety Foundation, formed in 1987, set up and coordinated the Australian Incident Monitoring Study (AIMS). The reports collected are both anonymous and voluntary. Although incidents are reported for patients of all ages, a subset of paediatric data are reported separately from this reporting system.[10]
- The Pediatric Perioperative Cardiac Arrest (POCA) Registry, created through analysis of closed malpractice, claims data from the ASA. Closed Claims Project is a voluntary effort that provided valuable insights into the cause and consequences of perioperative cardiac arrest in children.[10]
- The Pediatric Regional Anesthesia Network (PRAN) is collecting data from participating institutions on the risks and complications of regional techniques in children.[10]
- Lorinc et al. have identified airway/respiratory events, cardiovascular events, medication errors, handover communications, NORA anaesthesia and sedation and obesity as some important areas where QI initiatives are to be implemented.[11]

## UNDERSTANDING THE ETHICAL AND LEGAL CONSIDERATIONS IN PAEDIATRIC ANAESTHESIA

Ethical considerations in paediatric anaesthesia include:[12]

- Written informed consent and assent from patients/care providers
- Explanation of obligations towards the child and family
- Shared decision-making in the best interest of the paediatric patient
- Informed refusal and respecting the refusal of assent and avoiding coercion
- Considerations regarding paediatric end-of-life therapy
- Ethical and legal issues related to conducting research in paediatric patients.

Legal issues in paediatric anaesthesia include:

- *Informed consent:* Considering the time constraint as a limiting factor for patient–anaesthesiologist interaction, especially in paediatric cases admitted for day care surgery, it is the responsibility of the anaesthesiologist to give the complete disclosure of information in easy language for the parent to understand.[13]
- *Stringent maintenance of records:* Medical records should explain all details about the child's pre-anaesthetic checkup, informed consent or refusal, intraoperative anaesthesia records and post-operative course. It is essential to maintain records in legible form, preferably even in digital format, for sufficiently long duration since cases can be registered as later as 3 years after the surgery.
- *Consumer Protection Act (CPA):* Paediatric anaesthesiologists are most commonly tried for liability in scenarios such as hypoxic brain damage leading to death during general anaesthesia, neurological deficit after neuraxial or regional anaesthesia, inadequate monitoring during the procedure and awareness during anaesthesia.[14]

## FUTURE DIRECTIONS AND INNOVATIONS IN PAEDIATRIC ANAESTHESIA CURRICULUM

Teaching and learning during paediatric anaesthesia degree/fellowship courses in our nation are variable and are always centred around the patient in the operating theatre. The evaluation process also varies between institutions. It may include both formative and summative assessments, with theory and practical assessment in the form of long and short case discussions and table viva voce. There is a definite need to achieve a uniform level of knowledge and skill in paediatric anaesthesia training programmes. Though the literature in this regard is sparse, to achieve uniform competencies and technical skills, the strengths and scope of various training programmes across the globe need to be identified and amalgamated. Newer teaching–learning and assessment methods are emerging and can be adopted.

## Newer Teaching–Learning Methods

Some newer interactive teaching methods such as e-learning, blended learning, flipped classroom, hybrid system, simulation-based teaching, active classroom sessions, podcasts, vodcasts, social media and web-based collaborative education, problem-based discussions, reflective feedback and mentorship can be incorporated.[15]

### *E-learning*

E-learning can increase learner engagement and satisfaction. Learning management systems such as modular object-oriented dynamic learning environment (MOODLE) allow learners to study a topic to the depth that they desire and at a pace that suits them. App-based learning can be used as an alternative, e.g. in paediatric basic life support, instead of instructor-based education.[15]

### *Blended Learning*

Blended learning includes the use of both online media and two-way face-to-face communication.[16] For example, after understanding the basic idea of a topic online/through videos, a student can then attend the workshop/seminar physically to enhance knowledge and sharpen skills.

### *Flipped Classroom*

Flipped classroom is a model of blended learning in which online pre-recorded lectures of average 20-minutes duration/medium-length reading assignments are viewed by the trainees before the scheduled class so that basic concepts related to the topic are understood by them at their own pace and time. This is followed by live, active classroom sessions wherein teachers and peers engage the students in discussions around clinical applications and problem-based learning. The knowledge gained prior to the class can stimulate student interest and facilitate face-to-face learning.[15]

### *Hybrid System*

This is a novel platform for learning and performing skills. It provides an algorithm for peer-to-peer hands-on training in skill laboratories and also a direct feedback option from both the peers and the instructors.[17]

### *Webinars*

They are a powerful online tool to disseminate knowledge from experts to post-graduates and provide accessibility to students over a wide geographical area. However, they are teacher-centric, and interaction with students is limited.[15] The Indian Society of Anaesthesiologists National is doing yeoman service in this context by conducting regular weekly online teaching classes in the form of webinars for post-graduate students.

### *Simulation*

Paediatric anaesthesiology training should focus on handling dynamic situations, requiring a trainee to analyse the situation and make decisions with clinical expertise.[18] High fidelity simulation helps create countless scenarios of possible critical incidents, impossible otherwise, for a person to experience them clinically. Though an expensive tool, simulation offers a safe environment and assesses teamwork, communication skills and high cognitive skills. It can be useful for procedures such as securing an intravenous line and airway management in children.

### *SLICE (Structured Learning in Clinical Ethics) Model*

It can be used as a template to help medical professionals identify their own 'moral compass' to provide guidance in complex ethical areas. The model has five domains: (1) Conscience, (2) compliance, (3) concurrence, (4) conversation and (5) conversion. Settings include teaching ethical aspects of transplantation, legislation for undergraduates and consent in paediatric anaesthesia.[19]

## Newer Assessment Methods

Assessment should be both formative and summative to allow early identification of the students' weaknesses, ensuring timely corrective actions during the course of training.[20]

Assessment methods should include the assessment of both clinical and non-clinical professionally useful skills. Newer formative assessment tools include workplace-based assessment (WPBA) tools such as Mini-Clinical Evaluation Exercises (mini-CEX), direct observation of procedural skills (DOPS), logbook, Objective Structured Clinical Examination (OSCE) stations, Pediatrics Milestone Project, etc.[20] The Pediatric Anesthesiology Milestone Project is a joint initiative of the Accreditation Council for Graduate Medical Education (ACGME) and the American Board of Anesthesiology.[21] The milestones include knowledge, skills, attitudes and other attributes for each of the ACGME competencies organised in a developmental framework from less to more advanced. Arranged into numbered levels, tracking from levels 1 to 5 is synonymous with moving from novice to expert in the subspeciality. Selection of a level implies demonstration of milestones in that level, as well as those in lower levels.

## CONCLUSION

Paediatric surgery and paediatric anaesthesia have evolved in parallel with the times. Paediatric anaesthesia is a routine part of the post-graduate curriculum in anaesthesiology and is delved into deeper along with dissertation work in the fellowship courses. Several challenges are to be faced in paediatric anaesthesia, and the paediatric anaesthesia training has to be geared up to meet these challenges. There is scope for the integration of newer teaching-learning methods such as e-learning, blended learning, simulation, hybrid learning and SLICE model and the application of assessment methods such as WPBA tools, OSCE and Pediatric Anesthesiology Milestone Project in paediatric anaesthesia education. Newer curricula in paediatric anaesthesia should be devised keeping in mind the ethical and legal considerations specific to paediatric anaesthesia and the ultimate goal of the delivery of quality and safe anaesthesia.

## ACKNOWLEDGEMENT

The authors thank the authors of the article Sen I, Dave N, Bhardwaj N, Juwarkar C, Beegum S. Specialised training in paediatric anaesthesia: Need of the hour. Indian J Anaesth. 2021;65:17-22 for giving permission to allow publication of **Table 1**, after modifications.

## REFERENCES

1. Malde AD, Prabhu SS, Sundaram S, Bajwa SJS. Paediatric anaesthesia practice: has it really changed over the times? Indian J Anaesth. 2022;66:621-4.
2. Frank JR, Hall AK, Oswald A, Dagnone JD, Brand PLP, Reznick R. From competence by time to competence by design: lessons from a national transformation initiative. Perspec Med Educ. 2024;13(1):224-8.
3. National Medical Commission. (2019). Guidelines for competency based postgraduate training programme for MD in anaesthesiology. [online] Available from https://www.nmc.org.in/wp-content/uploads/2019/09/MD-Anesthesia.pdf. [Last accessed June, 2025].
4. Sen I, Dave N, Bhardwaj N, Juwarkar C, Beegum S. Specialised training in paediatric anaesthesia: Need of the hour. Indian J Anaesth. 2021;65:17-22.
5. Shih G, Bailey PD. Nonoperating room anesthesia for children. Curr Opin Anaesthesiol. 2020;33(4):584-8.
6. Tesoro S, Gamba P, Bertozzi M, Borgogni R, Caramelli F, Cobellis G, et al. Pediatric robotic surgery: issues in management-expert consensus from the Italian Society of Pediatric and Neonatal Anesthesia and Intensive Care (SARNePI) and the Italian Society of Pediatric Surgery (SICP). Surg Endosc. 2022;36(11):7877-97.
7. Barbour R, Deka P. Paediatric anaesthesia for low-resource settings. BJA Educ. 2017;17(11):351-6.
8. Khan FA, Haider S, Abbas N, Akhtar N, Haq NU, Khaskheli MS, et al. Challenges of pediatric anesthesia services and training infrastructure in tertiary care teaching institutions in Pakistan: a perspective from the province of Sindh. Anesth Analg. 2022;134(3):653-60.

9. Tjia I, Rampersad S, Varughese A, Heitmiller E, Tyler DC, Lee AC, et al. Wake up safe and root cause analysis: quality improvement in pediatric anesthesia. Anesth Analg. 2014;119(1):122-36.
10. Varughese AM, Rampersad SE, Whitney GM, Flick RP, Anton B, Heitmiller ES. Quality and safety in pediatric anesthesia. Anesth Analg 2013;117(6):1408-18.
11. Lorinc AN, Walters CB, Lovejoy HK, Crockett CJ, Reddy SK. Hot topics in safety for pediatric anesthesia. Children (Basel). 2020;7(11):242.
12. Shah M, Waisel D. Ethics in pediatric anesthesiology. In: Lalwani K, Cohen IT, Choi EY, Raman VT, Lalwani K, Cohen IT (Eds). Pediatric Anesthesia: A Problem-Based Learning Approach. England: Oxford University Press; 2018.
13. Rai E, Chen RYY, Noi CS, Hee HI. Evaluation of anesthesia informed consent in pediatric practice-An observation cohort study. J Anaesthesiol Clin Pharmacol. 2019;35(4):515-21.
14. Shinde SS, Parak SC, Bhati S, Sahay N, Battu GS. Medico-legal and ethical issues in anaesthesiology profession. Indian J Anaesth. 2021;65(1):54-60.
15. Kundra P, Kurdi M, Mehrotra S, Jahan N, Kiran S, Vadhanan P. Newer teaching-learning methods and assessment modules in anaesthesia education. Indian J Anaesth. 2022;66(01):47-57.
16. Banditvilai C. Enhancing students' language skills through blended learning. Electronic J e-Learning. 2016;14:220-9.
17. Ignatavicius P, Gudaityte R, Dobozinskas P, Vaitkaitis D, Krikscionaitiene K, Dambrauskas Z. The novel platform for self-directed peer-to-peer medical simulation for development of the technical and non-technical competences. Ann Surg Edu. 2019;1:1001.
18. Bhagwat M. Simulation and anaesthesia. Indian J Anaesth. 2012;56(1):14-20.
19. Logarajah S, Roff S. Structured learning for clinical ethics in anaesthesia. Clin Ethics. 2016;11(4):200-9.
20. Lagoo JY, Joshi SB. Introduction of direct observation of procedural skills (DOPS) as a formative assessment tool during postgraduate training in anaesthesiology: exploration of perceptions. Indian J Anaesth. 2021;65(3):202-9.
21. The American Board of Anesthesiology. (2015). The Pediatric Anesthesiology Milestone Project–A Joint Initiative of The Accreditation Council for Graduate Medical Education. [online] Available from https://www.acgme.org/globalassets/PDFs/Milestones/PediatricAnesthesiology.pdf. [Last accessed June, 2025].

CHAPTER 22

# The Rights of Children in Anaesthesia: Ensure You're Providing Ethical and Appropriate Care!

*Navdeep Sethi, Anjolie Chhabra, Rakhee Goyal, Parul Jindal*

## ABSTRACT

Paediatric patients are a heterogeneous group, ranging from preemies to adolescents below 18 years of age. Following the initiative of the United Nations Convention on the Rights of the Child (UNCRC) 1989 and Safetots.org (Safe Anaesthesia for Every Tot), there is now an increasing stress on the right of every surgical child for safe and quality anaesthesia. Infants and sick children undergoing complex surgery are at the highest risk for perioperative complications and need to be cared for in specialised paediatric centres. In India, parental consent is essential for procedures performed in children <18 years of age. As per the UNCRC mandate and Indian Council of Medical Research biomedical research guidelines 2017, informed consent and age-appropriate assent must be obtained before providing anaesthesia to a child. End-of-life (EOL) care is emerging as a new albeit essential corollary to the larger issue of ensuring the rights of the child. During the EOL period, paediatric patients primarily experience significant pain and discomfort. Paediatric anaesthesiologists are an integral part of paediatric palliative care during EOL and should aim to relieve pain and suffering of the child and family.

***Keywords:*** Anaesthesia, Child, Consent, Protection, Rights.

## INTRODUCTION

Rights of the child in anaesthesia are still in evolution since 1948, when the United Nations (UN) General Assembly adopted the Universal Declaration of Human Rights (UDHR) as the first legal document that would protect fundamental human rights universally. Later in 1989, the United Nations Convention on the Rights of the Child (UNCRC) established the rights of children to enjoy the highest attainable standard of health (ratified by all UN members with the exception of the United States).[1] These rights are directly applicable to all children coming for surgery under any kind of anaesthesia. Different countries may have different protocols or even different legislation, but the basic rights to safe and quality health care are the same universally and must be respected and practised in letter and spirit.

Even in the most advanced countries, there are increased complications related to anaesthesia in children.[2,3] This increased morbidity in paediatric anaesthesia is possible even in otherwise healthy children coming for surgical procedures.[4] Children need specialised centres with trained paediatric teams that cater to their specific needs and ensure better outcomes and more satisfaction. With this aim in mind, the international paediatric anaesthesia community, through its initiative of SAFETOTS (Safe Anaesthesia for Every Tot, www.safetots.org), has derived 10 rights (10Rs) from the UNCRC charter that are applicable to all children undergoing surgery and anaesthesia **(Box 1)**.[4,5]

## Right to the Highest Possible Standard of Medical Care

This is the most critical right that should be made available to every child. Children undergoing complex procedures, suffering from significant comorbidities, those belonging to American Society of Anesthesiologists (ASA) physical status ≥ III and those under 3 years of age are more susceptible to anaesthesia-related complications.[2] The APRICOT (Incidence of Severe Critical Events in Paediatric Anaesthesia) study further revealed that there was increased airway and cardiovascular morbidity in children who were cared for by less experienced staff.[6] Therefore, children need to be cared for by qualified, well-trained teams in specialised paediatric centres. India has a diverse healthcare system with state-of-the-art facilities at one end and primary health centres at the other. Universal access to specialised paediatric centres for surgery and anaesthesia is very limited. However, academic institutions and anaesthesia societies such as Indian Society of Anaesthesiologists (ISA), Indian Society of Paediatric Anaesthesia (IAPA) and Research Society of Anaesthesiology Clinical Pharmacology (RSACP) are promoting awareness about rights of children, besides pushing the government to bring policy changes and educate anaesthesiologists about child safety. There are an increasing number of opportunities for further specialisation in paediatric anaesthesia such as 6-month training, 1-year fellowship under IAPA or 2-year fellowships under the National Board of Examinations, besides 3-year Doctorate of Medicine (DM) degree courses.

**BOX 1:** The 10Rs of SAFETOTS.[4,5]

1. Right to the highest possible standard of medical care
2. Right to non-discrimination
3. Right to protection from economic exploitation
4. Right to protection from unnecessary treatment and examination
5. Right to avoid pain, fear and stress
6. Right to parental guidance
7. Right to privacy
8. Right to information
9. Right to be heard
10. Right to be cared for with children with the same needs

### Right to Non-discrimination, Right to Protection from Economic Exploitation and Right to Protection from Unnecessary Treatment and Examination

All children, irrespective of their race, gender, religion, nationality and social and financial status, must enjoy equal right to the best possible care in anaesthesia. Each child should be treated with sensitivity and empathy by every member of the surgical team at all times. Unnecessary or profit-making investigations or interventions should strictly be avoided. Children should be carefully involved and supervised in any research project or training workshop. Government policies play an important role in ensuring this goal of child safety, e.g. National Ethical Guidelines for Biomedical Research Involving Children, Indian Council of Medical Research (ICMR) 2017.[7]

### Right to Avoid Pain, Fear and Stress and Right to Parental Guidance

Not all children, especially those who are in non-verbal stage, can express their fear, pain or separation anxiety. It is important that they are treated with utmost sensitivity and provided adequate pre-medication and multimodal analgesia depending on the extent of procedure. Most paediatric centres allow parental presence in the pre- and post-anaesthesia care units, some during the induction of anaesthesia as well and in a child-friendly environment to allay separation anxiety.

### Right to Privacy, Right to Information, Right to be Heard and Right to be Cared for with Children with the Same Needs

The privacy of children should be respected at all times during the induction and maintenance of anaesthesia and recovery. This includes protection against exposure during physical examinations and personal hygiene activities, protection against treatment and behaviour which diminishes self-respect. They should be assured that no harm will come to them during surgery and anaesthesia. According to their age and level of understanding, they have the right to be involved in the medical decision-making process in anaesthesia, sedation and pain therapy.

## INFORMED CONSENT AND ASSENT IN PAEDIATRIC ANAESTHESIA

Paediatric patients are a diverse group, extending from pre-term to adolescents below 18 years of age. As children grow, their cognitive, social and emotional capacities increase. Children <7 years of age may be unaware that they are unwell and need treatment. Children aged 7–12 years may understand their illness and what the treatment entails; still, older children

(12 or more years old), though minors, may have the cognitive ability to understand and participate in the decision-making process.[7]

Traditionally, informed consent for any healthcare intervention was only obtained from a child's parents. However, this changed following the 1989 UNCRC. This convention aimed to provide greater autonomy to children as regards their health-related decisions.[1] Following this, it became acceptable to explain the procedure to children, especially those 7 years old or more, in an age-appropriate manner, and obtain their informal, verbal assent in parental presence. In case of children, a written informed consent is usually taken from the parent/legal guardian of the child after explaining all the risks and benefits of the procedure. It is done based on the premise that the parent will act in the best interest of the child, who may not have the capacity to give consent.[8-10]

Sometimes, despite parental consent and the child's assent, a child may refuse induction of anaesthesia, say just outside the operating room. In this situation, if there is no intravenous cannula in place, doing a forcible inhalational or intramuscular induction may seem to be a fast and easy option. However, it is advisable not to do so, and in case of an elective surgery, it may be better to reschedule the surgery. This will give the parent time to convince and explain the procedure to the child (right to information).[11] Prior to rescheduling, the anaesthesiologist can try and develop a rapport with the child, use oral pre-medication, or distract the child with games and videos so that the child does not resist induction. Parental presence during induction can also be tried. For emergency life-threatening surgery, parental consent with pre-medication suffices even if the child refuses assent.[11]

Another scenario commonly encountered is refusal of consent for regional anaesthesia (procedure to be performed after the child is anaesthetised). In this situation, the advantages and side effects of the block should be explained to the child and parents in simple, age-appropriate language, i.e. following the right to inform. In case they refuse, they should not be forced; instead, alternative methods for providing analgesia should be adopted.[12]

## END-OF-LIFE ISSUES IN PAEDIATRIC PATIENTS

The death of a child is heart-wrenching for a parent. The parents may think they are 'giving up' on their child if the treatment is stopped and may continue treatment beyond significant hope of recovery. During the end-of-life (EOL) period, paediatric patients primarily experience significant pain and discomfort along with symptoms such as dyspnoea, fatigue, irritability, loss of appetite, nausea, vomiting and constipation or diarrhoea which may not be managed effectively. Paediatric palliative care (PPC) during the EOL aims to relieve suffering and improve the quality of life of the child, besides providing physical, emotional and spiritual support to the child and family.[13,14]

**BOX 2:** The rights of the dying child—the Trieste Charter proposal.[16]

1. To be considered as a 'person' until death, irrespective of age, location, illness and care setting
2. To receive effective treatment for pain and for physical and psychological symptoms causing suffering through qualified, comprehensive and continuous care
3. To be listened to and properly informed about his/her illness with consideration for his/her wishes, age and ability to understand
4. To participate, on the basis of his/her abilities, values and wishes, in care choices about his/her life, illness and death
5. To express and, whenever possible, have his/her feelings, wishes and expectations taken into account
6. To have his/her cultural, spiritual and religious beliefs respected and receive spiritual care and support in accordance with his/her wishes and choices
7. To have a social and relational life suitable to his/her age, illness and expectations
8. To be surrounded by family members and loved ones who are adequately supported and protected from the emotional and financial burden of the child's illness
9. To be cared for in a setting appropriate for his/her age, needs and wishes, and that allows the proximity of the family
10. To have access to child-specific palliative care programmes that avoid futile or excessively burdensome practices and therapeutic abandonment

Palliative sedation therapy (PST) may be instituted when traditional symptom management is not sufficient to relieve suffering. Continuous intravenous infusion of midazolam/propofol/dexmedetomidine under strict protocols is commenced within 2 weeks of anticipated death. Clinical algorithms for identifying appropriate patients for PST have been developed.[15]

The Trieste Charter proposes fundamental rights for children who are approaching the end of their lives. This proposal consists of 10 rights and duties which can be applied in such clinical situations and help professionals and families to take care of these terminally ill children **(Box 2)**.[16]

## CASE SCENARIOS ILLUSTRATING THE APPLICATION OF A CHILD'S RIGHTS IN CLINICAL SITUATIONS

### Case Scenario 1: Tanisha's Elective Surgery

Tanisha, a 13-year-old girl (*hypothetical*), has mild scoliosis. It is not life-threatening, but elective corrective surgery can prevent future complications and improve her quality of life. However, the surgery involves significant recovery time and potential risks. The parents are ready for the surgery, but Tanisha is hesitant as she is scared of post-operative pain and the recovery process, and she has final examinations in the next 3 months. The health professionals sit together with Tanisha and her parents and explain to them the procedure and post-operative management with videos of some previous patients. Finally, all agree for surgery after 3 months.

In this case, Tanisha expressed her views (*right to participate and right to be heard*), the entire procedure was explained (*right to information*), and testimonials of previously treated patients were shown to her (*right to be cared for like children with the same needs*). The case was operated after 3 months, taking care of her immediate concerns, pain and recovery time (*right to avoid pain, fear and stress*) whilst providing her with the long-term benefits of the surgery (*right to the highest possible standard of medical care*).

## Case Scenario 2: Monica's Emergency Surgery

Monica, an 8-year-old girl (*hypothetical*), is rushed to the emergency department after a car accident. She has sustained a severe head injury, intra-abdominal bleeding and multiple fractures. She is in critical condition and needs to be stabilised as early as possible to prevent further deterioration. Her parents are hesitant about giving immediate consent for an emergency surgery, asking for more time to consult other family members. Monica, though semiconscious, is anxious and afraid of the surgery. She is explained the necessity of the surgery (in age-appropriate terms) along with her parents. Her father urges the team to proceed with whatever is necessary to save her life. The medical team quickly does emergency surgery to stabilise Monica.

In this case, the *right to the highest possible standard of medical care* was provided by prioritising lifesaving measures, as delay could be life-threatening. *Right to information and right to avoid pain, fear and stress* were maintained by explaining the need for surgery to Monica, alleviating her fear of pain. The medical professionals can proceed with lifesaving surgery if the consent is delayed or unclear in the *child's best interests*, emphasising to the parents that their priority is saving her life.

## Case Scenario 3: Ayush's Journey

Ayush, a 12-year-old boy (*hypothetical*), has been battling an aggressive form of leukaemia for 4 years. Despite multiple rounds of chemotherapy, immunotherapy and a bone marrow transplant, the cancer has returned. The medical team has concluded that further curative treatment is unlikely to succeed, and the focus now is switched to palliative care to ensure a pain-free, comfortable and dignified remaining life. Though Ayush's father wishes to continue and explore experimental treatment, expecting some miracle for him, his mother wants him to be comfortable at home, on palliative care. Ayush, on the other hand, quite aware of the current situation, is not willing to continue painful treatment; instead, he wishes to spend time with his siblings at home. The medical team hears Ayush's wishes, counsels the parents and keeps him at home, providing him the best palliative care available.

The current scenario protected Ayush's *right to information* about his illness, *right to be heard* about his wishes and *right to participate* in decision-making. His parents were counselled, giving him the *right to protection from unnecessary treatment and examination* and the *right to the highest possible standard of medical care*. He was provided with the best palliative care at home, protecting his *right to avoid pain, fear and stress*. The treating team emphasised what was in the *best interests of the child* and provided *right to protection from harm* by avoiding experimental treatments that would prolong suffering and by giving pain management, emotional and psychological support and fulfilling his wishes to be with his siblings.

## CONCLUSION

The rights of children in anaesthesia are paramount and should be upheld to ensure their safety, dignity and well-being. These rights include informed consent and age-appropriate assent, the presence of a trusted caregiver whenever feasible, the mitigation of pain and anxiety and the assurance of high-quality care based on established medical guidelines. Anaesthesia providers must adopt a child-centred approach, respecting the physical, emotional and psychological needs of the child whilst advocating their best interests.

## REFERENCES

1. Jensen KN, Hansen TG. Children undergoing anaesthesia: what are the rights of the child? Signa Vitae. 2021;17(4):203-7.
2. Disma N, Veyckemans F, Virag K, Hansen TG, Becke K, Harlet P, et al. Morbidity and mortality after anaesthesia in early life: results of the European prospective multicentre observational study, neonate and children audit of anaesthesia practice in Europe (NECTARINE). Br J Anaesth. 2021;126:1157-72.
3. Koppenberg J, Stoevesandt D, Watzke S, Schwappach D, Bucher M. Analysis of 30 anaesthesia-related deaths in Germany between 2006 and 2015: an analysis of a closed claims database. Eur J Anaesthesiol. 2022;39:33-41.
4. Weiss M, Vutskits L, Hansen TG, Engelhardt T. Safe anaesthesia for every Tot: the SAFETOTS initiative. Curr Opin Anaesthesiol. 2015;28:302-7.
5. SAFETOTS. (2024). Rights of the Child (10Rs). [online] Available from https://www.safetots.org/rights-of-the-child-10r/. [Last accessed June, 2025].
6. Habre W, Disma N, Virag K, Becke-Jacob K, Hansen TG, Johr M, et al. Incidence of severe critical events in paediatric anaesthesia (APRICOT): a prospective multicentre observational study in 261 hospitals in Europe. Lancet Respir Med. 2017;5:412-25.
7. Indian Council of Medical Research. (2017). National ethical guidelines for biomedical research involving children, 2017. [online] Available from https://ethics.ncdirindia.org//asset/pdf/National_Ethical_Guidelines_for_BioMedical_Research_Involving_Children.pdf. [Last accessed June, 2025].
8. McCombe K, Bogod DG. Consent and capacity: issues for paediatric anaesthesia. BJA Educ. 2020;20(11):377-81.

9. Katz AL, Webb SA. Informed consent in decision-making in pediatric practice. Pediatrics. 2016;138(2):e20161485.
10. Casby C, Lyons B. Anaesthesia consent considerations in children and young people. Anaesth Intensive Care Med. 2021;22(11):718-22.
11. Massie J, Skinner A, McKenzie I, Gillam L. A practical and ethical toolkit for last-minute refusal of anesthetic in children. Pediatr Anesth. 2021;31(8):834-38.
12. Lönnqvist PA, Morton NS, Ross AK. Consent issues and pediatric regional anesthesia. Pediatr Anesth. 2009;19(10):958-60.
13. Hauer JM, Wolfe J. Supportive and palliative care of children with metabolic and neurological diseases. Curr Opin Support Palliat Care. 2014;8(3):296-302.
14. Erondu MU, Mahoney DP. Palliative care, resuscitation status and end-of-life considerations in pediatric anesthesia. Curr Opin Anaesthesiol. 2020;33(3):354-60.
15. Cuviello A, Johnson, LM, Morgan KJ, Anghelescu DL, Baker JN. Palliative sedation therapy in pediatrics: an algorithm and clinical practice update. Children (Basel). 2022;9:1887.
16. Benini F, Vecchi R, Lazzarin P, Jankovic M, Orsi L, Manfredini L, et al. The rights of the dying child and the duties of healthcare providers: the "Trieste Charter". Tumori. 2017;103(1):33-9.

CHAPTER 23

# Ethics of Research and Training in Paediatrics: Ensure you are Conducting Ethical Research and Taking Appropriate Measures in Training

*Neerja Bhardwaj, Divya Jain, Nandini Dave, Banashree Mandal*

## ABSTRACT

Imparting ethical clinical training as well as conducting ethical scientific research is an integral part of medicine. This is extremely challenging to accomplish for the specialty of anaesthesia, especially paediatric anaesthesia where the patients cannot give consent by virtue of their immaturity. The need of the hour is to develop teaching modules which incorporate options such as simulation or virtual patients, thereby allowing the practice of important skills without causing harm to the patient. The National Medical Commission has recommended that post-graduate training in medicine should be skill-oriented and, therefore, has made provision of skill laboratories mandatory. At the same time, students need to be aware of the ethical principles involved in research, and this should be the part of the core curriculum.

***Keywords:*** Anaesthesia, Ethics, Postgraduate, Research, Training.

## INTRODUCTION

'Ethics' is derived from the Greek word 'ethos' meaning 'character' or 'conduct'. Whilst ethical conduct in medicine has mainly been associated with research, its role in teaching and training is also important particularly in children where it is more related to good practice. If a medical educator follows ethical clinical practice, ethical research automatically follows.

The concern of teaching and training in children takes its foundation from the fact that the margin of error is minuscule as opposed to adults. Moreover, autonomy needs to be respected in an age-appropriate manner, even though the subjects are under the legal age to consent. Anaesthesia training is even more complicated when the child loses consciousness and is nowhere in a position to dissent or withdraw from care.

Teaching methodologies are varied; they include didactic lectures, bedside teaching, procedural training under supervision and simulation-based modules conducted in skill laboratories. All these methods vary greatly amongst countries and regions, depending on the availability of technology and expertise but may be useful for ethical teaching and training.

Biomedical research forms the cornerstone of evidence-based medicine, guiding clinical practice and decision-making to ensure effective and safe patient care. According to the Belmont Report, research on human participants should ideally be guided by three basic principles: (1) Respect of person, (2) justice and (3) beneficence.[1] The principle of respect for persons includes the moral requirement to protect those with diminished autonomy, including children.[1] On the other hand, the principle of beneficence and justice entails an obligation to act impartially and ensure the benefit of research to all subjects, including those in the vulnerable category. As a result, maintaining a balance and fulfilling key principles of conduct of research involving children are both challenging and crucial.

This chapter aims to put forth the ethical principles governing research in children in India as well as mechanisms to prevent harm when training physicians in paediatric anaesthesia. It will also discuss the training of students in an ethical manner, teaching ethics in post-graduate programmes and comparing training in India and other countries.

## Training Students in an Ethical Manner

Enhancing paediatric anaesthesia education and training is crucial to grooming future generations of 'safe and skilled' paediatric anaesthesiologists. Ethics in education includes five basic principles: (1) Ethics of care, (2) justice, (3) critique, (4) profession and (5) community.[2] Educators should consider the 'best interests of the student' on the basis of professional principles, codes and standards. In medical education, especially when vulnerable subjects such as children are involved, the educator faces the dichotomy of ensuring that the best interests of the patient are also protected whilst maintaining the highest professional standards.

Educating trainees is an art form which is always challenging, especially so in the branch of anaesthesia, where we administer multiple drugs and perform interventional procedures, e.g. endotracheal intubation, insert invasive lines and perform central neuraxial and peripheral nerve blocks during the perioperative period. When the patient is a child, the ramifications increase manyfold.

The patient as a 'subject to learn skills' is no longer acceptable, and, therefore, hospitals which train clinicians need to look beyond the traditional teaching methodologies. In a recent review, Kundra et al. detailed the new teaching–learning methods in anaesthesia education and advocated for a major change in the existing practice.[3] Novel approaches and technologies, such as simulation-based training, telemedicine, online learning, mobile applications and advanced monitoring, offer exciting opportunities to address the challenges in this field.[4]

Simulation-based teaching is beneficial in teaching core competencies which are less feasible on patients, thereby avoiding risks to patients and students. Simulation offers the opportunity for repeated practice and the freedom to learn from errors in a safe manner. One can create

**TABLE 1:** Framework of training.

| | |
|---|---|
| Phase 1 | Simulation-based training in skill laboratories, with emphasis on both technical and non-technical skills |
| Phase 2 | Observation of delivery of anaesthesia by expert faculty and anaesthetic delivery under supervision for low-risk surgery and low-risk patients |
| Phase 3 | High-risk patient care under supervision |
| Phase 4 | Bridge between independent trainee and preparation for grooming of an independent faculty |

real-life situations in operation theatres by using artificial intelligence (AI) and machine learning (ML) technologies. This bio-like feedback in anaesthesiology helps to develop cognition, as well as psychomotor and affective domains, thereby helping in making correct decisions in patients with complicated physiology.[5]

Simulators may be of various types ranging from low fidelity, part trainers which are low cost, full-body trainers, high fidelity simulators or virtual reality simulators. For many skills such as intravenous cannulation, part-task trainers are more than adequate, and high-fidelity trainers may not be required for simulation training. For effective teaching, the choice of type of simulator is based on the learning outcomes. Equally important is the role of the instructor; effective debriefing is imperative, since this is where learning occurs. A stepwise approach and framework for training has to be adopted **(Table 1)**.

To improve students' clinical skills and assess learning outcomes, medical teachers may use standardised patients (SPs). However, is it ethical to request parents to allow their child to be utilised for evaluating the clinical competence of students? Are there any situations where this process should be permitted? It is an educational challenge to involve minors as SPs and should include a child advocacy team as well as logistics. One should consider what is best for the child and whether there is any risk of harm. It is essential to consider the well-being of the child, and they should be allowed to withdraw at any time. A minor's assent as well as dissent is required and should be respected. The 'rule of 7' can be used to assess the capability of a minor. Minors aged $<7$ years, minors aged 7–13 years and minors aged $\geq 14$ years are important cutoffs to assess the capability and maturity of the children to make a decision as well as understand consent.[6] Use of technology may obliterate the need for minors to be used as SPs. Advances in technology have made virtual humans and other forms of AI much more lifelike. Paediatric virtual patients have been created and are being used in some centres since many years.[7]

Ethical considerations must guide the development and implementation of these innovations to maintain the highest standards of care for paediatric patients. To understand the ethical issues involved, teachers should have easy access to the training required for this purpose. Ongoing professional development courses can provide support as well as opportunities for reflection, so that they can be a part of communities, where learning and collaboration with colleagues are encouraged. This will help them to create a strong ethical culture in their day-to-day working. The 'anaesthetist educator' should also be aware of legislation and good practice guidelines as relevant to children in accordance with national and institutional policies. The continued exploration and integration of these approaches will contribute to better outcomes and safer anaesthesia care for children.

## Teaching Ethics in Post-graduate Programmes

The curriculum of post-graduate programmes includes teaching ethics and related topics. The goal is to refresh and reinforce the important ethical principles which have been taught in medical colleges so as to prepare the post-graduate students to handle ethical issues encountered in their day-to-day practice as consultants. In a review, Hong et al. elucidated the teaching of ethics in the post-graduate programmes.[8] The educational content of such programmes includes ethical theories and the Hippocratic Oath, respect for patients' autonomy, the principles of beneficence and non-maleficence and justice, care at end-of-life, communication skills, doctor–patient relationship, law of ethics, etc. Ethics of research and ethical dilemmas which may be different for different specialities should be included in the curriculum. The methodology is variable and includes a case-based approach, online ethics modules and group discussions. Some universities offer Master's programmes or fellowships in Medical Ethics.

The task of shaping clinicians capable of applying ethical principles in their clinical practice is difficult and challenging. The changing of medical students to healthcare professionals involves a combination of knowledge of ethics and skills which are built over time with ongoing exposure to clinical work. The programmes must create an environment where medical personnel can proactively incorporate these into their daily work in healthcare organisations.

## Comparison of Training in India and Other Countries

The previous medical education system in India was subject-centric, its curriculum lacked uniformity, and it was time-based. The activity of teaching and learning and the ways of assessment were focused more on knowledge than on aptitude and practical skills. This patient-based training was the standard method of training as it was thought that the motor skill development and assessment of learning outcomes are far better when trainees are dealing with actual patients.

Training is largely focussed on skill development, and there is not enough emphasis on acquisition of non-technical skills required to make an all-round clinician based on the humanitarian and ethical factors. Opportunities for skill and knowledge acquisition are also very variable, depending on the workload and patient footfall in the training institution.[9] Based on the results of a recent survey, inclusion of simulation techniques in post-graduate training in anaesthesia is extremely low (20%) in some states in our country.[10] The latest National Medical Commission Post-graduate Medical Education Board guidelines recommend that during the training programme, patient safety should be considered most important. For this, the relevant clinical skills should be initially learnt on the models, followed by their performance under supervision and ultimately independent performance. Since acquisition of competencies is the keystone of post-graduate medical education, such training should be skills-oriented and provision of skills laboratories in medical colleges is mandatory.[11]

The time has now come when we need to uniformly upgrade the post-graduate programme across our nation. Quality improvement initiatives such as physician exchange programmes, for both the students and teachers, can change the mindset. The grooming of medical personnel in ethics is the need of the hour so that they can adapt to varying clinical situations so as to enhance perioperative care which is safe.

## CONCERNS OF ETHICAL RESEARCH IN CHILDREN

Children form a unique population, characterised with developmental and physiological parameters different from adults. Therefore, clinical trials are necessary to invent treatments specific for age and interventions that specifically target diseases and conditions prevalent in the paediatric population. However, conduct of biomedical research in children has been fraught with ethical issues. Children, especially the neonates, have increased chances of being harmed in the conduct of research because of their developmental, physiological and pharmacological immaturity. Moreover, they may not be able to safeguard their own interests due to their inability to give autonomous consent. The Declaration of Helsinki, therefore, has placed children under the vulnerable category.[12]

### Regulatory Bodies for Ethical Conduct of Medical Research

The ethical principles governing clinical research are based on various guidelines and policies to ensure safe and scientifically sound investigations. These guidelines outline specific protocols and considerations tailored to the unique vulnerabilities and needs of children involved in research studies.

The Declaration of Helsinki (latest version, 2013), published by the World Medical Association, is the most important document in research ethics.[12]

Along with it, the guidelines formulated by the Council for International Organizations of Medical Sciences (CIOMS) in association with the World Health Organization (WHO; latest version, 2016) act as a basic format for ethical conduct in biomedical research involving human subjects, including children worldwide.[13] Although there are no separate international guidelines for research in children, the United Nations Children's Fund (UNICEF) has initiated a global project called Ethical Research Involving Children (ERIC), to support researchers to carry out ethical research involving children from diverse geographical, social or cultural backgrounds.[14] In addition, the majority of the countries have formulated their own guidelines in accordance with the local laws and cultural values, e.g. Common Rule in the United States, European Union Guidelines and the Medical Research Council Guidelines in the United Kingdom, with minor deviations in the co-consent or age.[15,16]

In India, the Drugs Controller General and Drugs and Cosmetics Rules, 1945 give approval for newer drugs, vaccines and devices. The Indian Council of Medical Research (ICMR) is the apex regulatory body responsible for the coordination of biomedical research involving human participants. ICMR first issued the 'Policy Statement on Ethical Considerations involved in Research on Human Subjects' in 1980, which was later updated to 'Ethical Guidelines for Biomedical Research on Human Subjects' in 2000 and 2006.[17-20] In 2017, for the first time, ICMR made a significant advancement and published national ethical guidelines for biomedical research involving children from 0 to 18 years of age.[21,22] These guidelines provide recommendations on various aspects of research in children, including risk assessment, informed consent, assent, participant selection and confidentiality to ensure their rights, safety and well-being and further uphold ethical standards for the responsible conduct of research in children.

## Recommendations for Ethical Approval Based on Degree of Risk

It is important that the assessment of any risk of the study protocol should focus on the procedures over and above the standard care which the child would receive. The recent Indian ethical research guidelines involving children have updated the classification of risk into four categories **(Box 1)**.

**BOX 1:** Classification of risk.

- Less than minimal risk involves research on anonymous or non-identified data/samples, data available in the public domain
- Minimal risk involves questioning, observing and measuring the anthropometric parameters (such as height and weight) in a child-friendly manner
- Minor increase over minimal or low risk includes blood test, oral sedation for diagnostic procedures, etc.
- More than minimal or high-risk procedures such as lumbar puncture, lung or liver biopsy and intravenous sedation for diagnostic procedures

However, these risk categories are relative, as they are determined based on age, development and the underlying medical condition of the child; for example, lumbar puncture in a child with leukaemia would be minimal risk compared to a healthy child.

These guidelines in accordance with the international guidelines, clearly state that:

- For research procedures that offer direct benefit to the individual child participant, it may be justified to allocate it a risk category higher than minimal risk.
- However, for research procedures, where there is no direct benefit to the individual child participant, the risk levels should be confined to minimum risk or low risk.

## Recommendations on Informed Consent and Assent

One of the most challenging aspects in paediatric research is when and how to involve the children in making a decision regarding participation in the research trial. The concept of informed consent (IC) and assent has been introduced so that the child (competent minor) and the concerned adult can make a joint decision regarding this aspect.

The permission obtained from parents or the legally acceptable representative (LAR) of the child for participation in the research is termed 'consent'. The three key elements to be followed for taking IC are:

1. *Competence of the parent/LAR:* In case the parent/LAR is illiterate, verbal/oral consent may be taken and signed by an impartial witness.
2. *Information is easily comprehended:* The information provided should be concise and communicated in simple local language.
3. *Voluntariness of participation:* The participant has the freedom to participate or withdraw from research at any time during the study.

There are certain conditions such as when the research involves maintaining confidentiality, e.g. human immunodeficiency virus-infected patients, or research involving publicly available information or retrospective studies, where parental consent may be waived.

Assent refers to the child's voluntary agreement to participate in research, considering their developmental level and capability of understanding. The information provided should be simplified and tailored according to the child's developmental and cognitive abilities.

According to the recent ICMR guidelines, children between 7 and 11 years of age are required to give oral assent in the presence of a parent/LAR, whilst children between 12 and 18 years of age have to give a written assent. If a child attains 13 years of age during the study, then one should obtain a written assent in addition to parent/LAR consent.

The age at which assent can be given differs in different countries, with majority allowing assent above the age of 7 years along with parental consent.

In certain jurisdictions, minors below the age of consent may be considered 'emancipated' or 'mature' minors, and they have the authority to give consent for certain low-risk research without the involvement of their parents or guardians.[23]

### Recommendations on Safeguard Systems

Various new amendments have been made to the existing practices, to safeguard the rights of children participating in research in the recent updated guidelines of the ICMR.

- *Ethical committee:* Member with paediatric expertise should be a part of the Ethics Committee that evaluates a study involving children.
- *Investigator experience:* The research team should include an investigator(s) having expertise in paediatric care.
- *Data and Safety Monitoring Board (DSMB):* The DSMB conducting review should have members with paediatric experience. In addition, anaesthesia research studies in particular should have robust monitoring and safety protocols in place to promptly identify and address any adverse events or complications related to the administration of anaesthesia.

### Recommendations Regarding Compensation

Expenses incurred by children or their caregivers during the research process should be reimbursed, and they should receive financial compensation for any impairment or disability resulting from their involvement in research.

### Recommendations for Special Situations

- *Neonates:* Neonates are the most vulnerable subset of the paediatric population; therefore, research involving neonates needs to be thoroughly examined regarding the risk-benefit by the Institutional Ethics Committee that has an additional advisory member with expertise in neonatal care. Whenever feasible, children of older age group should be studied prior to planning studies in infants or neonates. Continuous consent from the parents can be sought where there is uncertainty about whether the parental consent has been freely given.[24]
- *Emergency situation:* Research in emergency settings such as neonatal resuscitation requires additional safeguards. In emergency situations, deferred consent involving minimum verbal information initially, followed by formal consent later can be obtained, where formal consent is not feasible.

## TRIAL REGISTRATION

Clinical trial registration in a public registry before enrolment of the first patient is essential not only to remove publication bias but also to ensure accountability and transparency. This is especially necessary in children, where the interest of the vulnerable population needs to be safeguarded.

## CONCLUSION

Anaesthesia training is unique since it requires expertise in cognitive (knowledge), psychomotor (procedural skills) and affective (non-technical skills) domains of learning. Incorporating ethical principles in the curriculum is a necessity for the teaching and training of future budding clinicians. Research involving children poses challenges in balancing the ethical principles of research. The recent ethical guidelines involving children by ICMR will serve as a guide for the paediatric investigators and researchers conducting clinical research in India.

## REFERENCES

1. The National Commission for the Protection of Human Subjects of Biomedical and Behavioral Research. The Belmont Report: Ethical Principles and Guidelines for the Protection of Human Subjects of Research. Washington DC: Department of Health, Education and Welfare; 1979.
2. Furman G. The ethic of community. J Edu Admin. 2004;42:215-35.
3. Kundra P, Kurdi M, Mehrotra S, Jahan N, Kiran S, Vadhanan P. Newer teaching-learning methods and assessment modules in anaesthesia education. Indian J Anaesth. 2022;66(1):47-57.
4. Feldman A. Enhancing pediatric anesthesia education and training: Novel approaches and technologies. J Clin Anesthesiol. 2023;7(4):183.
5. Kundra P, Senthilnathan M. Amalgamation of artificial intelligence and simulation in anaesthesia training: much-needed future endeavour. Indian J Anaesth. 2024;68(1):8-10.
6. Wendler DS. Assent in paediatric research: theoretical and practical considerations. J Med Ethics. 2006;32(4):229-34.
7. Hubal RC, Deterding RR, Frank GA, Schwetzke HF, Kizakevich PN. Lessons learned in modeling virtual pediatric patients. Stud Health Technol Inform. 2003;94:127-30.
8. Hong DZ, Goh JL, Ong ZY, Ting JJQ, Wong MK, Wu J, et al. Postgraduate ethics training programs: a systematic scoping review. BMC Med Educ. 2021;21(1):338.
9. Mehdiratta L, Dave NM, Sahni N, Johnson E, Bidkar PU, Grewal A. Comparing postgraduate anaesthesia education in India and abroad: strengths and scope. Indian J Anaesth. 2022;66(1):70-6.
10. Pavithran P, Kaniyil S, Rajesh MC, Venugopal V, Jitin TN, Davul A. The clinical learning environment in anaesthesiology in Kerala: is it good enough? A web-based survey. Indian J Anaesth. 2021;65(3):234-40.
11. National Medical Commission. (2019). Guidelines for competency-based postgraduate training programme for MD in anaesthesiology. [online] Available from https://nmc.org.in/wp-content /uploads/2019/09/MD-Anesthesia.pdf. [Last accessed June, 2025].
12. World Medical Association. Declaration of Helsinki: ethical principles for medical research involving human subjects. JAMA. 2013;310(20):2191-4.

13. Council for International Organizations of Medical Sciences (CIOMS). (2016). International ethical guidelines for health-related research involving humans. [online] Available from https://cioms.ch/wp-content/uploads/2017/01/WEB-CIOMS-EthicalGuidelines.pdf. [Last accessed June, 2025].
14. Child Ethics. (2013). Ethical Research Involving Children, ERIC Project. Available from https://childethics.com/resources/. [Last accessed June, 2025].
15. U.S. Department of Health and Human Services. (1991). Federal Policy for the Protection of Human Subjects ('Common Rule'). [online] Available from https://www.hhs.gov/ohrp/regulations-and-policy/regulations/common-rule/index.html. [Last accessed June, 2025].
16. Dorscheidt JH, Hein IM. Medical research involving children–giving weight to children's views. Int J Child Rights. 2018;26(1):93-116.
17. Indian Council of Medical Research. (1980). Policy statement on ethical considerations involved in research on human subjects. [online] Available from http://ethics.ncdirindia.org//asset/pdf/Policy_Statement_1980.pdf. [Last accessed June, 2025].
18. Indian Council of Medical Research. (2000). Ethical guidelines for biomedical research on human subjects. [online] Available from http://ethics.ncdirindia.org//asset/pdf/Ethical_guidelines_for_biomedical_research_on_human_subject-2000.pdf. [Last accessed June, 2025].
19. Indian Council of Medical Research. (2006). Ethical guidelines for biomedical research on human participants. [online] Available from https://ethics.ncdirindia.org//asset/pdf/ICMR_ethical_guidelines_for_biomedical_research_for_human_participants_2006.pdf. [Last accessed June, 2025].
20. Indian Council of Medical Research. (2018). National ethical guidelines for biomedical and health research involving human participants. [online] Available from https://ethics.ncdirindia.org//asset/pdf/Handbook_on_ICMR_Ethical_Guidelines.pdf. [Last accessed June, 2025].
21. Behera SK, Das S, Xavier AS, Selvarajan S, Anandabaskar N. Indian Council of Medical Research's National Ethical Guidelines for biomedical and health research involving human participants: the way forward from 2006 to 2017. Perspect Clin Res 2019;10(3):108-14.
22. Indian Council of Medical Research. (2017). National ethical guidelines for bio-medical research involving children. [online] Available from https://ethics.ncdirindia.org/asset/pdf/National_Ethical_Guidelines_for_BioMedical_Research_Involving_Children.pdf. [Last accessed June, 2025].
23. Spriggs M. Children and bioethics: clarifying consent and assent in medical and research settings. Br Med Bull. 2023;145(1):110-9.
24. Allmark P, Spedding M. Clinical trials in neonates: ethical issues. Semin Fetal Neonatal Med. 2007;12(4):318-23.

# Index

Page numbers followed by *b* refer to box, *f* refer to figure, *fc* refer to flowchart, and *t* refer to table.

## B

## C

## D

## I

## J



## K



## L

## M